PRAISE FOR

PANIC PROOF

"*Panic Proof* is jam-packed with comprehensive, practical, science-backed advice and holistic tools for anyone suffering with panic disorders. Dr. Nicole Cain is a force of wisdom, compassion, and empowerment, and I hope this book gets into as many hands as possible."

—Dr. Nicole LePera, author of the #1 *New York Times* bestsellers *How to Do the Work* and *How to Be the Love You Seek*

"In *Panic Proof,* Dr. Cain delivers a groundbreaking approach to understanding and managing panic disorders. Her emphasis on the body's role in panic attacks, coupled with her compassionate and relatable writing style, makes this book a must-read for anyone seeking lasting relief from anxiety."

—Jolene Brighten, NMD, FABNE, certified sex counselor and bestselling author

"As a clinician working for the past thirty years with patients who have panic disorders, I understand the deep struggle these people face. They need resources that not only educate but also offer an integrative, holistic approach to their conditions. Dr. Cain's expertise shines through in this truly unique resource for patients. *Panic Proof* is a valuable book that will empower readers to take control of their anxiety and live panic-free lives."

—Paul S. Anderson, NMD

"*Panic Proof* is a deeply researched and well-written book that shows distinct anxiety presentations and offers very thorough approaches to addressing anxiety and panic disorders."

—Russell Kennedy, MD, author of *Anxiety Rx*

"Dr. Cain's *Panic Proof* is a beacon of hope for those struggling with panic disorders. Her focus on the body's cues and the root causes of panic sets this book apart from others in the field. This is an invaluable resource for anyone seeking a holistic and sustainable path to panic freedom."

—Ellen Vora, MD, author of *The Anatomy of Anxiety*

"*Panic Proof* is the book we've all been waiting for. Dr. Nicole Cain challenges conventional wisdom about panic disorders with a trauma-informed approach that helps you finally hear what your body is trying to tell you and helps you understand that your body is trying to keep you safe with anxiety. With its practical exercises and research-backed solutions, this book provides hope and healing. . . . An invaluable resource for anyone seeking lasting relief."

—Claire Bidwell Smith, LCPC, author of
Anxiety: The Missing Stage of Grief and *Conscious Grieving*

PANIC PROOF

PANIC PROOF

The New Holistic Solution to End Your Anxiety Forever

DR. NICOLE CAIN

RODALE
NEW YORK

No book can replace the diagnostic expertise and medical advice of a trusted physician. Please be certain to consult with your doctor before making any decisions that affect your health, particularly if you suffer from any medical condition or have any symptom that may require treatment.

A Rodale Trade Paperback Original

Published in the United States by Rodale Books, an imprint of Random House, a division of Penguin Random House LLC, New York.

Illustrations by Haylee Masteller

ISBN 978-0-593-58257-2
Ebook ISBN 978-0-593-58258-9

Printed in Canada on acid-free paper

RodaleBooks.com | RandomHouseBooks.com

2 4 6 8 9 7 5 3 1

FIRST PAPERBACK EDITION

Book design by Barbara M. Bachman

To every Charlotte, Aria, Matthew, Esme,
Jenny, and David.
Your stories are powerful and important.
I dedicate this book to you.

CONTENTS

PART III

HOW TO BE PANIC PROOF

INTRODUCTION

The Truth About Panic and the Lies You've Been Told

If you're reading this book, you're likely struggling with panic. Maybe you're newly diagnosed with panic and anxiety, or maybe you've been struggling with panic for many years. Either way, I know it may seem hard right now to imagine a life where anxiety isn't running the show.

Maybe you were told that anxiety is pretty common (it is) and that anxiety doesn't heal, it's just managed (that's a myth).

Maybe you're just beginning to heal from panic and anxiety, or maybe you've been around the block a time or two and feel stuck. Regardless of whether you're relatively new to the panic game, or you've tried everything under the sun to make panic stop, I want you to know three things:

1. I've been there,
2. I've got your back, and
3. *You can* heal from anxiety and panic!

But before we go any further: you have likely heard two big lies, and I want to address them straight out of the gate.

Lie 1: Symptoms are bad; we're here to make them go away.

Lie 2: The experts likely know more about your brain and body than you do.

Let's just dig into each of these for a moment.

LIE 1: SYMPTOMS ARE BAD; WE'RE HERE TO MAKE THEM GO AWAY.

This could be the official slogan for the medical profession. You go to the doctor when you are suffering, and your doctor wants to relieve that suffering. Symptoms are seen as problems to be solved.

But what if our symptoms are actually trying to tell us something? What if they're not problems but solutions?

Let's say you're in the market for a car. You find one you really like, and you get in the driver's seat to take it for a spin. Once you shut the door, you get hit by the overpowering scent of a tree-shaped air freshener hanging from the rearview mirror. Even so, the car works great and so you buy it and take it home. A week later, as the tree loses its scent, you notice a different aroma. This one, however, is quite offensive.

SCENARIO 1: You get a new air freshener and don't investigate further.

SCENARIO 2: You explore *why* there's a smell and, after further investigation, discover the remains of a rotten burrito in the glove box.

In Scenario 1, you've simply masked the symptom. The problem is still there—it's just not as noticeable.

In Scenario 2, you've addressed the root cause of the symptom. The problem is gone, and you've actually made your car better in the process.

The same is true for our bodies. Symptoms are not problems, they are solutions. They are our bodies' way of telling us that something is wrong and we need to make a change.

When we ignore our symptoms, we're only making the problem worse. We're like the person who buys a new air freshener instead of cleaning out the rotten burrito.

IT'S THE SAME STORY if you've been experiencing panic attacks. Panic attacks are a symptom, and you can try to cope your way out of the problem (using medications, supplements, meditation, etc.). You'll succeed for a while. But if you can't keep up your coping strategies for a short period of time (and let's face it, it's impossible to always be on top of them), the panic returns.

Similar to finding the rotten burrito, you can instead explore the *why* behind the panic. Whether the symptom is a yucky smell or a feeling of panic, it is a sign pointing to a deeper issue. The symptom is not the problem but instead is part of the *solution* to the problem. Realizing and understanding that something is off gives you the opportunity to heal not just your panic but your energy and health on a deeper level.

The word *vitality* means energy, life, and health, while *resiliency* describes the ability to withstand or recover from challenges. Together these words describe a state of being fully alive and able to withstand stress. Your body is both vital and resilient, and it produces symptoms to tell you what needs healing and how.

LIE 2: THE EXPERTS LIKELY KNOW MORE ABOUT YOUR BRAIN AND BODY THAN YOU DO.

This is another common lie that we're told. We're told that doctors and therapists are the experts and that we should just listen to them.

But the truth is, we know our bodies better than anyone else does. We know what feels right and what feels wrong. We know what makes us feel better and what makes us feel worse.

Don't let anyone tell you that you know less about yourself than they do. (That's the definition of *gaslighting*.) My hope for you is that this book will help you learn to trust yourself so that you can become your own best advocate. Your doctors are experts in their respective fields, but you are the only person living inside your mind and body. And that's tough when you feel like your mind and body are at war.

This isn't my autobiography, so I am not going to get into my whole childhood, but I do want to share a little bit of my backstory. It's important that you know I've been through the dark circle of hell that is panic.

Not only have I been there, I've come out on the other side.

And you can too.

Not only have I healed myself, I have helped literally thousands of panic sufferers get their lives back. Helping you to become Panic Proof is what sets my soul on fire, and because of that, I'm going to be a little bit vulnerable.

MY STORY OF PANIC

It was 3:00 A.M. and my body was on fire. I hadn't gotten a good night's sleep in almost six months, and over the last three evenings, I had slept for only an hour. I was spiraling, and with the passing of every minute, I became more certain that I was going to die.

What began with a few bad nights of sleep due to stress had expanded into a full-fledged emotional crisis. As panic climbed, my level of functioning plummeted. My stomach was in knots, and I struggled to eat, which resulted in so much weight loss that my menstrual cycle stopped. Day and night, adrenaline surged, causing jerking and twitching of my muscles and violent pounding of my heart. The worst physical symptom was the constant burning pain—it felt as if coals from a fire had been placed beneath my skin in my back and chest.

"Your nervous system is stuck in autonomic arousal," my husband, a clinically trained psychotherapist, said. "You have to take a break and give your body time and space to let that adrenaline come down and re-equilibrate."

But I couldn't take time off. I was in repayment for over a quarter-million dollars in student loans, and I had just opened an integrative mental health practice with my business partner. The cost of rent plus overhead was double what I had budgeted, and I was panicking.

During the day I would show up as my best and most together self, and at night I would fall apart. Staring at the ceiling into the late hours of the night, I'd go over checklists of what I'd need to remember for the following day, and I'd do mental math, trying to calculate how many teaching and clinical hours I would need to work in order to cover my expenses.

After countless sleepless hours, the sun always rose again, illuminating the same realization: *You can't keep up. You're in severe financial trouble. Everything is falling apart.*

Objectively, the conclusions that my anxious brain had drawn were not true. I had a thriving private practice, I never came up short for a payment at home or in practice, and my loving husband was there to support me no matter what happened emotionally or financially. While my past had been fraught with financial insecurity and emotional deprivation, my current reality was emotionally and financially sound.

But that's the thing with anxiety: When our emotional brain detects uncertainty, danger, or cues that remind us of a past threat, it shuts down the logical part of our brain—namely, the prefrontal cortex. In an effort to ensure our survival, it does everything it can to fight, flight, or freeze (or fawn, flop, and fracture), and it logs that experience away for future reference.

Your cells have memory.

Since the moment you were conceived, your every thought, sensation, event, and emotion has been filtered through your brain. And today, as you go through your day-to-day life, your brain is continually processing, tossing, and integrating information via a process known as neuroplasticity.

Psychiatrist Bruce Perry, MD, PhD, teaches that the more frequently a circuit in your brain gets activated, the more automatic it can become. And the more automatic the firing of that neuron becomes, the more it feels like it's a part of who you are.

For many, this is how anxiety begins.

My anxiety began in childhood. I just didn't recognize what it was until many years later.

I was born in 1982 to two very young and isolated parents who recycled how they had been parented into their own child-rearing strategy: shaming us kids, with a hearty helping of corporal punishment, whenever we did anything that displeased or enraged them.

Starving for safety and love, I took on the roles of helper, peacemaker, and people-pleaser early on in life. This showed up in lots of different ways. I adopted the preferences and ideologies of my parents to garner acceptance and approval, I took responsibility for their moods and experimented with techniques to soothe their ire or lift their sadness, and I curated a *part* of myself that was particularly able to detect subtle warning signs that someone was upset or disapproving.

Parts Work is a therapeutic approach used by many trauma-informed clinicians. It teaches that in response to traumatic events, we develop "parts" of ourselves to shield us from future vulnerability to those types of experiences. A part of myself helped me by becoming more hypervigilant and attuned to others' moods, but that same hypervigilance also caused me to become anxious, self-critical, and prone to panic later in life.

Recent research has taught us that traumatic and aversive experiences did not take place only in the past. These events fundamentally change how our mind and body are organized, because the mind wants to—above all—stay alive. Unconsciously, it changes its behaviors, emotions, and thought patterns in order to continue surviving in the present.

In elementary school, I became very sick with laryngitis, bronchitis, and an upper respiratory infection. I was taken to a doctor who gave me an antibiotic and steroids, and after about a month, I was better. Except it happened again the next year. And the next. For the next *twenty years,* I would predictably fall ill for the entire month of November. I would be unable to speak, could breathe only with the aid of an albuterol inhaler, and was at the mercy of my doctor's prescription pad.

Years later I read a quote attributed to poet and writer Robert Bly:

"The body weeps the tears the eyes never shed." It struck me that I had learned to silence the voice of my own needs, but that something had changed and I was losing my actual voice as well.

My beacon of hope was our family doctor. He was the person in authority who could diagnose my ills and give me the medicine that I thought would bring back my health. When in doubt, I'd turn to the expert, and he would tell me what to do. I was drawn to the idea of the healing power of medicine. In my mind, doctors were the ultimate helpers and healers. And I wanted to be one.

Over the next few years, while the other kids played outside during recess, I sat in the school library devouring first aid books. I designed and assembled my very own first aid fanny pack, which consisted of Band-Aids, triple antibiotic cream, and gauze.

But my physical symptoms didn't stop. Next came chronic nasal congestion, for which I was prescribed a decongestant and two different types of nasal sprays. Then came chronic asthma, and two more inhalers and an increased dose of decongestant. Anxiety followed, and after only a quick interview, I was given an antidepressant.

By the time I started college, I was on more than six different medications, yet I was no healthier. In fact, my trajectory was moving away from health and toward disease. I was developing depression, brain fog, digestive upset, and difficulties sleeping.

Let down by the medical system's inability to help me, I made the decision not to go to medical school and instead become a mental health counselor. This fit into my big picture mission, which was to take care of my family, make them happy, and earn love.

LET'S REWIND, BACK TO the climax of my personal panic story. It's 3:00 A.M., and I'm wide awake and panicking.

As an expert in holistic remedies for mental health, I have a massive apothecary of remedies and solutions at my disposal, so I was as equipped as anyone to beat anxiety and panic. This was my zone of genius. I have worked with clients on more than three continents, helping them to utilize holistic and mind-body strategies to stabilize their moods and improve their well-being.

I had tried literally everything I could think of to make my own panic and anxiety go away. I went to see some of the best practitioners in their respective industries. I took thousands of dollars' worth of supplements, herbal medicines, amino acids, homeopathic remedies, Bach flower essences, traditional Chinese herbs, sedatives, and adrenal herbs. I went to qi gong and meditated; I did acupuncture, yoga, and massage; I tried hypnotherapy, neurofeedback, and biofeedback; and I saw a therapist, a chiropractor, and a psychiatrist who prescribed benzodiazepines and an antidepressant.

No matter what I did to sedate my nervous system, distract my thoughts, or suppress my body into submission, my symptoms persisted.

While the dominant medical system has revolutionized healthcare with the development of diagnostic assessment tools, powerful pharmaceutical medicines, and lifesaving surgical advancements, it has one major downfall: it has taught us to hand over our fate to the experts whom we employ.

From my earliest memories, I was trained to rely on the wise counsel of those who knew more than I did. As a child, adults taught me when, what, and how much to eat, when to go to sleep, and what time to wake up. As I grew older, my doctors told me how to take care of my body and what to do for symptoms if and when they arose. As an adult, when I achieved a master's in clinical psychology and later graduated from medical school, I stepped into that role of authority. I was trained to identify symptoms, run diagnostic testing, and create integrative treatment plans for my patients.

I became an expert at turning to experts, and then eventually I *became* the expert for other people.

In his famous book *The Body Keeps the Score,* Bessel van der Kolk, MD, writes, "As long as you keep secrets and suppress information, you are fundamentally at war with yourself. . . . The critical issue is allowing yourself to know what you know. That takes an enormous amount of courage."

You are courageous for reading this book. In a medical system designed to ease suffering, you are courageous for being willing to look at your symptoms and listen to their deeper messages.

Change came when I finally stopped trying to distract, suppress, ignore, and cope with my panic and anxiety and started asking my symptoms, *What are you trying to tell me?*

Healing took time, but it was worth it. Writing this chapter, as I reflect on my past life, it feels drastically different from where I am today.

I have learned that my symptoms are my messengers for what needs healing and how.

I have learned that profound healing is possible.

I have learned that I am fully capable of self-healing.

I have learned that my past does not have to dictate my future.

Healing means reorganizing years of panic-provoking circuitry in your brain and nervous system, restoring balance and health to your gut, hormones, and neurotransmitters, and creating a new relationship with your *self*.

You too can heal, and this book will show you how.

HOW THIS BOOK IS ORGANIZED

Panic Proof is divided into three parts:

1. Untangling what your anxiety and panic are trying to tell you;
2. Understanding that your panic is protective; and
3. Becoming an agent in your own rescue.

The three chapters in Part I will help you get crystal clear on what your panic is trying to do for you. Chapter 1 will help you shift your origin story from *What's wrong with me?* to a trauma-informed perspective that asks, *How am I adapting to my past and present experiences?* Then in Chapter 2, I explain how a mismatch between symptom severity and recommended treatments often results in persistent panic. Chapter 3 explores the nine types of panic and anxiety, which will shape your understanding of what your symptoms are trying to heal and how.

In Part II, I will argue that your panic is protective and that you can utilize this knowledge to move from panic to power. Each chapter will explore a different mechanism of how your body and mind are taking action to help protect you against perceived danger. Chapter 4 will introduce you to your brain, explaining the differences between a calm brain and an anxious one. In Chapter 5 we'll dig into the relationship between panic and the trillion mood-altering microbes (aka psychobiotics) that make up what is referred to as your second or gut brain. You will learn how to leverage your gut in healing your brain.

In Chapter 6 I will reveal the biggest myths about the relationship between panic and neurotransmitters, the teeny-tiny chemicals that your brain uses to relay information throughout your body. You'll discover that it's a whole lot more complicated than "low serotonin causes anxiety, and getting more serotonin makes anxiety go away." Chapter 7 will explore how your endocrine system may be a root cause of your panic, and how a shift in one hormone may result in a domino effect that affects your entire mind and body, including your sex, thyroid, and adrenal hormones.

Part III, "How to Be Panic Proof," is where the magic happens. It's all about teaching you how to take your power back! Chapter 8 teaches about removing the obstacles to panic freedom. In Chapter 9 you will learn about using bottom-up therapies to retrain your stress responses, which includes recalibrating your autonomic nervous system so that it is primed for calm, not for panic. In Chapter 10 you will learn how to become your own trauma-informed clinician, equipped with the skills for exploring the *who, what, how,* and *what now?* messages from your anxious and panicking parts of the self. In Chapter 11, you will be introduced to the latest research into holistic supplements, herbs, and psychobiotics for stopping panic and creating calm. You'll build your Panic Proof Protocol, which will include the template for the 90-day Panic Reset program.

While you are reading this book, you will meet Charlotte, Aria, Matthew, Esme, Jenny, and David. These six individuals represent the thousands of people I've worked with over the last decades as an integrative physician. While they are not real, their stories, feelings, and journeys are composites of true stories.

Throughout this book, you will find a quiz, worksheets, and self-assessment checklists as well as links to further reading and audiovisual materials that are available on my website. For example, did you know that there are nine types of anxiety, and that identifying which type of anxiety you're dealing with will help you identify treatments that are more likely to be effective? This quiz and these checklists are the gifts that keep on giving: every time you go back to retake them, and study your results, you will better understand your symptoms. Bookmark those pages, and check back often. As you understand the messages from your symptoms, you'll be able to meet your needs and create true and lasting healing.

Lastly, at the end of each chapter, you will find a section titled "TL;DR," which stands for "Too Long; Didn't Read." These are a list of the key concepts from the chapter that you can save in your phone, write on a Post-it, or share with a friend.

One of the panic survivors you'll meet in this book, Charlotte, was big into writing on her bathroom mirror in lipstick. Once she started to lean into panic, she wrote the following message on her vanity mirror in looping lipstick cursive and left it there: "All vibes welcome."

Your vibe is welcome here. So let's get started!

PART I

The Secret Messages from Anxiety and Panic

THE STORY OF THE

Weathered House

IMAGINE A HOUSE THAT HAS WEATHERED MANY SEASONS AND WITnessed the comings and goings of multitudes of people.

Over the years, the house has seen its fair share of storms. Some were traumatic and violent, breaking windows and eroding the foundation; others were filled with lightning that sparked the growth of beautiful flowers and trees. Some seasons were quiet and restful, while others felt lonely and still. Still others felt overwhelming and unsafe.

Every visitor makes a mark on the house. Some leave behind personal belongings, such as furniture, artwork, or photographs. Others make changes to the house's layout, by knocking down walls or adding new rooms. Some pass through the doors almost invisibly, leaving footprints that fade slowly over time. Some call the house their home, making the space a reflection of their own identity.

There are a lot of houses like this in the world. Some were built by caretakers who carefully selected a plot that was protected from the dangerous elements, and who were mindful to make the house light-filled, strong, and beautiful. These houses are resilient and sturdy, and they can withstand even the most perilous storms.

Other houses were built with light and love but by hands that had no skills. So those houses have fragile foundations and thin walls. These houses are still beautiful, but they are more vulnerable to deterioration or destruction.

Still other houses were built and deserted. These neglected houses are found in disrepair.

Every house, no matter its unique story, will settle, shift, groan, and adapt to the world outside and to the lives lived within its walls.

You Are Not Just Living in a House—You Are the House

Your physical, emotional, and mental space is constructed with materials passed down from your ancestors, influenced by the external factors you have been exposed to, and shaped by the people who have entered and exited your life. *Each person's house is unique.*

People often believe that there is a single, universal "normal" way to do things such as decorate a room, react to a stressor, or relate to peers. However, this is simply not true. There is no one right way to be, and everyone experiences the world in their own unique way.

The rigid belief in a singular "normal" can have devastating consequences. It fosters bias and discrimination against individuals who live differently from the perceived median. Imagine the devastating impact of labeling someone struggling with anxiety as "overly emotional" or dismissing an individual experiencing depression as "lazy." Such statements, rooted in a narrow view of "normal," are not only inaccurate but also deeply harmful, preventing individuals from feeling safe enough to share their experiences and seek the support they need.

The truth is that while all our brains share a basic structure, each mind functions in a unique and magnificent way. The concept of "normal" is subjective and fluid, influenced by factors like culture, age, gender, and personal experiences. What is considered normal in one context may be considered unusual in another. As such, viewing neurotypicality as the singular norm hinders our ability to appreciate the vast spectrum of human experience.

Instead, we have an incredible opportunity to embrace the breathtaking diversity of minds and experiences. By recognizing the multitude of ways human beings can exist within their own mental and emotional spaces, we open ourselves to a world of richness, understanding, and empathy. We celebrate the unique challenges and strengths that every individual brings to the table, fostering a more inclusive and supportive environment for all.

Remember, your experience of anxiety or stress is profoundly individual. There's no "one size fits all" approach to navigating these emotions. Embrace the fluidity of your being, explore various coping mechanisms, and, most important, be kind to yourself on this journey of self-discovery. You are not alone, and your unique way of being is valuable and deserving of respect.

All Vibes Are Welcome

Ever feel like you have to hide your sadness or anxiety because of the "good vibes only" culture? Let's ditch that! We're all wonderfully different, experiencing a kaleidoscope of emotions, which is part of what makes us human.

Instead of clinging to toxic positivity, let's actively encourage hope and honest conversations about all emotions, not just the positive ones.

By welcoming every emotion, we create a safe space where people feel supported, no matter their emotional ups and downs. We're all in this together. Let's support one another and create a world where everyone feels safe and accepted.

How do we do it? We start with presence.

The Power of Presence

When we are present, we are fully attuned to the present moment. We are not dwelling on the past or worrying about the future. We are simply here, right now, holding space for whatever is happening.

Presence is a powerful tool for healing. When we are present, we can accept our thoughts and feelings, without judgment. We can let go of the past and focus on the now. We can connect with our inner wisdom and strength. We can build resilience in the face of challenges.

When was the last time you stopped and were really present in your "house"?

For many, presence is terrifying. It can be difficult to be in the moment and walk around our metaphorical hallways and look at the peeling paint, the cracks in the foundation, or the decades of memories hidden in corners, beneath beds, or locked away in closets.

Neurobiologically, we enter this world with a binary view of good and bad, safe and unsafe, healthy and unhealthy. Children need such concrete thinking to safely form their ego. Concrete thinkers see the world in black and white, with no shades of gray. They have difficulty understanding complex concepts or ideas, and they often struggle to make decisions.

This limited perspective, rooted in concrete thinking, is gradually challenged as the prefrontal cortex matures. This area of the brain, responsible for complex thinking, decision-making, and empathy, begins to fully develop in late adolescence or the early twenties.

With its maturation, we become more acutely aware of our vibrant existence and the inevitable finiteness of our bodies. This awakening can be both liberating and terrifying. On the one hand, it frees us from the confines of childhood, granting us the autonomy to navigate the world and embrace the present moment with open hearts and minds. On the other hand, it forces us to confront the unyielding reality of our own mortality, a confrontation that can be a source of profound anxiety.

Death is a universal fear. We are all terrified of it, to some degree. We are haunted by fears of car accidents, plane crashes, the loss of loved ones, and illness. We fill our lives with distractions, coping mechanisms, and anything that can pull our minds away from the reality that we have a body that ages, can be injured, or gets sick.

Our consumer-driven culture encourages us to focus on future promises, taking us away from the present, and bombarding us with messages about youth, beauty, and eternal life.

However, despite our best efforts, symptoms and reminders of our mortality inevitably arise, forcing our awareness back to what we've been trying to avoid. We harbor worries, thoughts, and inner voices about these things, and we often refrain from discussing them out of a fear of judgment, as if speaking them aloud will somehow make them come true.

According to renowned psychologist and philosopher Carl Jung, beneath the surface of our conscious awareness lies a hidden world—a realm of thoughts, fears, beliefs, and images.

Jung asserted that these hidden aspects, if left unexamined, can manifest as compulsions, anxieties, and even physical ailments. Suppressed memories of childhood trauma, recurring dreams filled with cryptic symbols, or deeply held but unacknowledged beliefs about ourselves—all can subtly dictate our lives without our consent.

In other words, the more we deny and suppress what lies within us, the more control it has over us.

Jung proposed a different approach, advocating bringing the unconscious into conscious awareness through presence. By being present and speaking openly and honestly about our fears and thoughts, he taught, you can become crystal clear on what your panic is trying to do for you.

To be present, we need to embrace a new standard that encourages us to acknowledge our cultural conditioning and the habits that hinder our being present. We must be radically honest with ourselves and acknowledge our uniqueness, our true feelings and thoughts, even if they are uncomfortable or don't immediately make sense. Sometimes what seems confusing or unsettling in the darkness can gain clarity when brought into the light of awareness. It is through this process that we can become Panic Proof and find peace.

Top-down, Bottom-up

Your body and mind can heal themselves naturally if you listen to their signals and respond with solutions that meet their needs. In this book, you are going to learn just how to do that. When you're working with your body and mind in this way, you're learning vital resiliency.

This process can be broken down into two key parts: top-down, which we will focus on in Part I of this book, and bottom-up, which you will learn about in Parts II and III.

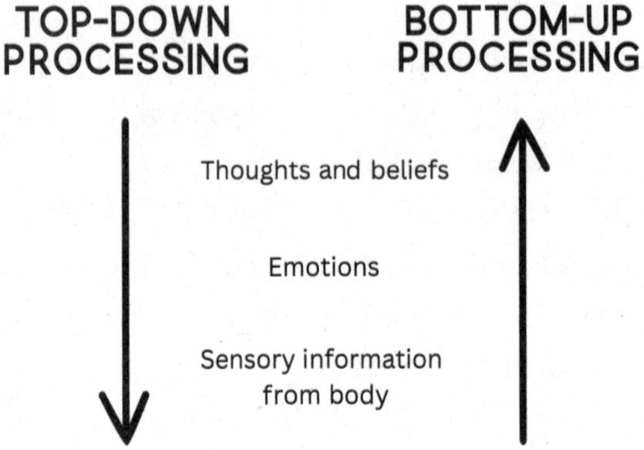

If you have ever seen a counselor or therapist, you have likely experienced some form of top-down therapy. Mental health treatments, such as Cognitive Behavioral Therapy (CBT), tend to start with the "top" of the brain, or cortex, known as the "analytical brain," and work their way down to the body. These treatments aim to change the way people *think* about their experiences in order to change how they *feel* emotionally and physically. And they can be effective! Treatments like CBT can help people to feel better and to behave in more helpful ways. CBT is a common approach for panic and anxiety and is an important foundation for deeper work.

However, for some individuals (myself included), top-down approaches are not enough. Sometimes we feel panic even when our thoughts are not logical, and despite our best efforts to change our thoughts, our body continues to pump out stress hormones, fueling anxiety and panic attacks.

Focusing solely on top-down approaches is akin to turning off the water to a leaky faucet without fixing the pipe that is causing the leak. The water may stop for a moment, but the underlying issue remains unresolved, leading to eventual overflow.

Bottom-up repatterning is a newer approach to mental health

treatment that focuses on regulating the body to heal the mind. It is based on the idea that the body and the brain are interconnected and that by working with the body, we can also heal the brain.

Bottom-up healing techniques, such as Somatic Experiencing, Mindfulness, Eye Movement Desensitization and Reprocessing, and Expressive Arts Therapy, can help us to:

- Become more aware of our body sensations
- Identify the needs of our different biological systems (explored in Part II)
- Process difficult emotions that are stored in the body and nonverbal parts of the brain
- Develop healthier ways of coping with stress (explored in Part III)

Bottom-up therapies are often more integrative and are designed to help people consider their whole body, connect with their own inner wisdom, and create their own path to healing.

In Part I, we will use top-down techniques to help you *understand* your panic. These strategies can also help you lay the groundwork for how you want to reorganize your experience around panic. Then, in Parts II and III, you will gain clarity about the role your body plays in panic and how to heal and recalibrate the body so that your lived experience is calm and empowered.

Are you ready to get started?

I am. Let's do this.

1

HOW DID YOU GET HERE?

IT WAS AN UNUSUALLY CRISP FALL DAY IN PHOENIX, ARIZONA, AND MY good friend Charlotte and I were sitting outside and catching up over tea. My Arizona blood turns into a solid block of ice when the temperature falls anywhere below 60 degrees. So I was wearing a heated vest, gloves, and my favorite fuzzy cobalt blue hat. Charlotte was wearing a light-gray hoodie, half unzipped over a T-shirt that read: SOMETIMES I WET MY PLANTS.

Charlotte is one of my favorite people. She is quirky, quick to smile, and about as "crunchy" as they come. She feeds her kids kale chips from Trader Joe's, wears organic cotton, and gets a thrill out of composting. She has a degree in physical therapy, she's a new mom of two adorable young girls, and she's married to the man of her dreams.

But over the last few months, Charlotte had changed, and she could see the worry all over my face.

"Nothing's wrong," she said as she took a big gulp from her mug of kava kava tea. "I just need to get the girls to bed on time so I can have at least an hour to myself, horizontal on the couch, with a brain-numbing show on."

I wasn't convinced. Nodding toward her drink, I asked, "How many of those have you had today?"

"Are you kidding? I live, eat, and breathe kava," Charlotte admitted with a smile. Her hands were jittery. "It's probably a little excessive, but I figure, 'go big or go home.'"

Kava kava tea is made from the root of the plant called *Piper methysticum,* and one of its superpowers is the temporary relief of anxiety.

Alarm bells were going off in the back of my mind. "Can we talk about this?" I asked.

Charlotte set down her tea. "I know you're worried about me. But it's not a big deal. I'm just a little stressed."

"I appreciate that you're trying to take care of me and reassure me right now." I reached out and touched her hand. "Would you let me take care of you, back?"

"This is why I love you." She sighed. "Okay. Lay it on me."

This is when I shared with Charlotte my concerns for her health. Her rapid drop in weight, her immunity to the cold, the tremors in her hands, her inability to sleep, and her need to drink excessive amounts of anti-anxiety tea.

She listened as I spoke, and when I finished, she squeezed my hand and said, "I hear you. But I'm not worried, and you shouldn't be either. I'm fine."

But she wasn't fine.

YOU CAN'T SOLVE A PROBLEM YOU'RE NOT WILLING TO HAVE

"Sensing, naming, and identifying what is going on inside is the first step to recovery."

—Dr. Bessel van der Kolk, *The Body Keeps the Score* (2014)

We live in a world that is constantly bombarding us with distractions. We are always plugged in, always connected, and always looking for the next thing to distract or entertain us. This constant stimulation can make it difficult for us to focus on the present moment and to confront the problems that lie within us. And before we know it, time has flown by, and we're scratching our heads, wondering, *How did I get here?*

Charlotte was a victim of distraction and avoidance. She wasn't in tune with the signals from her mind and body. She was so busy doing "all the things" that she either didn't notice what was going on with her or she chose not to acknowledge that she had any sort of actual problem.

If we want to heal from anxiety, we need to learn to slow down, to be present, and to listen to our minds and bodies. When you listen, your body will share. So let's talk about what comes next.

RADICAL ACKNOWLEDGMENT

Radical acknowledgment is the practice of accepting and respecting the messages from our mind and body, without judgment. When we radically acknowledge our anxiety, we learn its secret language and can leverage its power for good.

Here's an example of how radical acknowledgment might work. Let's say you're feeling anxious about giving a presentation. You notice physical symptoms, like a racing heart, sweating, and shaking. Instead of trying to push these sensations away or ignore them, you radically acknowledge them. You say to yourself, *I'm feeling anxious right now. My heart is racing, and I'm sweating. This is a normal reaction to stress. I'm going to allow myself to feel these emotions, and then I'm going to focus on giving my presentation.*

Radical acknowledgment is not about making your symptoms of fear go away. It's about changing your relationship with your thoughts, emotions, and sensations so that you are no longer afraid or anxious, but rather curious about what they have to say regarding what needs healing and how. When you practice radical acknowledgment, the signs and symptoms you attribute to anxiety become powerful messengers that are trying to tell you something. And when you learn to understand them, you can take steps to heal and move forward.

FEAR OF THE FEAR

One of the most common objections I hear from my clients, as we begin the process of radical acknowledgment, is that they're afraid of feeling afraid. They worry about the physical sensations of fear, like a racing heart or numbness in their scalp, and they're afraid that these sensations will get worse. Fear of fear can be so paralyzing that it can prevent people from doing things they enjoy or even from leaving their homes.

I know this feeling well, because I used to have it myself. For almost a decade, after a particularly stressful plane flight, I had a terrible phobia of flying. I was so afraid of feeling afraid that I would avoid flying at all costs. But I had to fly for work, and so despite feeling terrified and physically ill, I had to get back on that plane.

So I tried to "therapize" myself out of feeling anxious. I took the Fear of Flying course with Captain Ron at the Phoenix Sky Harbor International Airport (highly recommended!). I interviewed pilots, and I did a podcast with an aerospace engineer (thanks, AJ!). I followed Charlotte's lead and downed kava kava. I practiced deep breathing, meditated, and prayed. Eventually I resorted to taking a benzodiazepine medication and curling into the fetal position and trying not to cry until the plane finally reached its destination.

One of the most frustrating parts about this whole experience was that it made absolutely no logical sense.

I had nailed the top-down strategies, and my analytical brain was mostly on board. I *knew* that flying was safe. (Still, a part of me remained a work in progress. It would occasionally pipe in with anxious thoughts, such as *Well, okay, but what if . . . ?*)

But the big thing was that my *body* was still afraid. I wasn't afraid of flying; it was the lack of control over the intense emotions and physical sensations that arose during flying that made me anxious: fear of the fear.

HAVE YOU EVER FELT that way?

If you've been there, I want you to know three things:

- Fear is a normal human emotion. And like all emotions, it is temporary.
- Your emotions are not dangerous. Your emotions are great big loud expressions from your mind and body saying, *Hey! Pay attention to me!* Your most powerful tool in your toolbox is to sit down, thoughtfully attend, and listen to what your symptoms have to say.
- You can learn how to work with the body to create calm-on-command (Parts II and III).

I had to get myself into the right trauma-informed space that honored the messages from both my brain and my body. After doing a lot of work (much of which is covered in these pages), I booked another trip. And the flight was wonderful. And so I booked another, and another. It felt like my world simply opened up.

I feel emotional writing this section, because my fear of flying had held me back in so many ways over the years, and now that that fear is gone, I've had the opportunity to reclaim so much of my life. And I know deep in my bones that you can, too.

Let's dig into how you actually do this. First, we start by laying a foundation of top-down. That is what the remainder of Part I will be all about. Then, we'll move on to bottom-up in Parts II and III.

HOW TO LISTEN TO THE SECRET MESSAGES OF YOUR ANXIETY

In this next section, you're going to discover three exercises for learning how to simply listen to the secret messages of your anxiety. Try to practice one each day. The more you practice, the easier and more natural the skill of radical acknowledgment will become.

Exercise 1: The Art of Resisting Versus Receiving

The first step is to receive the information your mind and body are giving you without resisting. When we receive, we allow ourselves to fully experience our moment, without judgment or attachment. This can lead to feelings of peace, calm, and acceptance. When we resist, we try to push away or change our experience. But that will only result in greater feelings of frustration, anger, and even more anxiety. (Remember what Jung said about the importance of facing our fears in order to conquer them.)

SIGNS YOU ARE RESISTING THE MESSAGES

- You try to change your thoughts or feelings. You tell yourself that you shouldn't be feeling this way, or that you need to feel better right now.
- You try to avoid your experience. You distract yourself with activities or substances, or you try to numb your emotions with medication.
- You try to control your experience. You try to force yourself to feel happy, or you try to stop yourself from feeling sad.

When we resist our experience, we are essentially saying that our experience is wrong or bad. This can lead to a lot of unnecessary suffering.

Instead of resisting, we can choose to receive our experience with compassion and curiosity. This can help us to understand our experience and to find ways to cope with it in a healthy way.

SIGNS YOU ARE RECEIVING THE MESSAGES

- You acknowledge your thoughts and feelings without judgment. You say to yourself, *I'm feeling sad right now,* or *I'm having the thought that I'm not good enough*.
- You allow yourself to fully experience your emotions. You sit with your sadness, or you allow yourself to cry.
- You learn from your experience. You ask yourself, *What is*

this experience trying to teach me? or *What do I need to do to take care of myself right now?*

It can be challenging to sit with difficult emotions and feel them fully. However, it is worth it. When we receive our experience with compassion and curiosity, we can learn and grow from it.

RESISTING VS. RECEIVING

RESISTING	RECEIVING
• Refusing to tolerate the moment • Giving up on the process • Distracting yourself from the unpleasant sensations • Overfilling your schedule so you don't have time to be in your suffering • Trying to be in control • Attaching to your hurts • Trying to fix your suffering • Attaching to your thoughts	• Being in the moment • Holding the space even when the emotions become extremely powerful • Letting go of the need to control • Giving yourself space and time to listen • Letting go of the impulse to change your feelings • Giving your mind and body empathy • Noticing, releasing, noticing, releasing • Remembering that you are not your thoughts

Exercise 2: Writing Your Biography

Your current experience in your emotional and physical well-being is the sum of every single moment of your existence. Your biography, written account, or narrative of your life matters. Your origin story has clues about why you feel the way you feel. It includes your experiences and how your body adapted. By digging into those clues, we can begin the process of unwinding your anxiety.

For this exercise, you are going to write your biography. There's really no right or wrong way to tell your story, but in case you'd like a little guidance, I've got you.

Let's go back to our metaphor about the house.

Step 1: Discover how your house was built.

Let's begin by exploring the building materials that have gone into creating and sustaining your house. Those materials include your ancestors' experiences, their DNA, their nutrition, lifestyle, traumas, patterns, thoughts, and behaviors. It also includes where they built you, and whether they were skilled at being parents or were novices. It also includes patches, remodels, and fixes, which represent treatments, therapies, and skills that you have used or are currently using to maintain your house.

By understanding the building materials that went into creating you, you can start to understand how your embodied self was shaped. This can help you to become more aware of what is yours and what doesn't belong to you, acknowledge your strengths and weaknesses, and identify areas where you may need to heal or transform.

Self-Reflection

Here are some questions you can ask yourself to explore your building materials:

- What were my parents' experiences like?
- What were their hopes and dreams for me?
- What were their traumas and challenges?
- What were their thoughts and beliefs about parenting?
- How did they take care of themselves?
- What was their lifestyle like?
- What was their nutrition like?
- Where did they build me?
- Were they skilled at being parents?
- Did they use care and attention in raising me?
- As I look around my house, do I see any items that do not belong to me?
- What kinds of adaptations can I see in my house that are in response to what has transpired around me?

Step 2: Explore external and internal influences.

Every experience you've had has shaped your brain and body. Think of your brain as a secretary, faithfully documenting every event, making associations, drawing conclusions, and logging them away. These notes form the foundation of how you see the world.

In Step 2 you look back through your life and identify the weather patterns that have impacted you. In this metaphor, the weather represents the different types of experiences you have had. Nourishing rain and lightning can represent positive experiences that help you grow, learn, and become stronger and more resilient. Terrible storms can represent negative experiences that cause you pain and suffering. By identifying the different weather patterns you have experienced, you can start to understand how your embodied self has been shaped. This can help you become more aware of your strengths and weaknesses and to identify areas where you may need to heal or transform.

Self-Reflection

Here are some questions you can ask yourself to explore your weather patterns:

- As you reflect on your life experiences, ask yourself: What major events have happened in my life, both positive and negative?
- How have these events affected my thoughts, feelings, and behaviors?
- How did these experiences shape me?
- When I encounter certain situations or people, what physical sensations do I notice in my body (e.g., increased heart rate, sweating, muscle tension)? Where does stress show up in my body? (Check out the Nine Types of Anxiety Quiz in Chapter 3.)
- What is my relationship like with my body?
- What makes my anxiety better or worse, for example, diet, supplements, times of the month, days of the week?

If you get stuck with any of these questions, consider keeping a journal. Writing down your thoughts and emotions can help you track how you are reacting to different situations.

You might also consider keeping a journal of your dreams. Dreams can often be a way for our subconscious mind to communicate with us. Pay attention to the themes and symbols in your dreams, as they may be providing you with clues about how your mind and body are adapting to your stress and trauma.

You might also talk to a trusted friend, family member, or helper such as a therapist or doctor. Talking to someone you trust can help you to process your thoughts and feelings and get support.

Step 3: Explore how your mind, body, and nervous system adapted in ways that resulted in panic.

Over time, our minds and bodies can learn to overreact to even the smallest stressors. These adaptations can lead to a vicious cycle, in which our anxiety triggers physical symptoms, which then make us more anxious.

The first step to breaking this cycle is to identify the ways in which your mind and body have learned to overreact. Here are a few reflection questions to get you started:

- How do I cope with stress? Where did I learn these coping mechanisms? Are any of my coping mechanisms contributing to anxiety?
- What people or scenarios tend to be activating for me? What situations, thoughts, environments, or people contribute to my anxiety?
- What are my thinking patterns? Do I tend to think in negative or catastrophic ways? Do I have fear-based beliefs? What about my thinking patterns can I improve?
- What is my self-talk like? What do I say to myself when I'm feeling anxious? Am I being kind and compassionate to myself, or am I being critical and judgmental?

Once you've identified the ways in which your mind and body have adapted to panic and anxiety, you can start to work on breaking the cycle. This may involve changing your coping mechanisms, learning to manage your triggers, challenging your negative thinking patterns, and practicing self-compassion. It's important to remember that this is a process, and that it takes time and effort to change. With patience and persistence, you can overcome anxiety and live a more peaceful and fulfilling life.

To help you maintain momentum, I created a guided imagery that you can listen to while you practice radical acknowledgment. You can find it by going to InsightTimer.com, downloading the app, searching for *Dr. Nicole Cain,* and clicking on the recording entitled "Radical Acknowledgment Guided Meditation."

RADICAL ACKNOWLEDGMENT TL;DR

- Your mind and body are the house where you live. The story of why you experience panic is told within the walls.
- What you deny and suppress will ultimately amplify and express itself.
- Top-down approaches for anxiety start with your thoughts and work their way down to the body.
- Bottom-up approaches for treating anxiety focus on healing the body in order to regulate the mind.
- By receiving the messages from your mind and body in the form of symptoms, you can learn to identify what needs healing and how.

2

STOPLIGHT STRATEGIES: RED LIGHT, YELLOW LIGHT, GREEN LIGHT

"I HAD A PANIC ATTACK, AND I NEED TO KNOW WHAT I CAN DO TO make it never happen again."

Aria is a high-powered consultant for a Fortune 500 company. She is affluent, perfectionistic, and demanding. She has high expectations of those around her and even higher expectations of herself.

On the outside, she appears to be a composed woman in her early forties. She's wearing a tailored pencil skirt in black and a blouse that matches her dark blue eyes. Poised on the couch across from me in my office, she has a tablet in hand and is ready for my response.

"Tell me about the panic attack."

Aria hesitated. "It's mortifying."

"One of the worst parts about panic is the feeling of being out of control." I sympathized.

Aria set her tablet next to her on the couch and leaned forward. "Do you really believe people can get better from this?"

I nodded. "I believe the mind and body are capable of incredible healing."

Satisfied, Aria took a deep breath and told me the story.

"I was in bed with a gorgeous executive from one of the companies we consult for. He had been after me for months. Flowers, sexy texts, and the whole lot. I finally gave in and agreed to go out with him."

She paused, averting her gaze.

"We were having sex. It was fabulous. I was getting close . . . And then suddenly out of nowhere: Sheer terror!

"I shoved him off me and jumped out of bed. All I could think about was how I needed air. I just needed to get out. The next thing I knew, my body was running naked out of the room and down the stairwell. I was entering the hotel lobby before my brain had fully picked up on what was happening.

"I was frantic and confused and I didn't know where to go. Thankfully, some woman grabbed my arm and pulled me into the hotel bathroom. She gave me her coat so that I could cover myself, and she called 911. I cried in the bathroom stall until the paramedics came."

MAYBE YOU'VE HEARD THAT panic attacks occur for no reason, that they can come out of the blue, and there is little you can do except wait them out, do some deep breathing, or take a pill. You've resigned yourself to the fact that sometimes our nervous systems go haywire, and that's just life. But that's a myth.

DEBUNKING MYTHS ABOUT PANIC

PANIC MYTH 1: Panic attacks occur for no reason.

TRUTH: There is *always* a reason for panic. It's just a matter of identifying what your body is trying to tell you.

PANIC MYTH 2: Panic and anxiety attacks come out of the blue.

TRUTH: Rarely do panic and anxiety attacks come out of the blue. Typically, signs of panic start small, and if the cause is not addressed, they may increase in intensity over time.

PANIC MYTH 3: There isn't much you can do about panic.

TRUTH: There is *a ton* you can do to become Panic Proof.

The more fluent you are in the language of your body, the more easily you will hear its whispers before they turn to shouts. Are you ready to stop avoiding your symptoms and start facing them? I've got your back. This chapter will provide you with the best tools to help you.

THE SPECTRUM OF PANIC AND ANXIETY

If you think about your levels of stress at different times in your life, they vary, right? Some days you're a little overwhelmed, and other times you're straight-up panicking.

Anxiety occurs on a spectrum. At one end of the spectrum are calm and relaxed feelings. At the other end are feelings of stress and panic at its worst, like in Aria's experience.

Two of the most common statements I hear from my clients are:

> *"I was having bouts of anxiety bordering on panic, so my doctor gave me an emergency prescription for Xanax. But it knocks me out and then I can't function."*

> *"During a full-blown panic attack, I tried deep breathing and it didn't help."*

Here's the thing: While benzodiazepines and breathwork may be valuable across different parts of the spectrum of anxiety, they are going to work only when they're optimally utilized. For example, in Aria's situation: What if the woman who helped her had suggested doing breathwork instead of calling the hospital? Does that mean breathwork doesn't work? No. It just means that breathwork might not have been the right solution at that exact moment. Similarly, it wouldn't make sense for you to call 911 every time you start feeling a little bit stressed.

This brings us to the million-dollar question: How do you know what to do and when to take action?

I want to introduce you to the Stoplight Exercise, which will help you match your symptoms with the appropriate solutions (i.e., when to use breathwork and when to use your emergency resources).

THE SPECTRUM OF ANXIETY

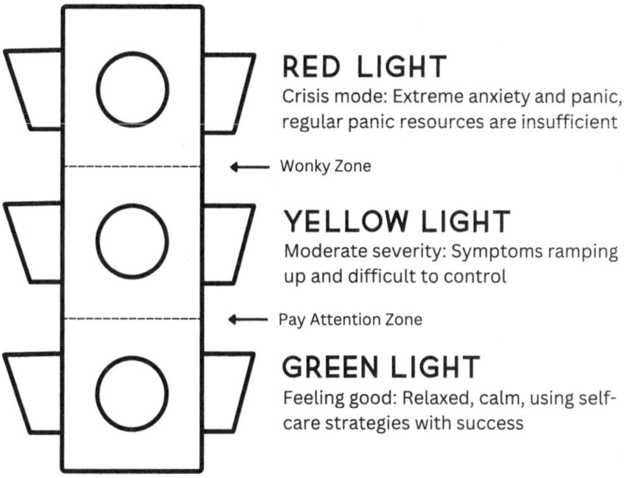
RED LIGHT
Crisis mode: Extreme anxiety and panic, regular panic resources are insufficient
Wonky Zone
YELLOW LIGHT
Moderate severity: Symptoms ramping up and difficult to control
Pay Attention Zone
GREEN LIGHT
Feeling good: Relaxed, calm, using self-care strategies with success

We start with the image of a stoplight with zones for a red light, a green light, and a yellow light. The Stoplight also has two zones that represent shifting from one color into the next: the Pay Attention Zone and the Wonky Zone.

- Green Light Zone
- Pay Attention Zone
- Yellow Light Zone
- Wonky Zone
- Red Light Zone

The goal of this chapter is to give you a much clearer understanding of what it feels like at each zone so that you can (1) learn how to stop panic before it starts and (2) identify the best solutions for the zone you're in.

Let's go back to Aria's story. Part of her healing process involved getting clear on her Stoplight Strategies. While Aria was adept in the skills she needed for her job—data analysis, customer relations, and company literacy—she did not possess the same level of skill when it came to being present with her emotions, not to mention her body's innate physical reactions to them. In fact, her modus operandi was to ignore and suppress anything uncomfortable.

That's why panic caught her by surprise, "suddenly, out of nowhere."

"I KNOW WHAT YOU'RE THINKING." The glimmer of vulnerability vanished from Aria's eyes. With a few smart clicks, she opened the document she had been taking notes in during our sessions. "You're thinking I have anxiety. But I don't. I'm just extremely stressed, and I had an episode. Which, as I said, cannot happen again."

"You described the panic attack as coming out of nowhere," I answered. "But often in retrospect, we can see that the body has been giving us little warnings all along.

"I like to visualize the process-to-panic with the imagery of a stoplight. The Green Light is a zone of calm. Then as stress rises you hit the Yellow Light Zone. And if your nervous system continues amping up, you will eventually hit the Red Light Zone, which represents panic or crisis.

"If you're open to it, doing the Stoplight Exercise together may help us identify your body's subtler signals of stress so that we can make a plan for you to take action before you reach the Red Light Zone or crisis."

"You're saying that my body may have given out warning signs before I went into this insane episode?"

"Possibly," I answered. "Let's walk through that evening together. Take me to the beginning of the date."

"I was actually feeling pretty good that day. Most of the time I'm stressed and at the edge of my rope."

"What was the difference between how you felt that day versus your usual level of stress?" I asked.

"When I'm calm, I feel like I can breathe more easily. My thoughts are in the moment instead of fixed on deadlines. I'm relaxed and feeling confident."

"Good." I nodded. "Those are descriptions of your Green Light Zone."

"Got it." Aria made notes in her workbook.

"So you're in the Green Light Zone, getting ready for your date. You're feeling calm and relaxed. What happened next?"

"I'm wearing a sexy little dress, we're at dinner, drinking champagne. Then I start to feel my brain slowing down." Aria shrugged. "When that happens, I take my Happy Pill.* It gives me the boost I need to feel like myself again."

"Got it. We're going to need to circle back to that, but first I want you to describe how the episode happened."

"Okay."

"Something changed. You were feeling good, but then you noticed your brain slowing down."

"Yes. I feel like I'm not quite there. A little less sharp."

"Okay, so that's one of the first signs that you're entering your Yellow Light Zone. What happened next?"

"After I take the Happy Pill, we finish the bottle of champagne and go to the hotel room. I am buzzed and on fire. I push him into the wall. We're taking our clothes off. My heart is racing. I'm tingling, I'm hot and frantic. It's really intense. It's not usually that intense, but I go with it."

"And then what happened?"

"We start to have sex, and I'm getting closer, and then suddenly I just freak out! It goes from fun and exciting to an absolute nightmare. One minute I'm feeling like a goddess, and the next I'm running naked into the lobby like an absolute lunatic."

"You were in the Green Light Zone, feeling good and happy. Then you felt your brain slowing down. This is the Pay-Attention Zone; this is when a shift is taking place. You went from green to yellow. You took your Happy Pill, and your brain sharpened up again, and you were drinking champagne. Next, you were in the hotel room, things were getting more intense, but you went with it. Then something drastically shifted—which is the Wonky Zone—and you snapped into the Red Light Zone."

"Exactly. Why did my body turn on me? How will I be able to stop it from happening again?"

* Her "Happy Pill" is Adderall, which she relies on anytime her mood drops.

"I hear your frustration, and I'm confident we can do just that. The first step is to help you make quick adjustments to effectively work with your nervous system. You start by increasing your awareness of your Green, Yellow, and Red Light Zones. Between today and our next session, your homework will be to walk through each stage and write down what you remember thinking and feeling in each of those phases. Once that is in place, we will have a foundation for the work that comes next."

"Tell me this: why now?" Aria's eyes flashed with anger. "I've been through way worse. Why did my body decide that now was a good time to go berserk?"

I paused and remembered an analogy that I've used in the past. "You mentioned you're a champagne girl. What about whiskey?"

Taken off guard, Aria raised her eyebrows. "Whiskey?"

I went on, "Stay with me on this one. Your body is designed to deal with stress, but the more stress you experience, the more its effects accumulate in your mind and body. We all start life with a big metaphorical barrel, like the ones they store whiskey in, and that barrel fills over time with each stressor we experience.

"What might have felt overwhelming and annoying years ago could cause more severe symptoms now. That same liquid that can be distilled into a fine beverage can just as easily overflow, encounter a spark, and explode, sending the entire warehouse of fine whiskey up in flames."

"Like in the episode," Aria concluded.

"Yes. Exactly." I nodded. "Your experience of panic gives us important information about what is going on in your mind and body, which will direct us to the best tools for emptying your barrel."

WE'LL LEARN ABOUT WHAT Aria shared in Chapter 8. But first: You probably noticed that Aria was using mood-altering substances in order to get through her day-to-day life. And that was a pretty big deal—considering it resulted, in part, in her running naked through a hotel lobby. This is an important part of her story, which we'll explore in more detail later.

But first, it's your turn to listen to your own anxiety.

THE STOPLIGHT EXERCISE

Green Light Zone

The Green Light Zone is a state in which you are happy, calm, confident, relaxed, motivated, centered, resilient, and connected with yourself and others. We cultivate our Green Light Zone by honoring our protective parts, engaging in self-care activities, resourcing, and doing frequent check-ins. Green Light Zones are eager, growing, honoring, protective, and directive. They are the deer happily grazing in a meadow: no worries, just resting and digesting. The Green Light Zone is mastered by your parasympathetic nervous system, which is all about relaxation.

Self-Reflection

Have you ever been in the Green Light Zone? What was it like for you? Describe your Green Light Zone in the space below.

Signs I'm in the Green Light Zone:

____

____

____

What makes you feel calm and relaxed? In the space below, jot down a few ideas or circumstances that help you feel relaxed, such as walking the dog, limiting caffeine, watching reruns of Bob Ross painting.

Things that make me feel calm and relaxed:

____

____

____

If you are struggling to come up with a time where you felt calm or safe, or are struggling to identify self-care strategies, you are not alone. Some of us have never felt truly safe. If you resonate with this, I will have some suggestions for you in the Panic Reset in Chapter 9. For now, try to come up with at least one thing you can think of that can help you relax, even just a little bit.

The Pay Attention Zone

In the Pay Attention Zone we shift from Green to Yellow. Your body will give you signs that you need to pause and pay attention. This zone is all about tuning in to the signals your body is sending. This is the moment when you switch from calmness to "something's up." Imagine a deer grazing in a field: it hears a noise, stops what it is doing, and looks up. The deer is assessing, *Am I in danger?*

When Aria entered her Pay Attention Zone, she experienced feelings of fogginess in her brain. For me, it's tightness in my chest. For others, this zone presents in the form of intuition, a knowing, or a gut instinct. Everybody's Pay Attention Zone is different. You will learn all about this in Chapter 3, which explores the nine types of anxiety. Once you figure out what your signals are, you will be more easily able to take action to stop anxiety before it even shows up.

Self-Reflection

What do you notice happening in your body, thoughts, or circumstances before stress or anxiety kicks in?

Signs I am in the Pay Attention Zone:

____

____

____

Yellow Light Zone

In the Yellow Light Zone, you are feeling amped up, with excess worry, anxiety, irritability, jaw clenching, and other sensations. When my Yellow Light Zone gets activated, I feel dread and constriction in my throat, and I clench my jaw. Aria described feeling buzzed, her heart rate sped up, and she was more amplified. The deer has decided that there is a probable danger and is moving away toward safety.

For some people, these feelings are positive and exciting, but as you will learn in Part II, the body produces the same chemical reactions in good stress as in bad stress. The major difference for us is context.

Self-Reflection

What does stress or anxiety feel like for you as it revs up? Try to remember thoughts and sensations that occur when you are in the Yellow Light Zone, and write them down in the space below.

Signs I am in the Yellow Light Zone:

____

____

____

We all have our triggers. They can be in the past, in our current circumstances, or even in the future. Write down your Yellow Light Zone triggers here. (Refer back to your notes from Chapter 1 about your history of stress.)

What pushes me toward the Yellow Light Zone?

____

____

____

The Wonky Zone

The Wonky Zone is where things are about to get real. The body is gearing up to switch into crisis mode. If you can zero in on the Wonky Zone, you'll have the chance to stop the cycle of panic before it starts. The first step is to become aware of what it is like when it happens for you.

Self-Reflection

Physical, mental, and emotional signs I am in the Wonky Zone:

____

____

____

Red Light Zone

The Red Light Zone is crisis mode, with the physical, mental, and emotional symptoms of autonomic arousal. You may have heard this described as "fight, flight, freeze, flop, fawn, and/or fracture" (which I'll refer to throughout this book as F6—you'll learn more about it in Chapter 4).

The Red Light Zone is panic, rage, dissociation, extreme pain, and whatever other experiences you may attribute to feeling out of control and at your wit's end. Aria's Red Light Zone was the panic attack that caused her body to go into literal flight.

Oftentimes people tell me that they tried deep breathing, meditation, herbs, and other great integrative tools in the Red Light Zone, without success. Perhaps it was not the right tool for that person. Or perhaps it was not the right tool for that particular Stoplight Zone.

Let me share an example. You drink water, right? (I sure hope so!) For general purposes, let's say you take a gulp every hour or so and that's enough. But now let's say that you're running in the middle of the hottest day of the summer, in Phoenix, Arizona. It is over 100 degrees, and you feel like the pavement is made of lava. You're sweltering hot, covered in sweat, and you realize that if you don't get a drink right away, you'll pass out. In this second scenario, will your typical single gulp be enough? Definitely not. That would be like a squirt bottle of water in a forest fire.

Self-Reflection

Things that push me into the Red Light Zone:

____

____

____

Signs that I am in the Red Light Zone:

____

____

____

When you are in the Red Light Zone, your body is in a state of crisis. Your nervous system is firing on all cylinders, and you're going to need crisis resources. The best resources will help you hold space for your anxiety and restore a sense of power over panic.

We'll dig into the treatments and solutions in Chapter 11. In the meantime, write down your go-to crisis resources, and after you read Chapter 11, jot down some of them here.

My Crisis Resources

____

____

____

____

STOPLIGHT STRATEGIES TL;DR

- There is *always* a reason for panic.
- Panic attacks rarely come out of the blue.
- There is *a ton* you can do to become Panic Proof.
- You will get the best results by selecting interventions that match the intensity of your symptoms.

3

THE NINE TYPES OF ANXIETY

"A MOVING TARGET."

That's how Esme describes her panic. As a second-generation immigrant, and the first member of her family to earn a college degree, Esme felt the stakes were high.

"When my anxiety began, it was all in my chest. In college, it just fluttered here and there. But after I graduated and left home, my stress got worse and my panic skyrocketed. It felt like a bolt of lightning shooting right into my heart making me dizzy and out of breath." She tried a medication, commonly prescribed for anxiety, called a beta-blocker.

"But it didn't make me less anxious," Esme said. "Instead, my symptoms just changed. Instead of centering right here"—she indicated her heart—"the panic moved to my gut. Everything makes me nauseated, and I throw up pretty regularly. My doctor added an antidepressant and a stomach pill, which definitely takes the edge off, but something I'm taking is giving me terrible headaches—especially around my cycle."

Despite a handful of prescriptions, what had begun as mild stress with the occasional heart palpitation had accelerated into full-blown panic so severe that Esme found herself contemplating her exit strategy. "It's not that I don't want to be here," Esme admits. "I just don't think I can live like this much longer."

* * *

DID YOU NOTICE HOW Esme's symptoms kept changing? Beginning with mild fluttering of her heart, transitioning to lightning-like chest pains, gastrointestinal upset, migraines, and then depression? One key aspect of her story of panic is that her symptoms are changeable, "a moving target."

But when her doctor tried to match the treatment to the symptom—a beta-blocker designed to stop palpitations in her Chest Anxiety, a "stomach pill" for the Gut Anxiety, and an antidepressant for overall anxiety and depression—she didn't get better.

HERE'S WHY:

- Her doctor mistook each symptom *as the problem* instead of the body's *solution to the problem.*
- They did not dive into the *why* of panic.
- Treatments were not aimed at building greater health of the mind and body.

Is there a better option? Yes. The solution has three parts, all equally important:

- Identify *why* Esme experiences symptoms of panic.
- Explore *what* her mind and body are doing to adapt.
- Learn *how* to restore vitality and resilience to equip the mind and body to heal.

ONE SIZE DOES NOT FIT ALL

A one-size-fits-all approach to panic and anxiety just doesn't make sense. But in our medical system, most people with anxiety and panic are thrown into the same small diagnostic bucket and thus receive similar treatments.

That's how I was trained. How we all were trained. Throughout both my master's degree in clinical psychology and medical school, my colleagues and I were instructed that mental health and brain health symptoms were problems to be organized into diagnostic categories and treated based on their categorization (usually involving a mix of counseling and some sort of prescription medication).

It felt like a conveyor belt: Patient comes in and gets a diagnosis and referral for treatment. Next! Rinse and repeat. Welcome to modern medicine!

By looking carefully at the symptoms of panic, we gain the ability to understand the nuance and meaning of each symptom. So far in this book, you've met Charlotte, whose panic presents with jittery hands, insomnia, and rapid weight loss. You've also met Aria, who has bouts of sheer terror with varying levels of dissociation, and Esme, who feels like she can't make heads or tails of her ever-changing symptoms.

Allow me to introduce you to the *nine different types* of panic and anxiety.

THE MANY VOICES OF PANIC

I'd like for you to put on your researcher hat. Imagine conducting a study where you go to the busiest city centers in your community and ask every person you see, "What does it feel like when you experience panic?" According to research, the most common answers you will hear are:

- Racing, pounding, or skipping of the heartbeat
- Chest pain
- Chest tightness or difficulty with breathing
- Flushes of heat or chills
- Dizziness or feeling disconnected
- Numbness or pins and needles
- A need to go to the toilet
- Churning or tightness, fluttering, or sick feeling in the pit of the stomach
- Racing, intrusive, disturbing, or anxious thoughts
- Terror

- Irritability or rage
- Hopelessness, despair, self-criticism
- Flashbacks, nightmares, or disturbing memories

While everyone's experience is unique, the most common symptoms of anxiety and panic can be divided into nine general categories.

Think about it this way: Imagine that each person is represented as a mountain, and their individualizing factors have formed ravines that flow from the top of the mountain all the way down to the base. Next, imagine standing at the top of the mountain and pouring water out of a pitcher. Pulled downward by gravity, the water follows the path(s) of least resistance through the ravines. Each grouping of ravines represents the different types of anxiety, how they got there, and how to heal.

If you have a fear of heights, your unmet need might be for safety or control. The ravine that represents this unmet need might be in your chest, with symptoms such as a racing heart or shortness of breath.

By understanding which form your panic takes, you can focus on treatments that address your unmet need that is being conveyed by that symptom, and you can identify more effective tools for the part of your body that manifests anxiety and panic symptoms.

Nine Types of Anxiety Quiz

CHEST ANXIETY

Circle the number that best describes you when you are experiencing panic and anxiety.

I feel tension and anxiety in my chest.

0	1	2	3	4
Not like me	Occasionally	Frequently, yes	Very much like me	Yes, very extreme

I experience shortness of breath or "air hunger."

0	1	2	3	4
Not like me	Occasionally	Frequently, yes	Very much like me	Yes, very extreme

I feel constriction at my chest like a band or a pressing heaviness.

0	1	2	3	4
Not like me	Occasionally	Frequently, yes	Very much like me	Yes, very extreme

My heart races, pounds, or skips beats.

0	1	2	3	4
Not like me	Occasionally	Frequently, yes	Very much like me	Yes, very extreme

I get a lump in my throat or feel the need to cough.

0	1	2	3	4
Not like me	Occasionally	Frequently, yes	Very much like me	Yes, very extreme

Total (out of 20) ____________

SCORING

NO TO LOW CHEST ANXIETY (0–6)

When panic strikes, you may get a symptom in your chest or throat, but Chest Anxiety is not your main thing.

MEDIUM CHEST ANXIETY (7–13)

Your symptoms tend to show up in your upper torso near your chest and heart. You may notice changes in your heartbeat and find it more difficult to get a satisfying breath. Notice how your symptoms fluctuate through time: is your Chest Anxiety an early indicator of panic, or does it emerge as your symptoms amplify? Journaling the process will help you identify the best solutions from the start.

HIGH CHEST ANXIETY (14–20)

Chest Anxiety is one of your body's main ways of communicating. Pay close attention to *how* you experience it. For example, does your heart pound, or do you experience shortness of breath? In Chapter 11 you are going to learn how to translate the nuanced messages of your Chest Anxiety into effective solutions.

NERVOUS SYSTEM ANXIETY

Circle the number that best describes you when you are experiencing panic and anxiety.

I experience stress-related muscle tension.

0	1	2	3	4
Not like me	Occasionally	Frequently, yes	Very much like me	Yes, very extreme

I have tension headaches or migraines.

0	1	2	3	4
Not like me	Occasionally	Frequently, yes	Very much like me	Yes, very extreme

I notice changes in my sensitivity to noise, light, and/or odors with panic and stress.

0	1	2	3	4
Not like me	Occasionally	Frequently, yes	Very much like me	Yes, very extreme

I feel dizzy, dissociated, or uncoordinated with panic or stress.

0	1	2	3	4
Not like me	Occasionally	Frequently, yes	Very much like me	Yes, very extreme

I feel nerve pains (tingling, shooting, burning, stinging, or even numbness).

0	1	2	3	4
Not like me	Occasionally	Frequently, yes	Very much like me	Yes, very extreme

Total (out of 20) ________________

SCORING

NO TO LOW NERVOUS SYSTEM ANXIETY (0-6)

When panic strikes, you may get symptoms in different parts of your nervous system such as your muscles, nerves, or head, but Nervous System Anxiety is not your main thing.

MEDIUM NERVOUS SYSTEM ANXIETY (7-13)

When you feel panic and anxiety, it may show up in your muscles, nerves, and/or head. You may experience numbness, tingling, or a feeling of detachment from your surroundings (derealization) or body (dissociation). Keep track of the different ways your nervous system reveals that it is stressed so that you can more quickly and easily catch the early signs that your body is shifting from calm to arousal.

HIGH NERVOUS SYSTEM ANXIETY (14-20)

Nervous System Anxiety is your body's main way of communicating. Pay close attention to how you experience it. For example, do you get tickling in your nerves or is the sensation more burning? In Chapter 11 you'll learn to translate your Nervous System Anxiety's nuanced messages into solutions that work.

IMMUNE SYSTEM ANXIETY

Circle the number that best describes you when you are experiencing panic and anxiety.

My anxiety symptoms change frequently, affecting different parts of my body (skin, pain, dizziness).

0	1	2	3	4
Not like me	Occasionally	Frequently, yes	Very much like me	Yes, very extreme

My anxiety symptoms are accompanied by other conditions like allergies, sensitivities, or chronic illnesses.

0	1	2	3	4
Not like me	Occasionally	Frequently, yes	Very much like me	Yes, very extreme

My anxiety symptoms started, or tend to worsen, during periods of high stress or change.

0	1	2	3	4
Not like me	Occasionally	Frequently, yes	Very much like me	Yes, very extreme

I have had past infections like strep, Epstein-Barr, or Lyme disease.

0	1	2	3	4
Not like me	Occasionally	Frequently, yes	Very much like me	Yes, very extreme

I tend to feel somewhat less anxious when taking anti-inflammatories or antihistamines.

0	1	2	3	4
Not like me	Occasionally	Frequently, yes	Very much like me	Yes, very extreme

Total (out of 20) ____________

SCORING

NO TO LOW IMMUNE SYSTEM ANXIETY (0–6)

Your risk factors and indicators of inflammation or imbalances in your immune system are low, suggesting that you are at low risk of Immune System Anxiety.

MEDIUM IMMUNE SYSTEM (7–13)

You may experience panic and anxiety as part of a bigger picture of symptoms that may range from head to toe. A common undercurrent is inflammation. When your inflammation levels rise your risk of anxiety increases, and as inflammation goes down, your risk for anxiety decreases.

HIGH IMMUNE SYSTEM (14–20)

Immune System Anxiety is one of the most prominent ways your body is communicating to you. Now that we have zeroed in on a possible root cause, you can zero in on treatments that include immune system balancing.

GUT ANXIETY

Circle the number that best describes you when you are experiencing panic and anxiety.

I struggle with digestive upset (gas, bloating, diarrhea, constipation, nausea, IBS).

0	1	2	3	4
Not like me	Occasionally	Frequently, yes	Very much like me	Yes, very extreme

I feel butterflies or a pit in my stomach.

0	1	2	3	4
Not like me	Occasionally	Frequently, yes	Very much like me	Yes, very extreme

My appetite changes (overeating, undereating, changes in food cravings).

0	1	2	3	4
Not like me	Occasionally	Frequently, yes	Very much like me	Yes, very extreme

I often find myself needing digestive support like antacids or enzymes.

0	1	2	3	4
Not like me	Occasionally	Frequently, yes	Very much like me	Yes, very extreme

I often deal with cramping or pain in my stomach or abdomen.

0	1	2	3	4
Not like me	Occasionally	Frequently, yes	Very much like me	Yes, very extreme

Total (out of 20) ______________

SCORING

NO TO LOW GUT ANXIETY (0–6)

When panic strikes, you may experience some distress in your digestive tract with gas, bloating, or changes in your bowel habits, but Gut Anxiety is not your main thing.

MEDIUM GUT ANXIETY (7–13)

When you feel panic and anxiety, you experience symptoms in your digestive tract. You may experience a pit in your stomach, nausea, vomiting, diarrhea, gas, or bloating. Do your symptoms start in your gut, or do they emerge as your anxiety amplifies? Journaling the process will help you identify the best solutions before your symptoms spiral into full-fledged panic.

HIGH GUT ANXIETY (14–20)

Gut Anxiety is one of the most prominent ways your body is communicating to you. Your gut is filled with trillions of mood-altering microbes that are in constant communication with your brain, and they have something to say to you. As you build your Panic Proof Protocol, you're going to want to put gut healing at the top of your list, which you'll learn a lot more about in Chapter 5, about the gut-brain axis.

THOUGHT ANXIETY

Circle the number that best describes you when you are experiencing panic and anxiety.

My thoughts can be intrusive, obsessive, disturbing, and unwanted.

0	1	2	3	4
Not like me	Occasionally	Frequently, yes	Very much like me	Yes, very extreme

My thoughts can often be "sticky" and hard to ignore or get away from.

0	1	2	3	4
Not like me	Occasionally	Frequently, yes	Very much like me	Yes, very extreme

My panic and anxiety can be provoked or worsened by my thoughts.

0	1	2	3	4
Not like me	Occasionally	Frequently, yes	Very much like me	Yes, very extreme

My thoughts hold me back from putting myself out there.

0	1	2	3	4
Not like me	Occasionally	Frequently, yes	Very much like me	Yes, very extreme

My thoughts interfere with things I want or need to do such as work or sleep.

0	1	2	3	4
Not like me	Occasionally	Frequently, yes	Very much like me	Yes, very extreme

Total (out of 20) ________________

SCORING

NO TO LOW THOUGHT ANXIETY (0–6)

When panic strikes, you may find it somewhat harder to concentrate, struggle with brain fog, or deal with low levels of distressing or intrusive thoughts, but Thought Anxiety is not your main thing.

MEDIUM THOUGHT ANXIETY (7–13)

Panic and anxiety definitely affect your thoughts. They may become more anxious, obsessive, repetitive, disturbing, confused, or distractible, or you may struggle to find words, or you're forgetful, scattered, inattentive, or you experience brain fog. These are the key characteristics of Thought Anxiety.

HIGH THOUGHT ANXIETY (14–20)

Thought Anxiety is one of the most prominent ways your body is communicating to you. Read through the subtypes of Thought Anxiety and circle what subtype is the most prominent when your anxiety is the worst. You'll want to know that for creating your Panic Proof Protocol in Chapter 11.

ANGER ANXIETY

Circle the number that best describes you when you are experiencing panic and anxiety.

I often feel annoyed by "little" things.

0	1	2	3	4
Not like me	Occasionally	Frequently, yes	Very much like me	Yes, very extreme

I often feel overwhelmed by my life circumstances.

0	1	2	3	4
Not like me	Occasionally	Frequently, yes	Very much like me	Yes, very extreme

I clench my jaw or grind my teeth.

0	1	2	3	4
Not lik me	Occasionally	Frequently, yes	Very much like me	Yes, very extreme

My fuse may be described as short and I can become easily angered.

0	1	2	3	4
Not like me	Occasionally	Frequently, yes	Very much like me	Yes, very extreme

I often feel the need to lash out—either verbally or physically—from frustration.

0	1	2	3	4
Not like me	Occasionally	Frequently, yes	Very much like me	Yes, very extreme

Total (out of 20) ________________

SCORING

NO TO LOW ANGER ANXIETY (0-6)

When panic strikes, you may experience feeling more easily annoyed or frustrated, but Anger Anxiety is not your main thing.

MEDIUM ANGER ANXIETY (7-13)

You experience moderate levels of Anger Anxiety with feelings of irritability, frustration, and overwhelm. Anger Anxiety refers to the *fight* part of fight, flight, freeze. Mapping out your cycles of anger can help you understand the process of how your nervous system is getting activated, and responds to stressful situations. With this data, you will be able to better recruit solutions that match your particular symptoms before they spiral out of your control.

HIGH ANGER ANXIETY (14-20)

Anger Anxiety is one of the most prominent ways your body and mind are communicating to you. Your nervous system is in autonomic arousal, and in its attempt to protect you, it may be producing stress hormones, such as adrenaline and cortisol, but this process is taking its toll on your emotional and physical health. Check out Chapter 11, which elaborates on symptoms associated with pitta imbalances, a common cause of Anger Anxiety.

DEPRESSIVE ANXIETY

Circle the number that best describes you when you are experiencing panic and anxiety.

I feel sad or low more days than not.

0	1	2	3	4
Not like me	Occasionally	Frequently, yes	Very much like me	Yes, very extreme

I struggle with low self-worth.

0	1	2	3	4
Not like me	Occasionally	Frequently, yes	Very much like me	Yes, very extreme

I feel depressed and discouraged as a result of my anxiety and panic.

0	1	2	3	4
Not like me	Occasionally	Frequently, yes	Very much like me	Yes, very extreme

I often feel sad and want to cry (whether I am able to cry or not).

0	1	2	3	4
Not like me	Occasionally	Frequently, yes	Very much like me	Yes, very extreme

I am hard on myself and overly critical of myself.

0	1	2	3	4
Not like me	Occasionally	Frequently, yes	Very much like me	Yes, very extreme

Total (out of 20) ________________

SCORING

NO TO LOW DEPRESSIVE ANXIETY (0–6)

When panic strikes, you may experience drops in your mood, causing you to feel mildly depressed, but Depressive Anxiety is not your main thing.

MEDIUM DEPRESSIVE ANXIETY (7–13)

When you feel panic and anxiety, you may also experience moderate feelings of sadness, discouragement, feelings of inadequacy, and/or hopelessness. Keeping a mood log and exploring your particular patterns of Depressive Anxiety will help offer clarity for when your symptoms ebb and flow. In your mood log, be sure to note how you feel, being mindful to include: triggers, thoughts, patterns, and accompanying mental and physical symptoms.

HIGH DEPRESSIVE ANXIETY (14–20)

When anxiety spikes, you tend to get a mix of anxiety and depressive symptoms. For some, this can show up with feelings of lethargy and collapse, and for others it can present with urgency and despair. The key is identifying the particularities of *how* you experience Depressive Anxiety. This will be particularly useful when selecting botanical remedies in Chapter 11.

HORMONE ANXIETY

Circle the number that best describes you when you are experiencing panic and anxiety.

I have noticed a relationship between my moods and my hormone levels or changes.

0	1	2	3	4
Not like me	Occasionally	Frequently, yes	Very much like me	Yes, very extreme

I struggle with my sex drive (desire and/or performance).

0	1	2	3	4
Not like me	Occasionally	Frequently, yes	Very much like me	Yes, very extreme

My blood sugar levels are unstable, and I find myself getting "hangry" or nauseated between meals.

0	1	2	3	4
Not like me	Occasionally	Frequently, yes	Very much like me	Yes, very extreme

My energy levels are unstable and are not where I want them to be.

0	1	2	3	4
Not like me	Occasionally	Frequently, yes	Very much like me	Yes, very extreme

It is difficult for me to maintain my optimal weight.

0	1	2	3	4
Not like me	Occasionally	Frequently, yes	Very much like me	Yes, very extreme

Total (out of 20) ____________

SCORING

NO TO LOW HORMONE ANXIETY (0–6)

You may see some subtle patterns related to your mood and potential changes in your hormone levels, but it's not quite clear. You may want to consider getting basic endocrine testing done to rule out endocrine-related causes of panic. We will explore these tests in Chapter 7.

MEDIUM HORMONE ANXIETY (7–13)

It is very likely that there is a relationship between your endocrine system and your symptoms of panic. You'll learn more about the endocrine system in Chapter 7. In addition to getting basic endocrine testing done, you may consider a deeper dive into more specific functional testing, which you'll learn about throughout this book.

HIGH HORMONE ANXIETY (14–20)

It is extremely likely that an imbalance in your endocrine system is playing a role in your panic. If you've had your hormones tested (thyroid, adrenals, sex hormones), you might consider doing a deeper dive into root causes of endocrine imbalances. To learn more, check out Chapter 8, on obstacles to cure.

TRAUMA ANXIETY

Circle the number that best describes you when you are experiencing panic and anxiety.

I have endured or witnessed an event that caused me to fear for my life or someone else's.

0	1	2	3	4
Not like me	Occasionally	Frequently, yes	Very much like me	Yes, very extreme

I endured abuse such as being struck, mocked, or neglected as a child or adult.

0	1	2	3	4
Not like me	Occasionally	Frequently, yes	Very much like me	Yes, very extreme

When I am awake, I have thoughts or daydreams about the traumatic event(s).

0	1	2	3	4
Not like me	Occasionally	Frequently, yes	Very much like me	Yes, very extreme

I have recurrent nightmares.

0	1	2	3	4
Not like me	Occasionally	Frequently, yes	Very much like me	Yes, very extreme

I feel like the world is generally unsafe and that I need to be hypervigilant.

0	1	2	3	4
Not like me	Occasionally	Frequently, yes	Very much like me	Yes, very extreme

Total (out of 20) ______________

SCORING

NO TO LOW TRAUMA ANXIETY (0-6)

While you've gone through stress, you're more resilient to the effects of aversive events in your life, and Trauma Anxiety may not be your main thing. It is important to note, however, that trauma shows up in many different ways that cannot be completely encompassed by this quiz.

MEDIUM TRAUMA ANXIETY (7-13)

You experience moderate levels of Trauma Anxiety. Your brain and body have adapted to aversive events, or traumas, which are very likely contributing to your symptoms of panic. Doing inner work can help offer clarity and deep healing. It is important to note, however, that sometimes healing occurs in layers. So be patient with yourself, and take your time doing the exercises in this book and, if needed, consider enlisting help.

HIGH TRAUMA ANXIETY (14-20)

Trauma and aversive experiences are very likely to be a central part of your anxiety and panic. In an attempt to protect you from the effects of trauma, your body has adapted, which can cause symptoms from head to toe. But the good news is that you can heal—the research has proven this again and again. In Chapter 10, you are going to learn how to be your own trauma-informed therapist, and I've also included resources for finding a trauma-informed therapist in Appendix B.

THE NINE TYPES OF ANXIETY

Now that you know your predominant type of anxiety, let's get to know them a bit better. As you read, make notes on how your symptoms *start* and *change* over time. You might even add some of these notes to your Panic Proof Protocol in Chapter 11. With practice over time, it'll become easier for you to detect subtle clues right away so that you can use your tools to stop panic before it starts.

CHEST ANXIETY

HOW ANXIETY MIGHT IMPACT YOUR HEART

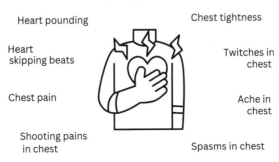

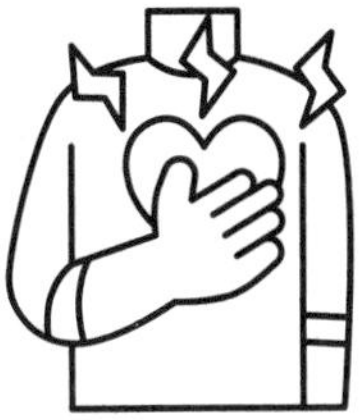
Squeezing sensation
Heart pounding
Chest tightness
Heart skipping beats
Twitches in chest
Chest pain
Ache in chest
Shooting pains in chest
Spasms in chest
Feeling pressure on chest

CHEST ANXIETY. Have you ever experienced heart palpitations so intense, it feels like your heart is going to burst right out of your chest?

It's as if you're being chased by a tiger, or you're running a marathon, or you've drunk six gallons of caffeine. But in actuality, you're sitting in a meeting, trying to fall asleep at night, or having dinner with your friends.

Symptoms of stress that present with tightness in your chest, racing heart, difficulties breathing, skipping beats, and even chest pains are associated with a type of anxiety called Chest Anxiety. Chest Anxiety is anxiety that shows up in . . . yep, you guessed it: your chest.

While Chest Anxiety is one of the most common places panic presents, symptoms manifesting in the heart and lungs can be particularly alarming. This is why so many Chest Anxiety sufferers wind up going to the emergency department, afraid that they're having a heart attack.

TWO THINGS YOU NEED TO KNOW:

1. If you have been thoroughly worked up by your doctors and have been given a clean bill of lung and heart health, you are in the fine company of patients seeking emergency care for chest pain who do not actually have any cardiac or

respiratory health issues but rather are suffering from episodes of panic and anxiety.

2. Your heart and lungs are doing exactly what they're designed to do.

I want you to think about it this way: when your brain detects danger, its main agenda is to get you to safety.

During panic your body responds in much the same way as it does when you're in actual danger: your brain triggers a state of activation, called autonomic arousal, which includes fight, flight, freeze, fawn, flop, and fracture (F6).

During F6, your breathing will speed up so your lungs can take in more oxygen, and your heart will beat faster so it can more quickly send that oxygen to the runaway muscles in your body such as your legs and feet. The better your heart and lungs can respond, the more likely you are to run away from danger.

While it's great to know that your heart and lungs are in tip-top shape, these changes can feel really frightening when they occur for seemingly no apparent reason. But know this: if you suffer with a racing and pounding heart during panic and anxiety, your heart is doing exactly what it's supposed to be doing.

Throughout this book, you are going to learn how to decode *why* you experience certain symptoms of panic, and *how* to heal. We will explore root-cause functional testing for Chest Anxiety and dive into Chest Anxiety–specific solutions later in Chapter 11.

NERVOUS SYSTEM ANXIETY. Do you know that feeling you get when you sit on your foot and it "goes to sleep"? You stand up after sitting in a funny position, take a step, and are flooded with feelings of pins and needles that can range from mild to pretty extreme.

You easily identify the cause of these funny sensations: *Sat on foot, cut off blood supply, foot now feels like it's being bitten by a thousand fire ants.* Check.

But what if you're minding your own business, taking an exam, or

NERVOUS SYSTEM ANXIETY

HOW ANXIETY MIGHT IMPACT YOUR NERVES

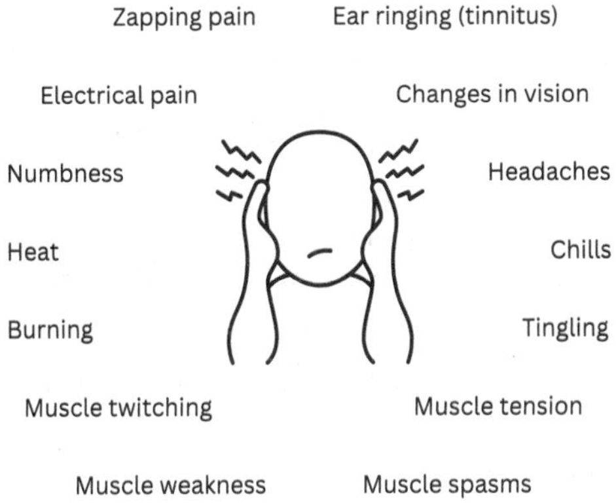

giving a presentation, and your nervous system starts to go haywire? You might experience all sorts of sensations such as pins and needles, numbness, or tingling in your hands, feet, or even face. If you're not already experiencing anxiety, these kinds of sensations can be pretty alarming.

Nervous System Anxiety manifests in symptoms associated with the nervous system. The nervous system is composed of your brain, nerves, and muscles. Here are the four main ways Nervous System Anxiety may show up in your body:

1. Brain: Headaches, migraines, dizziness or vertigo, brain fog, disorientation, seizures, a feeling of detachment from your surroundings (derealization) and/or your body (dissociation)
2. Nerves: Tingling, numbness, burning, buzzing, vibrating, shooting, stabbing, zapping, sweating, or chills
3. Muscles: Soreness, spasm, twitching, jerking, weakness, and/or pain
4. Mind: Depersonalization—feeling detached from oneself, or derealization—feeling detached from the world around you

We will take a deeper dive into the reasons for the different sensations of panic in Part II, but for now remember this: when the body is under stress, the nervous system shifts into a state of autonomic arousal. In autonomic arousal, a cascade of changes occurs from head to toe, gearing you up to combat danger.

We'll explore Nervous System Anxiety–specific solutions in Chapter 11.

IMMUNE SYSTEM ANXIETY

SIGNS ANXIETY MIGHT BE DUE TO AN IMBALANCED IMMUNE SYSTEM

IMMUNE SYSTEM ANXIETY. Do your anxieties feel like a constantly shifting puzzle? One minute you're drained and achy, the next you're jittery and overwhelmed. Doctors are stumped, leaving you feeling helpless and lost. This is the reality for many struggling with Immune System Anxiety.

Immune System Anxiety is a type of anxiety intricately linked to imbalances within your immune system. It often manifests after an illness or life change, and symptoms can affect you head to toe. Unfortunately, there's no single diagnostic test, making it challenging to pinpoint.

Symptoms can vary widely, but here are some of the most common:

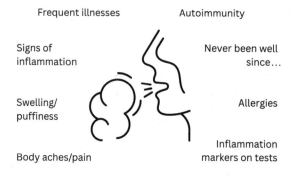

- **SKIN.** Redness, sensitivity (think eczema, psoriasis, or hives)
- **PAIN.** Fibromyalgia-like aches, headaches
- **DIZZINESS.** Lightheadedness, especially when standing
- **COGNITIVE.** Difficulty concentrating (similar to Thought Anxiety)
- **SENSITIVITY.** Reactions to foods, medications, or the environment (like chemical sensitivities)

The immune system and your nervous system (including the brain) are deeply intertwined. The field of Psychoneuroimmunology explores this complex relationship, revealing how mood, emotions, and the immune system influence one another.

While still in development, research suggests a two-way street:

- **STRESS AND TRAUMA.** High levels of stress, whether acute or chronic, can weaken the immune system and contribute to anxiety.
- **THE GUT-BRAIN-IMMUNE CONNECTION.** Studies on mast cells (immune cells) suggest they might regulate the blood-brain barrier, influencing what enters your brain and affecting your mood.
- **HISTAMINE.** This chemical plays a role both in the immune system and as a neurotransmitter. High levels are linked to anxiety.

There are risk factors for developing Immune System Anxiety, some of which include:

- **EMOTIONAL STRESS.** Both acute and chronic stress can play a role.
- **VIRAL ILLNESS HISTORY.** Epstein-Barr, strep, Lyme disease, etc., might be linked.
- **GENETIC FACTORS.** Mutations related to immune function might be involved.

- **IMMUNE SYSTEM IMBALANCES.** Allergies, autoimmunity, etc., might be indicators.
- **LIFESTYLE.** Pro-inflammatory habits such as poor diet, lack of sleep, and exposure to toxins might contribute.

GUT ANXIETY

HOW ANXIETY MIGHT IMPACT YOUR GUT AND DIGESTION

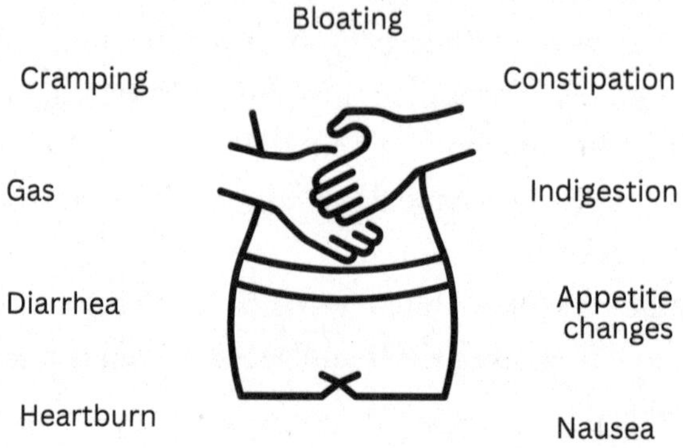

GUT ANXIETY. The term *gut wrenching* is more than a mere metaphor. You may get butterflies in your stomach with anxiety. You may experience gas, bloating, nausea, vomiting, indigestion, or pain with panic.

If you resonate with any of these symptoms, you might be experiencing Gut Anxiety.

Gut Anxiety is anxiety that manifests in symptoms in your digestive tract. It can relate to symptoms in your upper digestive tract, such as reflux/heartburn, burping, fullness or constriction in your throat and esophagus, nausea, stomach ulcers, and appetite changes, as well as symptoms in your lower digestive tract, like gas, bloating, cramps, diarrhea, constipation, butterflies, churning, and even digestive disorders like irritable bowel syndrome.

There are two primary reasons that anxiety can manifest in your gut:

1. Your gut and your brain are intimately connected via what is referred to as the enteric nervous system. The enteric ner-

vous system is often referred to as the "second brain" because it comprises millions of nerves whose jobs are to communicate back and forth with your brain.

2. It is well established that the microflora in your gut are responsible for maintaining your emotions, concentration, and moods. In fact, your gut bacteria can produce mood-altering chemicals such as dopamine, adrenaline, and gamma-aminobutyric acid (GABA), and they even produce approximately 95 percent of your serotonin levels.

In Chapter 5, you are going to meet Matthew, whose Gut Anxiety was so severe, it took over his life. You'll learn how his symptoms were his body's solutions to a traumatic event and how holistic treatments ended his anxiety.

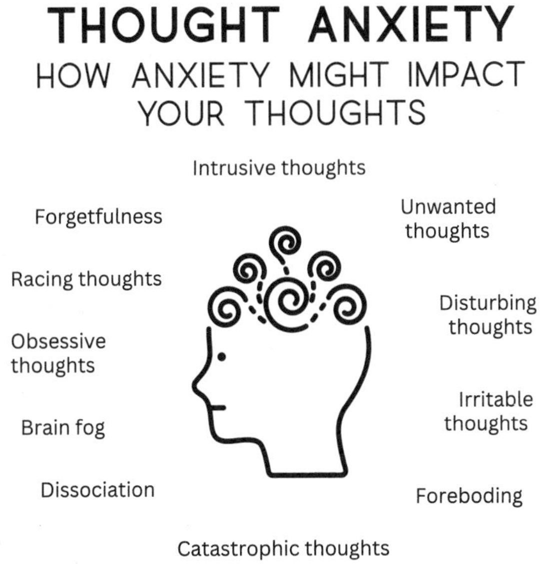

THOUGHT ANXIETY. Does it ever feel like your brain is relentlessly tormenting you with intrusive, persistent, and obsessive thoughts? This is one of the most frustrating anxiety symptoms because these thoughts can crush our confidence, distract us from what really matters, and hijack our happiness. These are symptoms of Thought Anxiety.

Thought Anxiety is particularly tricky, because no matter where we go and what we do, our brains are with us. And where our brains are, our thoughts will be too. You'll need to look at *how* you experience your thoughts as well as the *content* of your thoughts to figure out what needs healing.

There are four subtypes of Thought Anxiety, and they are differentiated by the *amount of thoughts* your brain is thinking (productivity of thoughts) and the *speed* of your thoughts (acceleration or deceleration).

Knowing which *subtype* of Thought Anxiety you deal with will help you zero in on solutions that will work best.

To get started, let's go through each of the four subtypes together, using the following scenario as an example. You are sitting in class or at a meeting, when unexpectedly, the presenter calls on you for input. Your stress response activates: your heart is racing, your breathing speeds up, and Thought Anxiety kicks in. What your thoughts do depends on your type.

THE FOUR SUBTYPES OF THOUGHT ANXIETY

- **THE AUCTIONEER:** Have you ever heard auctioneers speak? They say a lot, and they say it fast. Like, really fast. If you're the Auctioneer subtype, you will experience a *greater amount* of thoughts that are *faster*. Your brain will accelerate into thinking about anything and everything all together at once—like an auctioneer. But on caffeine.
- **THE RUMINATOR:** Do you get stuck in rumination? You're dwelling, obsessing, and can't move on or come to any conclusions. This can show up when you're trying to resolve a conflict or make an important decision. As a Ruminator subtype, your *amount of thoughts* increases, but the time it takes you to process, or create conclusions, will be *slower* and *longer*.
- **THE BROKEN RECORD:** Have you ever gotten a word, phrase, or short melody stuck in your head? It's like listening to a

broken record, and thoughts are going around and around in circles, making it hard to think about anything else. If so, you're dealing with the Broken Record subtype of Thought Anxiety. While the Broken Record has *few thoughts,* when they come, they are *rapid* and *repetitive.*

- **THE FOG:** When you're in the Fog, your thoughts will be *slow* and *few*. You will notice your mind is foggy, confused, slow, or even blank. When the Fog rolls in, you will find yourself forgetting words, phrases, or what you were about to say. This may be accompanied by feelings of dissociation and shutting down (dissociation is also seen in Nervous System Anxiety, we'll learn how to differentiate these later in Part II).

Now it's your turn. Based on the description of each subtype of Thought Anxiety, which do you resonate with the most? Circle the subtype of Thought Anxiety in the table below and bookmark this page. We'll be referring back to this section in Chapter 11, during our discussion about solutions based on your subtype of Thought Anxiety.

THOUGHT ANXIETY SUBTYPES

	VOLUME OVERPRODUCTION OF THOUGHTS	VOLUME UNDERPRODUCTION OF THOUGHTS
ACCELERATION: FASTER THOUGHTS	**THE AUCTIONEER** Too many thoughts processed too rapidly.	**THE BROKEN RECORD** Not a lot of variety in thoughts. They're looping, repetitive, and rapid.
ACCELERATION: SLOWER THOUGHTS	**THE RUMINATOR** Lots of thoughts processed, but slow to come to any conclusions or resolution.	**THE FOG** Too few thoughts processed, too slowly. May even lose thoughts altogether.

ANGER ANXIETY

HOW ANXIETY MIGHT MAKE YOU ANGRY

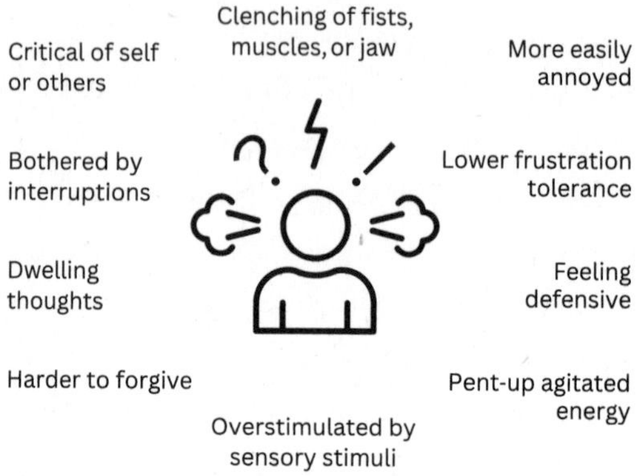

ANGER ANXIETY. When you're overwhelmed, do you ever feel irritated and annoyed? If you're on a deadline and someone interrupts you, do you want to lash out? If you feel like your stress, overwhelm, anxiety, and anger often merge into each other, you are likely dealing with a type of anxiety called Anger Anxiety.

For the purposes of this conversation, I am defining anger as an intense perception of feeling hurt, frustrated, disappointed, or even threatened. Anger is a natural response that the body and mind use to help move us out of those negative experiences and into those where we feel greater control or protection.

Anger and anxiety often go hand in hand. One of the reasons for this is that the neurochemicals that your body releases when anxious are quite similar to those released in anger.

One of the key chemicals that leads to anger is called adrenaline (otherwise known as epinephrine or norepinephrine).

Remember, anger is one of the key responses to stress—fight, flight, freeze, flop, fawn, and fracture. Here are some reasons your nervous system may shift toward anger in particular:

- You witnessed or were exposed to anger and/or violence while growing up.

- You had to fight for survival during childhood and adolescence, or later in life in conflict, combat, or war.
- You felt (and still feel) heard only when you expressed anger.
- Your sympathetic nervous system produces fight, while your parasympathetic drives freeze; with chronic activation, you may have less freeze and more fight.
- Emotions other than anger, such as sadness and fear, were not respected in your household growing up.
- Changes in the brain such as the amygdala (the emotional part of the brain) and the prefrontal cortex (the part of the brain responsible for logic and your ability to put on the brakes). Fun fact: The prefrontal cortex does not fully develop until a person's mid- to late twenties.

DEPRESSIVE ANXIETY

HOW ANXIETY MIGHT MAKE YOU DEPRESSED

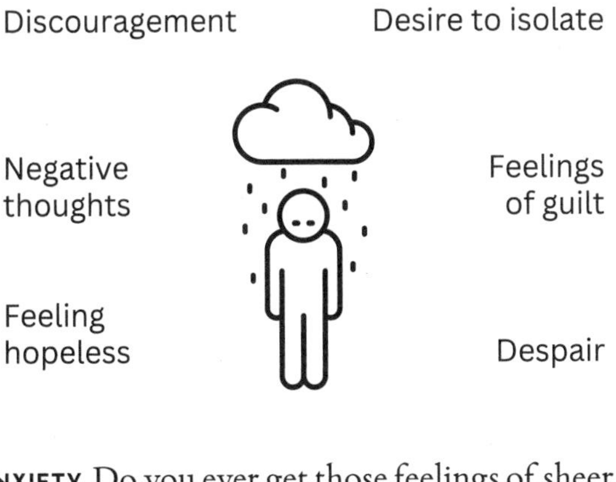

DEPRESSIVE ANXIETY. Do you ever get those feelings of sheer panic mixed with hopelessness and despair? You've been doing everything you can to combat the anxiety, but the longer it lasts, the more defeated you become. Or maybe the depression has sunk so low that feelings of losing control provoke panic.

Depression and anxiety have a complicated relationship. They feed into each other, creating a vicious cycle where depression aggravates anxiety, anxiety aggravates depression, and so on and so forth. Depression mixed with panic and anxiety is called Depressive Anxiety, and the loop where one feeds into the other is called the Depressive Anxiety Cycle.

Depressive Anxiety is very common. In fact, 85 percent of people with depression also experience significant anxiety, and 90 percent of people with anxiety also experience depression.

The following checklist explores the symptoms of depression and anxiety. As you read through it, ask yourself how your depression and anxiety interrelate. For example, how do your symptoms start? What makes them better and worse? Does one tend to lead into the other, and if so, how? These details will be important in Chapter 11.

DEPRESSIVE ANXIETY CHECKLIST

SYMPTOMS OF DEPRESSION	SYMPTOMS OF ANXIETY
• Sadness, emptiness, hopelessness • Loss of interest in activities or people • Sleep disturbances • Tiredness, weariness, fatigue • Changes in appetite (increased or decreased) • Difficulties with concentration and memory • Feelings of worthlessness • Guilty feelings even when you've done nothing wrong • Low self-confidence • Thoughts of suicide and death • Muscle weakness or soreness	• Persistent worry and fear • Feelings of foreboding or doom • Overthinking worst-case possibilities • Struggling with uncertainty or lack of control • Indecisiveness • Being keyed up or on edge • Feelings of detachment from self or surroundings • Sleep disturbances • Restlessness of mind and body • Digestive upset (nausea, bloating, diarrhea) • Numbness, tingling, or nerve pain • Muscle tension or spasms

If you've been to the doctor for treatment of depression and/or anxiety, likely you were given the option to try an antidepressant such as an SSRI (selective serotonin reuptake inhibitor) or SNRI (selective serotonin and norepinephrine reuptake inhibitor). Both types of medicine target serotonin levels in the brain. (SNRIs also affect norepinephrine levels.) However, there are two problems with taking antidepressants for Depressive Anxiety:

1. **FOR MANY, THEY AREN'T VERY EFFECTIVE.** Even though serotonin-modifying medicines are the standard treatment, only about 50 percent of people report lessened anxiety and depression with them.
2. **LOW SEROTONIN DOES NOT NECESSARILY CAUSE DEPRESSIVE ANXIETY.** Yeah, you read that right. Despite what many doctors say, recent research asserts that there is no clear evidence that low serotonin levels cause depression or anxiety.

You may be thinking: *But wait, my doctor told me the opposite! That antidepressants were useful for treating panic, anxiety, depression, and all sorts of other mental health symptoms!*

I hear you. I was told the very same thing. And I have seen how antidepressants can be helpful for certain people, and as an instructor at a medical school, I taught the chemical imbalance theory (CIT) to my students.

The CIT is the belief that an imbalance in the chemicals in your brain causes mood changes. It has dominated the interpretation and treatment of depression and anxiety for decades; however, this is about to change.

We're going to dig into the topic of neurotransmitters and the latest thinking about what causes mood changes in Chapter 6. Get ready to learn the truth about your brain that has been evading scientists and researchers for over 60 years.

HORMONE ANXIETY. Hormone Anxiety is anxiety that is caused by an imbalance in your endocrine system. Your endocrine system is a series of glands that release hormones all over your body to carry out all sorts of functions.

HORMONE ANXIETY

SIGNS YOUR ANXIETY IS RELATED TO YOUR HORMONES

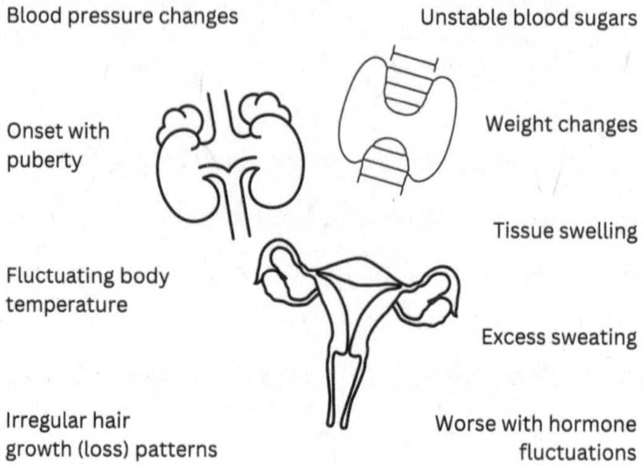

Examples of endocrine glands are: thyroid, adrenals, pituitary, hypothalamus, pancreas, ovaries, testicles, and parathyroid. These glands release all sorts of hormones that work hard to keep you healthy and balanced. Thyroid endocrine hormone comes from the thyroid gland, epinephrine and norepinephrine come from both adrenal glands, and luteinizing hormone (LH) and follicle-stimulating hormone (FSH) come from the pituitary gland. In a state of optimal health, your endocrine system—which is composed of both the endocrine glands and their hormones—balances your entire body and mind. But when something goes awry and your levels shift out of optimal ranges, you develop symptoms (e.g., panic and anxiety).

If you're wondering if your thyroid, adrenals, or hormonal balance is causing your panic attacks, check out Chapter 7.

TRAUMA ANXIETY. Have you ever gone through something so upsetting, disturbing, or overwhelming that you feel like it changed you? Perhaps you grew up in a tumultuous household, were the victim of abuse or assault, were bullied on the playground or at work, did not get your needs met by your caretakers, or witnessed something that terrified you.

Whatever did or did *not* happen was ingrained into the complex

TRAUMA ANXIETY

SIGNS TRAUMA MIGHT BE IMPACTING YOUR ANXIETY

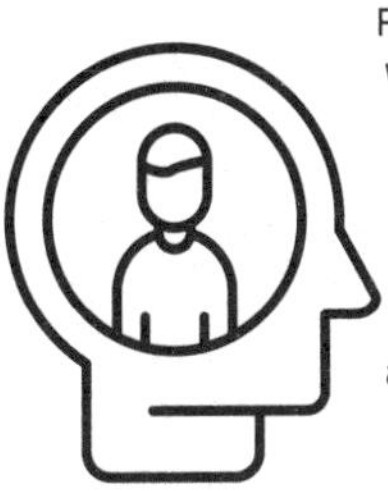
Avoiding anxious triggers
Extreme mood swings
Difficulty sleeping
Feeling like the world is unsafe
History of neglect
Panic attacks
Flashbacks
Unexplained aches and pains
Nightmares
History of abuse
Dissociation
Increased use of substances like alcohol
Depersonalization

network comprising your brain and nervous system. In an effort to protect you, your brain and nervous system respond via a series of nuanced adaptations and adjustments involving your hormones, neurotransmitters, inflammation levels, gut, behaviors, and emotions.

These are the roots of a type of anxiety called Trauma Anxiety. Trauma Anxiety occurs as a result of *adverse experiences,* whether a single event or a series of experiences, also known as trauma.

There are two important things you need to know about Trauma Anxiety:

First, Trauma Anxiety can lead to symptoms seen in the other types of anxiety.

This is because events that trigger the brain's stored associations with aversive events cause a ripple effect of changes throughout your entire brain and body. Even though adversity affects each person differently, typical symptoms of Trauma Anxiety include heart racing, high blood pressure, restlessness, difficulty sleeping, anger, fear, intrusive thoughts and memories of the traumatic event(s), and feelings that certain people or places are unsafe.

Second, Trauma Anxiety can occur as a result of the other types of anxiety.

Have you ever had fear of fear itself? Do you ever get thoughts like *What if the panic comes back?* or *What if I don't sleep tonight?* or *What if I lose control?*

Sometimes panic and anxiety can become so severe that you find yourself suffering with feelings of terror about it coming back or happening again. You find yourself avoiding things that might trigger your anxiety, and you realize over time that your world is getting smaller and smaller.

That, my love, is a trauma response.

When you go through something difficult and painful, it is natural for your body and mind to be worried about it happening again. This is part of how you adapt to try to be safer: fear makes you a bit faster, more vigilant, aware, and ready for the next attack to strike.

But in its effort to protect you, your nervous system is unknowingly enlisting your entire body to jump into danger mode. Problems arise when those automatic responses get in the way of your own personal sense of power and agency.

We'll dive into this in a lot more detail in Chapter 4. For now, I want to leave you with this:

You can heal from trauma.

Read that again.

You *can* heal from trauma.

It's never too late, it's never too deep, it's never too dark.

So do whatever you need to do to remember that *you can heal.* Stick a Post-it note in your car, take a picture of this page and save it in your phone, or maybe go big and write it in bright red lipstick on your mirror.

Whatever you have to do, hold on to hope.

It's your time to become Panic Proof.

DID YOU GET MULTIPLE TYPES?

When you took the Nine Types of Anxiety Quiz, did you resonate with multiple types of anxiety? More than half of people do; in fact, scoring high on just one type of anxiety is relatively rare. This is because your whole mind, body, and nervous system coordinate to create an anxiety response, and everyone's experience is different.

Your symptoms of anxiety and panic come from multiple systems in your body. The key is to zero in on the category you most relate to and the symptoms that are most debilitating for you.

A client once emailed me saying, "My panic attacks always start with an unsettled sensation in the gut, and if I pay close enough attention, I can almost always prevent a full-on attack by quickly using my Gut Anxiety tools. Otherwise other systems jump on board, like my nervous system, which makes my body feel like it's on fire, and then Thought Anxiety kicks in, and my brain goes into overdrive."

It's important to pay attention to the type of anxiety that typically arrives first so that you can stop the process before it gets carried away. By leaning into the nuance of your symptoms, you will begin to familiarize yourself with your own personal process to reduce panic and identify solutions that work for you.

Scoring for multiple types means that you can say, *Wow, body! Thanks for giving me so much data to support me as I heal!* The more you understand your own unique experience of autonomic arousal, the better equipped you will be to manage it.

I'll elaborate more on the individual techniques in Part III.

IDENTIFYING PATTERNS

Your symptoms of anxiety may change and shift over time. This is because your body is constantly adapting to its environment. Your nervous system, gut, and other systems may be affected by changes in your sleep, supplements, hormones, stressors, or even the time of year.

For example, one day you might feel jittery and tingly because your nervous system is activated. The next day you might have digestive problems because your gut is affected. It's important to pay attention to the type of anxiety that typically arrives first. This will help you identify the most effective solutions for your individual needs.

You can use the Nine Types of Anxiety Quiz to track your symptoms and identify your unique pattern of anxiety. Bookmark the quiz and take it again anytime you notice a shift in your symptoms. Once you have a general idea of how your panic typically presents, you can map out solutions that will give you the most impact.

NEXT STEPS

STEP 1: Write down the top three or four most bothersome, intense, or extreme symptoms you are experiencing at the moment or during a panic attack. (If possible, list them in the order they show up.)

Main symptoms (current/ lately/ at worst panic):

____

____

____

____

STEP 2: If you haven't taken the Nine Types of Anxiety Quiz in Chapter 3, do so now. In the space provided below, list your top one to three type(s).

Anxiety types:

______________ ______________

______________ ______________

Note: If you want to take a more detailed version of this quiz, you can find it for free at drnicolecain.com.

EXAMPLE

This is what Aria wrote when she did this exercise:

Symptoms of anxiety: *My worst symptom of panic is the adrenaline causing me first to have feelings of suffocation and next an extreme need to escape. Then I dissociate from my body, and I can't control my behavior or thoughts.*

Quiz results: *Chest Anxiety and Nervous System Anxiety*

STEP 3: Diving deeper. Why are you experiencing symptoms of panic?

Your panic is an adaptation. An adaptation is a modification or change that your brain and body make to maximize fitness for survival. You inherited adaptations from your ancestors, and you make adaptations every day of your life. When no longer useful, those adaptations show up as symptoms.

Go back to your notes from Chapter 1 and identify at least three events, experiences, or circumstances that your mind, body, and/or nervous system had to adapt or adjust to.

EXAMPLE: ARIA

What have I adapted to? *I'm an Energizer Bunny. I have to be. My job depends on me being on my game, alert, energized, sharp, and fast. If I can't meet expectations naturally, I use medications to fill in the gaps. I know this has taken a toll on my body, and apparently my mental health. I have adapted to a fear of failure, the fear of falling behind, and terror at the risk of losing everything I've worked for. So I've been pushing harder and faster. I've adapted to being more hyper, more awake, and apparently more disposed to panic.*

STEP 4: Save these notes for later. You will need them when we get to Chapter 11, which is where you'll be building your Panic Proof Protocol.

ANXIETY TL;DR

- There are nine types of anxiety. They are Gut Anxiety, Thought Anxiety, Trauma Anxiety, Chest Anxiety, Nervous System Anxiety, Immune System Anxiety, Depressive Anxiety, Hormone Anxiety, and Anger Anxiety.
- Identifying the main type of anxiety will help you zero in on solutions that will work best.
- Nuances in symptoms offer clues about what needs healing and how.
- You can have more than one type of anxiety at a time.
- Your type(s) of anxiety can change over time.

PART II

How Your Panic Is Protective

SEVERAL MONTHS AGO I WAS INVITED TO SPEAK TO A GROUP OF medical residents about panic and anxiety. I started the session by asking, "Are anxiety and panic dangerous?"

The unanimous consensus was that, yes, anxiety and panic had the potential to be harmful to health. And if a group of physicians believes that, my guess is that at some time or another you have heard that, too.

I am often asked questions like: "Is my heart going to stop?" "Is it normal for anxiety to cause numbness in my face or am I having a stroke?" "What if I get so anxious, my body just gives up?"

The research is abundantly clear that panic is a response your body utilizes to keep you safe. However, if left unchecked, the roots of panic can become problematic. This can lead to you feeling out of control of your emotional and physical reactions (a hallmark symptom of anxiety).

A Vicious Cycle

Here's the tricky thing about dealing with adversity: the body's physical and emotional responses to difficult situations can be stored in the body and brain, even if we are not consciously aware of the adversity.

Our bodies are very good at automatically responding to stress by releasing hormones, activating the immune system, and changing the balance of gut bacteria. These automatic responses are designed to protect us. However, if they are not properly addressed once the stressor has passed, they can get stuck in disharmonious feedback loops, furthering the problem and leading to a variety of health problems.

Let's say, for example, you're under extreme stress. Your body will produce more cortisol to help you cope. Cortisol helps you shift into fight, flight, or freeze mode. It also raises your blood pressure and breaks down glycogen into sugar to give you energy. But the excess sugar counteracts the effects of insulin, and over time it can cause insulin resistance. This causes high blood sugar, which impairs your immune system and drives up inflammation, which then triggers further cortisol release, which further suppresses your immune system.

Your impaired immune system may not efficiently eliminate pathogens (harmful bacteria and viruses) that are hanging around in your gut. This negatively impacts your gut microbes, which changes the signals that your gut sends to your brain. These pathogens can multiply, change hormone metabolism and detoxification, and even damage your gut lining. Your immune system will try to fight back, but this will only cause your body to produce more cortisol.

Over time, pathogens, toxins, and other metabolites can leak out of the gut and into the bloodstream and ultimately flow up to the blood-brain barrier (BBB), which is a protective layer that separates the brain from the bloodstream. Their continual presence can cause damage to the BBB. When the BBB is compromised, harmful substances can enter the brain resulting in inflammation, leading to panic, and increasing the risk of different types of neurodegenerative diseases.

Additionally, in order to try to compensate for high cortisol, your body may shift your cortisol into a less active metabolite called cortisone. This may cause you to feel like your cortisol is low when it's actually elevated. As a result of high cortisol, your body may also start to shift active T3 thyroid hormone into the inactive form, reverse T3. So on top of everything else, you may now feel like you have hypothyroidism. You're exhausted and constipated, so you're not detoxing efficiently. You're gaining weight, and you have brain fog. Low T3 thyroid can cause low progesterone, which sets off a domino of changes involving your other sex hormones such as estrogen and testosterone.

And this is just part of the adaptive process that takes place when you experience stress, adversity, or trauma.

No wonder we experience symptoms, right?

For many people, chronic panic attacks are caused by coping mechanisms that were originally intended to protect them but have now become the very things that are keeping them in a state of anxiety.

By looking at your symptoms as clues, learning about what they mean, and in some cases running functional testing, you can become better equipped to actually address the root causes of your symptoms. And by using trauma-informed and holistic methods, you can put things back into balance.

This is why, over the next few chapters, you will learn a lot about the science behind panic and anxiety. Some of the following sections can be a bit complicated, but I've strived to make it all digestible by weaving in case studies, images, tables, and self-assessment checklists. While it's impossible to be completely exhaustive, I've done my best to glean the most important information from my experience in helping thousands of people find freedom from panic and anxiety.

Are you ready to learn about the complex interplay between your brain, gut, neurotransmitters, and hormones, and how they have worked together to protect you from stress and adversity throughout your life?

Let's explore some potential sources of your body's feedback loop breaking down and intensifying your anxiety and panic. Later, in Part III, we will dig into how to restore normal functioning to those feedback loops.

4

THE BRAIN AND PANIC

WHEN JENNY WAS IN THE THIRD GRADE, SHE WAS IN A CAR ACCIdent. She was sitting in the back passenger seat, and her mom was driving. It was a rainy night, and a pickup truck, with a snowplow hooked to the front bumper, ran a red light and T-boned their car.

The accident was so sudden and violent that Jenny's brain had no time to process what was happening. All she felt was a wave of fear and pain as the truck slammed into her side of the car. As a result of the impact, Jenny's door was jammed shut, and no matter how hard she tried to escape, she couldn't get out. She ended up being freed by the first responders.

In that moment, and the moments that followed, her brain made a series of connections that would stay with her for the rest of her life.

The rain, the dark, the truck, the sounds of the windshield wipers, being in the back seat, sitting on the right, her mom driving—all these things became potential danger cues for Jenny. Her brain learned to associate these things with pain and fear, and it would always be on alert for them.

From that moment on, anytime it rained, Jenny found herself feeling afraid to get into a car.

Many years later Jenny was on a road trip with friends. She was sitting in the back seat, singing along to the radio and having a wonderful time. But then they hit an unexpected storm. Jenny noticed her heart rate picking up speed, her palms started sweating, and she felt a tickle of anxiety. She tried to tell herself that there was nothing to be afraid of, but her body wouldn't listen. The feelings of fear intensified until she couldn't take it anymore. She had to get out of the car. She told her friends to pull over, and she got out and stood on the side of the road. She took a few deep breaths and tried to calm down.

Later in counseling, Jenny realized that her anxiety was her body reenacting the traumatic car accident from her childhood, in what is called somatic reenactment. Shifting into a state of autonomic arousal, her body sent her into a state of "flight," making her want to run away and escape, which she was unable to do as a child.

In Chapter 9, I'll walk you through the Panic Reset, a four-step process that we used to retrain her brain and nervous system so that she was no longer primed for panic in the car.

WHAT YOU'RE GOING TO LEARN

If you're struggling with anxiety or panic, you know that it can feel like your brain is working against you. This chapter will take a look at the brain and anxiety and how you can use this information to help yourself heal.

In this chapter, we'll talk about the different parts of the brain that are involved in anxiety and how they work. We'll also talk about how trauma can affect the brain and lead to anxiety symptoms. And finally, we'll talk about brain states and how you can use information about them to help change your brain in order to heal from anxiety.

WHAT YOU WILL LEARN IN THIS CHAPTER:

- The different parts of the brain that are involved in anxiety
- How trauma affects the brain and leads to anxiety symptoms
- Brain states and how you can use this information to help you change your brain
- How to calm your emotional amygdala and activate your logical and problem-solving prefrontal cortex

I know this may sound a little daunting, but don't worry. I will break it all down for you in a way that's easy to understand and enjoyable to read.

So what are you waiting for? Let's get started!

BRAIN PARTS INVOLVED IN PANIC

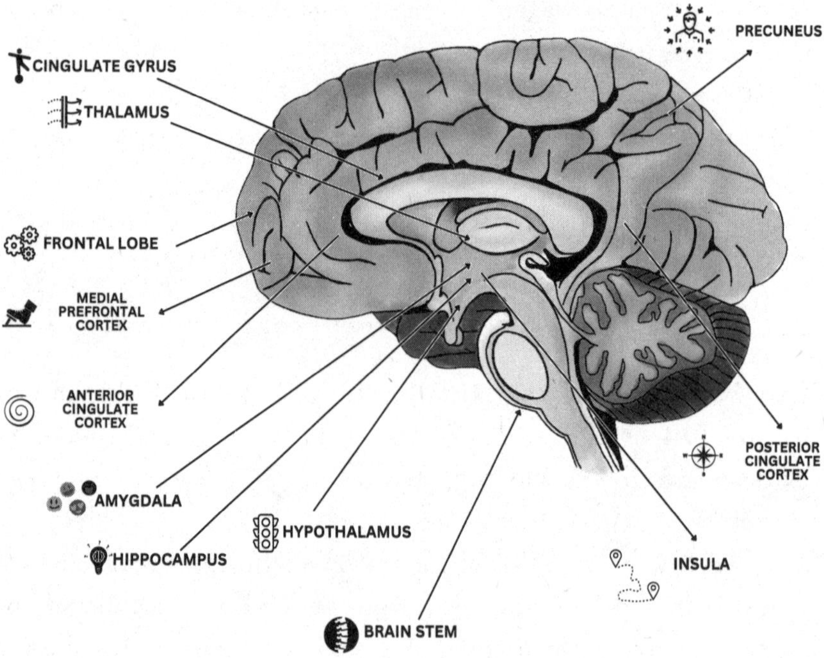

There are twelve main parts of the brain that are particularly important in the process of moving from calm to panic.

Let's start at the top left of this image and we'll work our way around it counterclockwise. You will notice that each part has a little icon next to it, which I hope will help you remember the main function of that part as it relates to panic and anxiety.

BRAIN PARTS INVOLVED IN PANIC

PART OF THE BRAIN	ITS NICKNAME	ITS MAIN JOB
Cingulate gyrus	The Balancer	Helps balance and process emotions via self-awareness and introspection
Thalamus	The Filter	Filters incoming sensory information as salient and relevant, or irrelevant
Frontal lobe	The Analyzer and Timekeeper	Analyzes information logically and differentiates time: "That was then, this is now"
Medial prefrontal cortex	The Brakes	Brakes big emotions, allowing us to be rational and in control of our emotions
Anterior cingu-late cortex	The Converter	Involved in processing emotions and decision-making
Amygdala	The Feeler	Responsible for processing emotions, especially fear and anxiety
Hippocampus	The Memory Keeper	Processes memories
Hypothalamus	The Traffic Cop	Regulates the body based on incoming data
Brain stem	The Relayer	Relays messages between the brain and body
Insula	The Internal Map	Creates a spatial internal map and facilitates awareness of self and body, and empathy
Posterior cingulate cortex	The Meta	Involved in metacognition (thinking about thinking) self-awareness, and the mind
Precuneus	The Physical Self	Anterior precuneus forms our physical sense of self or "I"

Each of these structures works collaboratively with the others in teams. Some teams help us focus and use logic, like the executive control network (ECN), which includes the prefrontal cortex. Other teams get activated when it's time to relax and let our minds wander, or when we need to go into danger mode or autopilot. This is called the default mode network (DMN), which includes the amygdala.

In anxiety, parts of the brain associated with the DMN often get activated, which shuts down the ECN and its logic-giving abilities. This can lead to feeling overly attuned to our internal thoughts and self-references, and behaving on impulse instead of thoughtfully. These are all cardinal features of panic.

HOW THE BRAIN COMMUNICATES

Your brain and nervous system are like a vast network of roads, with millions of signals traveling along them like cars on a crowded freeway. The roads are called *neurons,* and the cars are tiny little chemicals released by the neurons called *neurotransmitters*. Each neurotransmitter plays a unique role in regulating your thoughts, emotions, and behaviors. Check out Chapter 6 to read more about your different types of neurotransmitters, how they're made, what they do, how to identify if and how they're affecting your mood, and what you can do to get them back in balance.

When a neuron needs to send a signal to another neuron, it releases a neurotransmitter into a *synapse,* which is the gap or space between two neurons. The neurotransmitter crosses the synapse and then binds to a receptor on the next neuron, which causes the next neuron to fire—emit a slight electrical charge—allowing messages to be sent. This rapid-fire communication process continues throughout the brain, until the signals reach the spinal cord.

The *spinal cord* is a long and thin bundle of nerves that runs down your back in your spine. It acts as a relay station for signals traveling between your brain and the rest of your body.

MANY "NERVOUS SYSTEMS"

Together, your brain and spinal cord are called the *central nervous system,* aptly named because it is located in the center of your body. The nerves in the rest of your body are referred to as the *peripheral nervous system,* which is located on the periphery of your body.

The peripheral nervous system has three main subsystems:

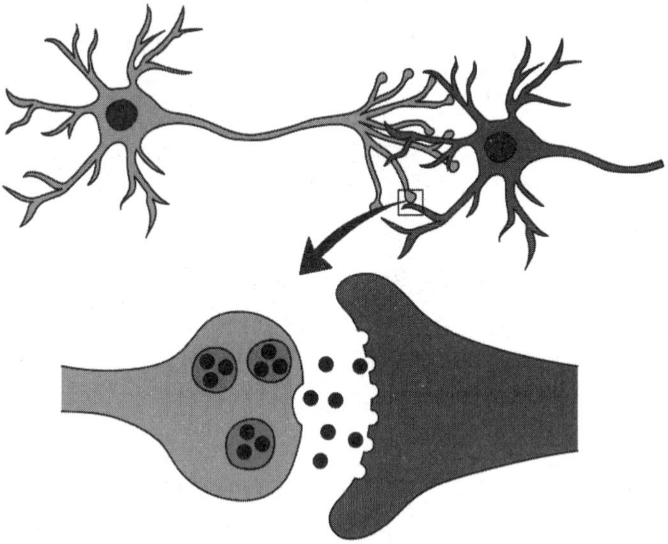

- **THE SOMATIC NERVOUS SYSTEM.** This system controls voluntary movements, such as moving your arms and legs, and sensory information, such as the softness you feel when you pet a puppy. When the somatic system gets amped up, you may find yourself feeling restless and fidgety. Bottom-up treatments (see Chapter 9) will teach you how to calm this system.
- **THE ENTERIC NERVOUS SYSTEM.** This system controls the muscles and glands in your digestive tract. Your gut regulates all sorts of factors that predispose you to panic. You will learn more about the nervous system of the gut, and how to leverage your gut to stop panic and anxiety, in much more detail in Chapter 5.
- **THE AUTONOMIC NERVOUS SYSTEM.** This system controls "involuntary" functions, such as heart rate, blood pressure, and breathing. You'll notice the quotation marks around the word *involuntary,* which are there because you actually have the ability to alter your heart rate, blood pressure, and breathing, which you'll learn a little more about next, and a ton more in Chapter 9.

THE NERVOUS SYSTEM DIAL

Let's expand a bit more on the autonomic nervous system (ANS), because this is where you have quite a lot of power to soothe the physical sensations of panic.

Remember, the ANS contains lots of nerves that regulate things like your heart rate, blood flow, breathing, and digestion.

Think of the ANS as a dial. When the dial is turned toward calm, your parasympathetic nervous system (PNS) takes over and you feel relaxed. Clinicians refer to this state as "rest, digest, and reproduce." Learning how to turn that dial to activate your PNS can help you feel the opposite of panicky. Instead, you will experience:

- Slowing down of your heart rate
- Reducing blood pressure
- Slowing down of your breathing
- Constricting pupils
- Reducing sweating
- Relaxing muscles

Turning the ANS dial in the other direction triggers your sympathetic nervous system to shift your body into a state called autonomic or sympathetic arousal. You may have heard it referred to as "fight-flight-freeze." Arousal of your nervous system causes a lot of physical symptoms that we often associate with panic, excitement, or agitation, such as:

- Increased heart rate
- Increased blood pressure
- Increased respiration
- Dilated pupils
- Sweating
- Muscle tension

These changes are designed to help you prepare either to fight or to flee from danger. But there are ways you can actually turn the dial when you want. Stay tuned; you'll learn how to do that in Chapter 9.

THE F6 OF AUTONOMIC AROUSAL

I've mentioned the fight, flight, freeze responses a few times; they are three of the main ways our bodies react to perceived threats. However, there are actually six ways our bodies commonly respond when activated. Which one do you connect with?

- **FIGHT.** This response manifests in changes in our body that make us more able to fight off danger. We may experience intense energy that comes out with the impulse to bite, kick, or strike. This is a common response to feeling threatened or attacked and is seen in Anger Anxiety.
- **FLIGHT.** This response is the urge to escape danger. Our body will direct blood to our running-away muscles, such as our legs and feet, and divert it away from small, less necessary groups of muscles, such as our fingertips or nose. This is why we sometimes feel Neurological Anxiety symptoms such as numbness when we're anxious.
- **FREEZE.** This response comes when we feel frozen in fear. Our brain may go blank (e.g., The Fog type of Thought Anxiety), or we may feel unable to move. Your heart rate will speed up, your breathing may quicken, and your blood pressure may spike.
- **FLOP.** This response happens when there is no hope for survival, and the brain and body simply give up. In flop, your heart rate, respiratory rate, and pulse all slow down, and your blood pressure drops.
- **FAWN.** This response is a survival mechanism, characterized by a feeling of submission or appeasement. People who fawn may try to please the person or thing that they perceive as a threat, and they may even apologize for their own

existence. This response is often seen in people who have experienced trauma or abuse.

- **FRACTURE.** This is the response in which our parts disintegrate from the present moment and break off. Have you ever felt dissociated, or as if you weren't quite in tune with your body or the environment? Maybe you felt you were "taken over" by a part of yourself that was behaving in direct opposition to your will. Maybe you found yourself zoning out, or you picked a fight with a loved one. Maybe you blacked out during a fit of rage. Maybe you became triggered and had a panic attack even though you logically realized you were safe. Sometimes a fracture can manifest in feeling like life is surreal or is not really happening. (We'll explore this more when we learn about Parts Work in Chapter 10.)

These six responses represent a fraction of the many ways that autonomic arousal (aka sympathetic arousal) can show up in your body. Everybody's experience of anxiety depends on a number of factors, including individual personality traits, environment, support systems, and biological differences.

HOW STRESS AND TRAUMA CHANGE YOUR BRAIN

As we discussed, the human brain processes a lot of information. In fact, your brain receives approximately 11 million bits of sensory data every second. That's a lot to manage! And as you may guess, your conscious mind is not aware of most of that input. In fact, researchers estimate that the conscious mind is able to process only around 50 bits per second (which is about 0.0045 percent).

Stress and trauma can change the way your brain processes content.

When we experience stress, our salience network (SN), including the thalamus, becomes more sensitive to environmental cues. This means we're more likely to notice hints that something might be dangerous, such as images, smells, tastes, sounds, or touch sensations.

So instead of sending on reasonable bite-size blasts of information, the SN bombards the amygdala, the brain's fear center, with a massive data overload. This can be incredibly overwhelming for the amygdala. If your SN is "leaky," meaning it transmits far more information than the amygdala can handle, you might experience symptoms of overstimulation, anxiety, and even panic attacks.

The amygdala, alarmed by the overwhelming data, signals the hypothalamus, which acts as a traffic cop, regulating your psychological reactions to stress. It coordinates the body's response, directly influencing functions like digestion, hormones, and others.

Throughout this process, the logical and analytical prefrontal cortex becomes less active. This is why you may become forgetful, struggle to recall words, or lose your ability to think clearly and make rational decisions. As a result, you may also overreact to things that are not actually dangerous.

Meanwhile, our memory-keeping hippocampus is working hard, along with other parts of our brain, to catalog and memorize all the relevant stimuli, to prepare us for future threats. However, because the logical brain is less active, the memories are stored as sensory fragments without a sense of time rather than as a coherent story.

This can be helpful in the context of actual danger, but it can also be problematic if the stress or trauma is prolonged. In this case, the brain's filter may become stuck in survival mode, making it difficult for us to focus on anything else and leading to anxiety, panic attacks, and other problems.

Here is an analogy that might help you understand how a leaky SN and the thalamus can predispose you to focus on things that are actually not important:

Imagine that you're walking down the street and you hear a loud noise. Your ears will pick it up and send it to the thalamus. The thalamus works with the other parts of the SN to decide whether the noise is important. If the noise is deemed unimportant it will be ignored. If, on the other hand, it is perceived as important (which is more likely if you have a history of stress or trauma), it will be sent onward for further processing.

In the case of past trauma, let's say you grew up in an area with a high crime rate, where loud noises on the street tended to indicate a threat. In this case, your thalamus would be more likely to respond to the loud noises as important, and activate autonomic arousal, even if they were not actually dangerous. This is because your brain would have learned to associate loud noises with danger.

Here is one of my favorite SN hacks for preventing and combating autonomic arousal:

THE SN HACK
A SIMPLE TRICK TO TURN OFF YOUR BRAIN'S "DANGER" ALARM

When you don't move your head for more than a few minutes at a time, your brain's salience network shifts into high alert. This can make you start to feel anxious. It's a natural evolutionary response. Think of a deer in headlights, frozen and not moving. Your brain interprets your frozen posture as a freeze response, even if you're just focused and staring at your phone or television.

A quick hack to calm the SN back down is to simply rotate your neck and eyes and to focus close and far every 20 minutes or so.

YOU CAN REPATTERN YOUR BRAIN AND BODY

Neuroscience teaches us that the human brain is very "plastic," which means that it can change and adapt. Just as your brain and body learned to protect you from harm's way, they can also learn how to keep you safe and calm when there is no danger.

One way to do this is to strengthen the medial prefrontal cortex. This part of the brain helps us regulate our emotions and control our impulses. When the medial prefrontal cortex is strong, it can help us to "hit the brakes" on our anxiety and panic responses, relieving us from continuously being activated by previous experiences.

There are many things you can do to strengthen your medial prefrontal cortex and to retrain your brain and nervous system so you can be more in the moment, instead of stuck in the past. You'll learn a bunch of strategies for this in Chapter 9, which explores bottom-up techniques.

But that's not the end of the story. Remember, panic doesn't just stop in the brain. Your body also has something to say. That is why I have dedicated chapters to each of the key bodily systems involved in panic, including signs that these systems have adapted to make you hypervigilant and thus panicky, and what to do about it, including identifying obstacles to cure, testing, habits, lifestyle changes, and holistic remedies.

NEXT STEPS

Now that you understand the role of the brain and the nervous systems, and how your experiences affect your feelings of anxiety, you may see how you have adapted to aversive events in order to be better protected from danger. And you've learned that your brain and nervous system are very malleable, meaning you can change your responses.

By practicing awareness of your brain, nervous systems, and body responses to different situations, you are strengthening the parts of your brain that are involved in helping you achieve agency and control over your emotions. Here are some of the strategies you will be learning throughout Parts II and III of this book:

- **HOW TO BECOME MORE AWARE OF WHAT IS HAPPENING IN YOUR BODY.** You can do this using techniques like meta-awareness, mindfulness, and Somatographic Imagery (see Chapter 9).
- **HOW TO INCREASE THE STRENGTH AND CONNECTIVITY BETWEEN YOUR THALAMUS AND PREFRONTAL CORTEX.** You can do this by increasing gray matter in your brain via neurofeedback and other brain-training exercises.

- **HOW TO IMPROVE THE FILTRATION SYSTEM OF THE SENSORY NETWORK.** You can do this by learning to identify and manage your stress responses.
- **HOW TO INTEGRATE YOUR EMOTIONAL BRAIN AND YOUR LOGICAL BRAIN:** You can do this by getting your physical and emotional body on the same page as your logical and analytical brain.
- **HOW TO REGULATE AND BALANCE YOUR AUTONOMIC NERVOUS SYSTEM.** You can do this using bottom-up strategies and holistic remedies, and by clearing and repatterning trauma reactions.

BRAIN AND PANIC TL;DR

- Your autonomic nervous system controls your body's involuntary responses to danger.
- You can learn to regulate your ANS so that you feel calm.
- There are six F's of autonomic arousal: freeze, flight, fight, flop, fawn, and fracture.
- Your brain has different networks that get activated based on different scenarios.
- Stress and trauma can change your brain's filtration system, making you panic more easily.

5

THE GUT-BRAIN AXIS

"Some of your deepest feelings, from your greatest joys to your darkest angst, turn out to be related to the bacteria in your gut."

—Scott C. Anderson, *The Psychobiotic Revolution* (2017)

MATTHEW HAD AN EXTREME PHOBIA OF PASSING GAS OR DEFECATING in his pants in public. The worry was so extreme that he built his life around his digestive tract. He never left the house without his emergency Xanax, he wore heavy amounts of cologne to cover any potential odors, he planned his trips around facilities that had private bathrooms—as opposed to those with stalls—and any time his guts felt uneasy, he canceled his plans.

Like many of us, Matthew's fear started after a very distressing event that happened to him when he was a child.

"I was a generally carefree third grader," he remembered aloud. "My class was about to go onstage to sing at a school-wide concert but I felt super anxious and sick to my stomach. I felt the gas building up in my abdomen, and I wanted to go to the restroom, but the teacher said it was time to go into the auditorium. So I just let the air release. But it wasn't just air that came out."

Matthew was not the first person who had told me about anxiety so severe that it caused stomach pain and diarrhea. In fact, it is extremely common for digestive and emotional symptoms to rise and fall in concert with each other.

"I soiled myself and the kid in line behind me had a fit." Matthew flushed with embarrassment. "I was traumatized. That event changed everything. My gut. My anxiety. I have never been the same since."

"Your brain, gut, and life experiences are intimately intertwined," I said. "Stressful or aversive experiences of all kinds can trip a series of responses that affect you head to toe, involving both your brain and your gut."

Like many, this was Matthew's first time learning about the relationship between the gut and the brain. "How is that even possible?" he asked.

This chapter will answer that question.

WHY PANIC MAKES YOU POOP

Do you ever feel the urge to poop when you're anxious? Panic poops can show up before, during, or even after a super stressful event. There are several reasons panic may send you rushing to the bathroom:

- **STRESS HORMONES.** During panic, the stress hormone adrenaline (aka norepinephrine) spikes and binds to different kinds of receptors on the intestines. When adrenaline binds to an alpha receptor, it causes the muscles to contract, causing acute diarrhea. Adrenaline can disrupt your immune system, impairing your gut bacteria from eliminating the bad bugs, which can cause long-term diarrhea.
- **INFLAMMATION.** Some individuals with anxiety also have high levels of a type of inflammatory cell called interleukin-1 beta (IL-1β). IL-1β can cause diarrhea in three ways: (1) It stimulates the smooth muscle of the colon, (2) it suppresses water and sodium absorption in the gut, (3) it can damage the gut's mucosal barrier.
- **CHOLECYSTOKININ.** This hormone is in your brain and your gut. A spike in cholecystokinin levels can cause panic and anxiety as well as stimulate your gallbladder to kick into ac-

tion, emptying its bile into your intestine and causing diarrhea. This is seen more commonly in people with irritable bowel syndrome.

- **GUT BUGS.** Your gut and brain are in constant communication. Anxiety in the brain provokes changes in your gut bugs (aka the microbiome), and changes in your gut bugs can change your mood and cravings. In certain panic sufferers, changes in the microbiome can result in increased amounts of diarrhea.

GUT ANXIETY

Many people find that their anxiety manifests as physical symptoms in the digestive system, such as nausea, vomiting, diarrhea, constipation, or abdominal pain. These symptoms of Gut Anxiety occur for good reason: the gut and the brain are closely connected. The two systems communicate with each other through a network of nerves, microbes, hormones, immune cells, and other chemicals.

Sometimes during panic, we don't *feel* symptoms in our gut, even when the gut is at the root of our symptoms. In Chapter 3, you completed the Nine Types of Anxiety Quiz, and now we're going to zero in on the type of Gut Anxiety you experience.

SELF-ASSESSMENT CHECKLIST: GUT ANXIETY SUBTYPES

STEP 1: Write down your Gut Anxiety score (from the quiz) in this blank: ________. If you scored >7, go to Step 2, where you'll zero in on your type of Gut Anxiety. If you scored <6 and do not resonate with this section, feel free to skip ahead!

STEP 2: Check the box(es) that relate to you when your stress and anxiety is at its highest.

VATA GUT

- ☐ I experience gassiness (burping) (passing wind).
- ☐ I tend to be more constipated (as opposed to diarrhea).
- ☐ I experience colicky abdominal pain especially after eating.

PITTA GUT

- ☐ I tend to deal with reflux/heartburn.
- ☐ I experience diarrhea more often than constipation.
- ☐ I have burning and acrid stool when I'm panicky.

KAPHA GUT

- ☐ I feel too full after eating small amounts of food.
- ☐ I feel like my bowels often do not fully eliminate when I go to the bathroom.
- ☐ My stool tends to be a bit greasy, heavy, or sticky.

SCORING

Circle the type that has the most checked boxes and set it aside. You'll need it for Chapter 11, where we will explore more about the meaning of vata, pitta, and kapha and how they relate to creating a Gut Healing Protocol.

THE GUT-BRAIN CONNECTION

"I KNEW IMMEDIATELY," EVE SAID. "ON PAPER I HAD MADE THE RIGHT choice, but as soon as I accepted the position, I knew it was the wrong move. I felt it in my gut . . . a sense of knowing." She shrugged. "There are no other words for it. As soon as my brain got out of the way, I just knew."

* * *

HAVE YOU EVER HAD that feeling in your gut? Maybe it speaks with butterflies, or a worrisome churning like Matthew's, or if you're like Eve, your gut is the source of intuition or knowing. It's so influential over our moods and thoughts that scientists have dubbed it our "second brain."

Your gut and brain are in constant communication, regulating your hormones, neurotransmitters, immune system, moods, thoughts, and cravings. And it is certainly involved in panic.

THE GUT-BRAIN AXIS

Let me introduce you to the gut-brain axis, a complex system of communication between the gut and the brain. A two-way street, its signals can travel from the gut to the brain and from the brain to the gut.

The gut contains trillions of bacteria, which are collectively known as the gut microbiota. They produce neurotransmitters, which are chemicals that send messages between nerve cells. They also produce hormones, which are chemicals that travel through the bloodstream to other parts of the body.

The gut-brain axis also includes the nervous system. The vagus nerve, the longest nerve in the body, carries signals back and forth between the gut and the brain, and the enteric nervous system is the nervous system of the gut.

THE MANY WAYS YOUR GUT COMMUNICATES

There are four main channels through which signals travel between the gut and brain:

- **GUT MICROBES.** These are the bacteria that live in your gut. Each strain of microbe/bacteria has its own unique effects on the mind and body. We will explore how they impact your mood and learn more about a specific class of mi-

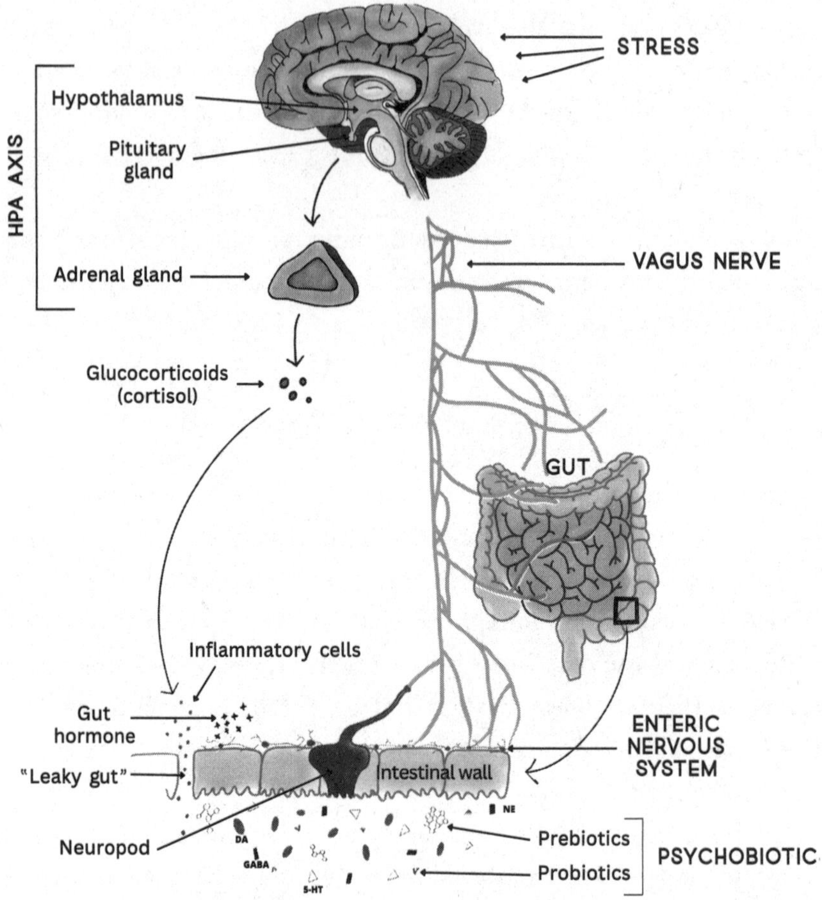

crobes, called psychobiotics, that have been shown to positively influence mood, including reducing episodes of panic and anxiety.

- **THE NERVOUS SYSTEM.** Your gut microbes directly influence your central nervous system (brain and spinal cord including the vagus nerve) and your enteric nervous system in the gut.
- **THE IMMUNE SYSTEM.** Your brain and gut keep a close eye on injuries and predators. If they detect danger, they communicate via inflammatory cells, called cytokines, which create a cascade of responses, including activating the amygdala (the part of the brain responsible for regulating emotions).
- **THE ENDOCRINE SYSTEM.** Your brain and gut use hormones to

get tasks taken care of. This process involves glandular release of hormone signals throughout the body, including activation of the hypothalamic-pituitary-adrenal (HPA) axis, causing cortisol to be released by the adrenal glands.

In the following sections, we'll explore the four primary gut-brain channels in more detail. You'll learn how to use psychobiotics to stop panic, receive tips for how to hack your vagus nerve in order to restore balance and calm to your gut and brain, dive into the world of inflammation and mental health, and explore the interplay among your gut, your hormones, and your mood.

THE DISCOVERY OF "LITTLE ANIMALS"

Our modern understanding of the relationship between gut microbes and human health stands on centuries upon centuries of thinkers and healers. For example, the Chinese physician Ge Hong (283–343 C.E.) was an eclectic philosopher, alchemist, and student of immortality. He was also a strong proponent of the therapeutic benefits of coprophagia, or the practice of eating feces. He observed this practice in certain animals, such as rabbits, and believed that it could be beneficial for humans as well. However, he did not know why it was useful, only that it seemed to be for some people.

Not until many decades later were scientists equipped with the tools to truly dig into the relationship between the components of our digestive tracts and our health. In 1677 scientist Antonie van Leeuwenhoek (1632–1723) peeked into his newly developed microscope and discovered "little animals" on the other end of the lens. Van Leeuwenhoek's revelation provided the scientific community its first glimpse into the tiny world of microorganisms. Approximately 200 years later researcher Louis Pasteur (1822–95) made the link between microorganisms and human disease.

Since the time of van Leeuwenhoek, Pasteur, and other brilliant researchers, the scientific community has made leaps and bounds in understanding the role our microbial companions play in the complex process that underpins health and wellness. It turns out, the stool itself wasn't therapeutic; rather, it was the "little animals," or healthy microorganisms, in Ge Hong's protocols that offered potential health benefits. Let's explore the human body's microorganisms in more detail.

THE MICROBIOTA

Over 100 trillion microorganisms are living in your body, collectively referred to as the gut microbiota. Your family of microbiota was passed down to you by your ancestors and is as unique as your fingerprint. With the ability to mutate every 20 minutes and change its composition in response to each meal it receives, your microbiota plays a key role in helping you quickly adapt to stressors by regulating your immune system, hormone levels, and neurotransmitters.

Some types of bacteria help us stay healthy and protect us from anxiety and stress, while others can make us feel sick or depressed. Each strain has its own unique set of characteristics, such as the types of nutrients it can metabolize, the neurotransmitters it can produce, and the diseases it can help prevent.

It is important to choose a probiotic supplement that contains strains that have been studied and shown to:

- Be therapeutically effective at doing the job you need done, and
- Work synergistically in combination with the other strains in the supplement.

Imagine that you have a garden. In your garden you have many types of plants, each with a different job to do. Some plants will keep the soil healthy, while others will help to attract pollinators. You want to be sure to keep invasive plants out of your garden, or plants that attract pests.

Strains of microbiota bacteria are like the different plants in your garden. Each strain has its own unique job to do, and you want to ensure that all of them work synergistically to keep your body healthy and protect you from pathogens.

PSYCHOBIOTICS

Over the last decade, pioneering researchers John Cryan and Ted Dinan have published more than 400 peer-reviewed articles on specific members of our gut microbial community that are involved in regulating mood and mind. They have named these beneficial bacteria *psychobiotics*.

"A healthy gut is connected to a healthy mind," Cryan said during an interview following the release of their book *The Psychobiotic Revolution: Mood, Food, and the New Science of the Gut-Brain Connection*, co-written with Scott Anderson. "We're talking about a paradigm shift in relation to how we conceptualize how our brains work."

Your gut microbes play an amazingly complex role in mood and mind. Psychobiotic microbes possess the ability to manufacture mood-altering neurotransmitters, such as relaxing GABA and acetylcholine, mood-boosting dopamine, and upward of 90 percent of the mood-regulating neurotransmitter serotonin.

It turns out, the community of microbes living in your gut are quite chatty, constantly communicating messages to your brain. But not all probiotics have the same effects, and not all probiotic supplements are created equal.

HOW TO SELECT A PSYCHOBIOTIC

Choosing the right psychobiotic can be a challenge due to the constantly evolving probiotic-manufacturing process. To ensure you're selecting the best possible product, consider these key factors.

The Old Approach: A Wide Net

For years, researchers have cast a wide net and combined as many beneficial bacteria as possible into commercial probiotic formulations, such as those from the genus *Bifidobacterium* or *Lactobacillus* and the yeast *Saccharomyces boulardii*. However, continued research has revealed that different probiotic strains within species of bacteria perform different functions in the management of health and specific disease.

In selecting the right probiotic for you, try to match your symptoms with the bacterial strains that have been studied to support those symptoms: for example, anxiety mixed with anger, or anxiety and inflammation, or anxiety associated with a high-stress work environment.

The better the match, the better success you will likely have using probiotics. Here is a guide to the best strains for different symptoms.

PROBIOTICS FOR ANXIETY*

PROBIOTIC	HELPFUL FOR THESE SYMPTOMS	STRAINS STUDIED
Bifidobacterium breve	Signs of high cortisol, signs of inflammation, overactive stress response; tends to be useful in those with chronic stress	CCFM1025
Bifidobacterium longum	Depressive Anxiety, Thought Anxiety especially with brain fog, signs of low GABA, emotional reactivity to negative stimuli	R0175, 1714, NCC3001
Lactobacillus plantarum	Feelings of burnout from high stress, sleep disturbances, emotional decision-making	PS128TM, W62
Lactobacillus helveticus	Anger Anxiety, signs of high cortisol, signs of inflammation	R0052
Lactobacillus casei	Difficulty with stress management, intestinal inflammation, signs of low GABA and acetylcholine	Shirota
Lactobacillus reuteri	Chronic stress to the brain, signs of low GABA and acetylcholine, signs of low serotonin	DSM 17938, JCM 1117
Lactobacillus rhamnosus	Postpartum symptoms, pathogens in the gut, chronic stress	GG, LC-705

* Please note that this table is not exhaustive. There may be other probiotics and strains of probiotics that are helpful for anxiety and panic.

Creating a Microbiome Dream Team

Choosing a probiotic with synergetic strains is like hiring a dream team for your gut. Some probiotics, like *Bifidobacterium breve* and *longum,* are power couples in the gut. Together, they've been shown to tackle anxiety like a tag team, achieving more than either could do solo. This secret weapon is called synergy, the art of choosing strains that amplify each other's benefits.

But not all probiotics play nice. Some clash, canceling out each other's effects. This is why it's important to choose a probiotic supplement that has been carefully formulated to include synergistic strains.

Why Clinical Trials Matter

When choosing a probiotic, look for one that has been studied in human clinical trials. These trials can provide evidence that the probiotic is effective and that it works synergistically.

For example, if you're looking for a probiotic to support gut-brain health, look for one with human clinical trials demonstrating improved gut health and brain function in the study participants. If your goal is to find a probiotic that alleviates anxiety by reducing histamine, search for clinical trials that specifically show reduced histamine levels.

It's very important to ensure that the formulation you purchase is the same as the one studied in the clinical trials. Some supplement manufacturers may modify their formulations, which can diminish the effectiveness of the product. A trustworthy manufacturer will not engage in such a bait-and-switch tactic.

The most convincing evidence includes multiple studies with positive outcomes, utilizing objective measures such as inflammatory markers, zonulin, and various laboratory markers (both blood and fecal samples). In some cases, fMRI data may also be used.

Quality Controls

Another way to identify a good probiotic is to look for one that has been certified by a third-party organization, such as the U.S. Pharmacopeia or NSF International. These organizations test probiotics to ensure that they meet certain quality standards.

Viability

In addition to clinical trials, look for a probiotic manufacturer that has studies on viability. *Viability* refers to the number of live bacteria in a probiotic supplement. Probiotics can lose their viability during manufacturing, storage, and transportation. Therefore, consider choosing a probiotic that has been shown to maintain its viability throughout the manufacturing process.

I know that's a lot to keep in mind, but I've done the work for you. Check out drnicolecain.com/book-resources for an up-to-date list of my favorite probiotic blends.

Now that we've talked about psychobiotics and strains, let's take a look at the vagus nerve and the enteric nervous system.

THE VAGUS NERVE AND THE ENTERIC NERVOUS SYSTEM

Your gut and brain are more connected than you might think. The vagus nerve (or cranial nerve 10) is a long nerve that relays information back and forth between your brain and the nervous system in your gut, the enteric nervous system, discussed in Chapter 4. This system is like a mini-brain in your gut. It controls everything from digestion to your mood, which is why it's often referred to as the "second brain."

Vagus nerve activation is one of the most powerful reset switches you have for shifting you out of a high-stress state (autonomic arousal) into one that is calm and relaxed (parasympathetic state).

Within your gut, your microbes are living their best lives producing neurotransmitters such as serotonin, acetylcholine, dopamine, and

GABA, and they are chitchatting with your nervous system impacting your feelings, hormone levels, and even organ function from moment to moment.

Stimulating your vagus nerve can shift your body out of sympathetic activation—you know, that state where your heart is pounding, nerves are tingling, stomach is clenching, and thoughts are racing—and into a parasympathetic state where you feel calm, grounded, and more relaxed.

The signal from the vagus nerve will tell your body to relax, and the composition of bacteria in your gut will respond in turn. Scientists have identified specific strains of gut bacteria that possess the ability to interface with the vagus nerve.

Within the walls of your intestinal tract are little cells called *neuropods*. These neuropods are surrounded by the network of nerves of your digestive tract, the enteric nervous system. Research suggests that chemical messages from your gut bacteria travel to the neuropods in the intestinal wall, stimulating them to relay that signal through your enteric nervous system and to your vagus nerve.

What happens next depends on the type of chemical message that gets sent by the gut bacteria. For example:

- *Bacillus* bacteria strains may release dopamine or noradrenaline.
- *Bifidobacteria* bacteria may secrete GABA.
- *Enterococcus* and *Streptococcus* families favor serotonin production.
- *Escherichia* family of bacteria is known for producing noradrenaline and serotonin.
- *Lactobacillus* bacterial family produces GABA and acetylcholine.

Each of these neurochemicals has different effects on how you feel physically and mentally.

Adrenaline is a neurotransmitter that can cause feelings of autonomic arousal or fear, while GABA does the opposite, making you feel relaxed and calm. If you're anxious, you may want to emphasize supplementing with bacteria from the *Bifidobacteria* family or *Lactobacillus* family so that you enjoy greater amounts of GABA.

Taking care of your gut health is an important part of managing anxiety. We'll dive a lot more into diet specifics in Chapter 11.

THE GUT-BRAIN IMMUNE SYSTEM

Did you know that inflammation in your body can lead to panic attacks and anxiety? This could be game-changing for your journey toward panic freedom.

The gut-brain immune system is a complex network of communication between the gut, the brain, and the immune system. As your body's defense system against infection, the immune system is made up of the lymphatic system, the spleen, the thymus, bone marrow, white blood cells, antibodies, and the complement system. When the immune system is activated, it releases chemicals such as histamines and cytokines. These inflammatory cells can travel throughout the body and affect other organs, including the brain.

According to David Heber, MD, PhD, professor emeritus of medicine at UCLA, "Seventy percent of the immune system is located in the gut." Your gut microbes regulate the entire process like musical conductors.

INFLAMMATION AND THE BRAIN

Inflammation, a natural response to injury or infection, protects us by recruiting specialized cells from the immune system to come to the scene of infection or injury, where they release chemicals that fight infection and repair damage. Brain inflammation can activate the amygdala, the brain's center for processing emotions like fear and anxiety. This activation, in turn, can lead to feelings of anxiety, stress, and depression.

LEAKY GUT, LEAKY BRAIN

Chronic inflammation wreaks havoc on both emotional and physical health. It can also damage gut cells, leading to increased intestinal permeability, often referred to as "leaky gut." This compromised barrier allows bacteria, toxins, and other unwanted substances to leak from the gut into the bloodstream, causing further problems.

Upon entering the circulatory system, these substances can wreak mayhem from head to toe, including damaging the blood-brain barrier, the semipermeable membrane that protects the brain from harmful substances in the bloodstream.

When the blood-brain barrier is damaged, harmful substances can "leak" through it and into the brain itself. The subsequent damage to the brain may result in myriad symptoms ranging from panic attacks to neurodegenerative diseases.

LEAKY GUT = LEAKY BRAIN

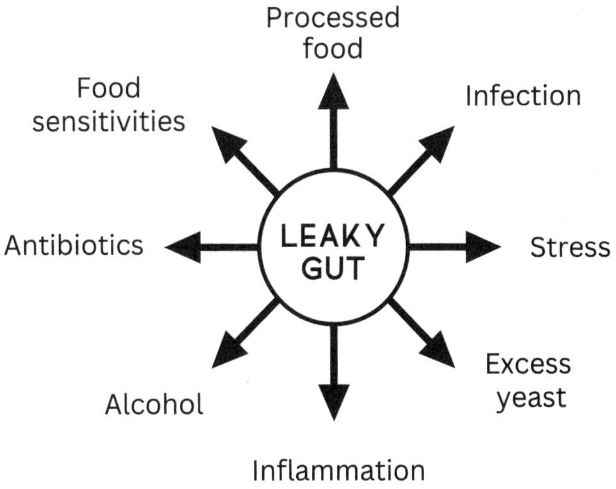

Sophia

AS A SEMIRETIRED CONSULTANT FOR AN ENGINEERING FIRM, SOPHIA was often invited to speak at conferences. However, there was just one problem: she had a phobia of public speaking.

Every time she agreed to a new contract, her stomach revolted, resulting in anticipatory gas, bloating, abdominal pain, and bouts of unrelenting diarrhea.

It hadn't always been so debilitating for Sophia. Initially, she struggled with what she described as "butterflies" in her stomach, but over time her symptoms got worse. Her doctors recommended pill after pill after pill, but antidepressants eliminated her libido, benzodiazepines gave her brain fog, beta-blockers crashed her blood pressure, antacids did not touch the pain, and antihistamines just made her sleepy.

Sophia's symptoms are consistent with Gut Anxiety (see Chapter 3). One of the tests that can be run to identify the root cause of Gut Anxiety is a comprehensive stool analysis. Sophia agreed to do this test in hopes that the result would yield some answers to why she felt the way she did and what to do about it. It did, in spades.

The particular test that Sophia used screened for dysbiosis, inflammation, gut microbiome health markers, and pathogens. Her results revealed that she had excess levels of candida, a form of yeast that is associated with digestive symptoms and anxiety; and excess methane-producing bacteria, which cause flatulence, gas buildup, and significant levels of inflammation and dysbiosis. These findings align with the symptoms of Gut Anxiety.

Sophia delved into the list of anxiety-reducing probiotics and selected these strains: *Bifidobacterium longum,* known to ease anxiety, improve mood, and boost cognitive function; *Lactobacillus rhamnosus,* helpful for recovering from chronic stress and gut imbalances; and *Lactobacillus casei,* which can combat inflammation, reduce stress, and elevate mood.

DYSBIOSIS: THE HIDDEN CAUSE OF ANXIETY

Dysbiosis is a condition in which the balance of bacteria in the gut is disrupted. It may be associated with loss of beneficial bacteria in the gut, excess growth of harmful bacteria, or a loss of microbial diversity. This can be caused by a number of factors, including stress, environmental toxicity, diet, hormonal imbalances, and medication. Dysbiosis has been linked to a number of health problems, including anxiety and panic.

DYSBIOSIS & PANIC

8 SIGNS YOUR PANIC MIGHT BE RELATED TO DYSBIOSIS

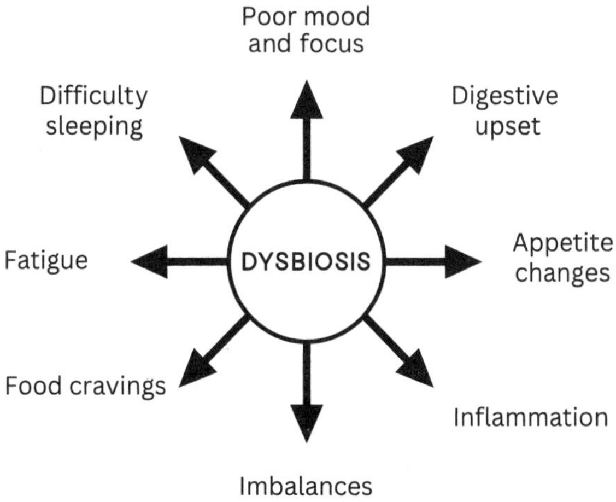

When it comes to dysbiosis, one thing is clear: the longer it lasts, the worse and more widespread the symptoms may become. As seen in Sophia's experience, seemingly mild inattention or anxiety can morph into more severe symptoms as gut dysbiosis worsens, potentially culminating in full-blown panic attacks.

In Part III, you are going to learn my favorite protocols for quickly healing leaky gut and leaky brain, and for combating dysbiosis.

THE GUT-BRAIN ENDOCRINE SYSTEM

Have you ever been told that your hormones are "off"? You have a diagnosis of hypothyroidism, or your estrogen is out of whack, or perhaps your cortisol is low. If we do a little digging, you'll often find that the gut is, in part, to blame.

Your gut performs a delicate dance, constantly working to keep you prepared for whatever life throws your way. But when faced with chronic stress, this delicate balance can tip, leaving you more reactive to stressful situations.

THE GUT AND SEX HORMONES. Believe it or not, your gut bacteria might be even more interested in your sex hormones than you are! These tiny microbes interact with your hormones in a lot of ways. For instance, some gut bacteria, like those belonging to the *Clostridia, Escherichia coli,* and *Bacteroides* species, produce an enzyme called beta-glucuronidase. This enzyme can reactivate and reabsorb estrogen in the intestines, influencing your overall estrogen levels. This explains, in part, why antibiotics can disrupt the gut microbiome and contribute to lower estrogen levels.

THE GUT AND THYROID HORMONES. Your gut has a lot to say when it comes to thyroid hormones. Here are three ways your gut can affect your thyroid hormones:

- **DYSBIOSIS.** Imbalances in your gut flora, or dysbiosis, are associated with nonceliac wheat sensitivity and celiac disease, which often co-occur with autoimmune thyroid diseases such as Hashimoto's thyroiditis and Graves' disease.
- **NUTRIENTS.** Your body needs specific micronutrients to make thyroid hormone, such as iodine, iron, copper, selenium, and zinc, all of which are absorbed and processed by your gut.
- **HELPFUL BUGS.** Some strains of bacteria, like *Lactobacillus reuteri,* can improve thyroid function by increasing levels of free T4.

THE GUT AND ADRENAL HORMONES. Your gut and your adrenal glands work together to help you cope with whatever stressors life throws your way.

A 2021 study published in the *International Journal of Molecular Sciences* revealed that the gut microbiota can change the expression of genes involved in making cortisol, a stress hormone. This means that your gut bacteria can help your adrenals meet your body's demands by actually changing your genetic expression. In addition to helping you respond to stress, cortisol also counteracts excessive inflammation.

As you can see, your gut and your hormones are intimately connected. This means that if you are struggling with panic, taking care of your gut health can help to improve your overall health and reduce your risk of panic attacks. Be sure to check out Chapter 11, which has all sorts of tips for improving gut health, including foods, supplements, and habits.

GUT ANXIETY TESTING

Functional testing can help identify imbalances in the gut microbiome, the immune system, and the nervous system that may be contributing to gut-related symptoms, such as anxiety, depression, and fatigue. Here are my favorite tests:

- **STOOL ANALYSIS.** Different stool tests offer insights into various aspects of gut health. Some tests assess the diversity of gut bacteria (microbiome), identify digestive enzyme deficiencies, and pinpoint sources of inflammation. Others may focus on measuring specific bacterial or viral levels.
- **ORGANIC ACIDS TESTING.** Organic acids are produced by your body as part of your normal metabolism. The levels of these acids in your urine can help you assess the function of the gut, the immune system, and the nervous system.
- **IMMUNE TESTING.** IgG food antibodies are produced when the body's immune system is exposed to a food protein, but we

don't know if that exposure is causing a problematic reaction. So elimination and reintroduction testing is a much more accurate way to determine if a food may be contributing to your symptoms. Food elimination and reintroduction are explained in Chapter 11.

There are a lot of functional medicine tests on the market, and not all are created equal. Here are a few tips for finding the right tests:

- Lean toward companies that are more thorough in their methods and use a combination of PCR, culture, and microscopic testing.
- Not all biomarkers are created equal. Select tests that use research-based biomarkers.
- Whenever possible, seek tests from companies endorsed by reputable organizations in the field, such as the American College of Gastroenterology.

How do you know if a particular company or test checks these boxes? They should report it on their website for starters. I've done the legwork for you—you can access my favorite physician-grade tests at drnicolecain.com/book-resources.

HAPPY GUT BASICS

If you have a happy gut, you're going to be a lot more likely to have a happy mind. While we talk a lot more about gut healing in Chapter 11, there are two key changes you can make today to get your gut back on track.

- **GET ENOUGH FIBER.** Everyone's fiber needs vary, and depending on your current gut health, you may need to slowly increase your fiber amount. Maybe start with 5 grams per day for a few days, then increase to 10 grams, then to 20. Aim for a maintenance daily dose of 20 to 30 grams of fiber per day. Tip: You can find a great fiber calculator by going to OmniCalculator.com.

Examples of high-fiber foods that your gut bacteria love include:

- Whole grains, such as cooked oats, barley, quinoa, and brown and wild rice
- Veggies such as broccoli and kale
- Legumes such as lentils, peas, and beans
- Fruit such as bananas and apples

- **EAT FERMENTED FOODS.** Your gut bacteria love them. My go-to fermented food is unsweetened yogurt. If you're vegan, there are a lot of wonderful new plant-based options you can try. You can also try other fermented foods such as kimchi, sauerkraut, kombucha, and kefir, but keep in mind that they may also increase histamine (which you'll learn more about in Chapter 6).

There are hundreds of different species in your gut, all with their unique tastes, preferences, and behaviors. Eating a diverse range of foods is one of the best ways to keep all your gut bugs happy and healthy.

Matthew

YOU MIGHT BE WONDERING WHAT MATTHEW DID TO HEAL HIS GUT Anxiety. He created a plan that was uniquely tailored to his individual needs, and by following the steps outlined in this book, you can learn how to do the same. Below is Matthew's plan. You'll notice that he refers to items that we haven't discussed yet, but don't worry, we'll cover all of these concepts and more!

Also, keep in mind that everyone's treatment plan is different, just as everyone's panic is different. Trust your body to tell you what it needs. Matthew, Esme, David, Aria, Jenny, and Charlotte all healed in their own unique ways, and so will you.

MATTHEW'S PANIC PROOF PROTOCOL:

My Stoplight Strategies:

HABITS THAT KEEP ME IN THE GREEN LIGHT ZONE: *Practicing jujitsu, getting regular sleep, going to counseling, sticking to my healthy food protocol, doing vagus nerve practices.*

SIGNS I AM TRANSITIONING INTO THE YELLOW LIGHT ZONE: *Unsettled "knowing" in my gut, thoughts shift toward over-analyzing my health and what I'm feeling in my body.*

SIGNS I AM IN THE YELLOW LIGHT ZONE: *I feel anxious about my health, I'm preoccupied with every little sensation I feel, and I'm isolating.*

HABITS, SUPPLEMENTS, AND MEDICINES TO GET ME BACK INTO THE GREEN LIGHT ZONE: *A psychobiotic + Saccharomyces boulardii 250 mg per day. Soluble fiber 6 grams per day.*

SIGNS I AM TRANSITIONING INTO THE RED LIGHT ZONE: *Pacing, racing thoughts, bubbling in my gut, urging of my bowels.*

SIGNS I AM IN THE RED LIGHT ZONE: *Extreme panic, horrible gut pain, diarrhea, isolating from other people.*

MY CRISIS RESOURCES: *My sister, the crisis hotline 988, and my counselor. Use my Panic Pack. Take my emergency prescription from my doctor.*

My Dosha:

- **SIGNS AND SYMPTOMS INDICATING MY DOSHA IS OUT OF BALANCE:** *Vata Gut Anxiety, super gassiness, bloat, racing thoughts, distractibility, restlessness*
- **FOODS TO BALANCE MY DOSHA:** *Sesame oil, cooked greens, root vegetables*
- **SPICES TO BALANCE MY DOSHA:** *Curry, ginger, clove, nutmeg, cinnamon*

- **HABITS TO BALANCE MY DOSHA:** *Walk in the grass barefoot, sit against a tree, eat slowly and mindfully, breathe in through top of my head down to my feet and back out through my head, always end coming into my feet. Weighted blanket. Heated blanket.*

THE PANIC RESET

STEP 1: Nervous System Calming Habits. *Make a Panic Pack with earthy rooted spices, sandalwood, cinnamon, and clove. Include a hot and cold pack. Include a spiky fidget toy. Practice extending the exhale when doing my grounding breath.*

STEP 2: Wise Mind Habits. *Practice focused attention meditation. Do Sudoku puzzles. Learn Japanese. Spend 10 minutes each night on this.*

STEP 3: Reintegration Habits. *Practice self-massage and kindness to my body and/or practice paying attention to my body. Practice interoception 30 minutes per day. Listen to Somatographic Imagery meditation weekly.*

STEP 4: Restructuring Habits. *Jujitsu practice. Therapy, focus on my "house audit" and Parts Work. Practice Firecracker three times every three hours when sitting at my computer and working at home.*

NUTRITION: Panic Proof foods I am emphasizing: *Stool testing said I needed more microbial diversity and fiber and to reduce inflammation. Add Costco salmon to weekly menu. Eat steamed salad or other cooked greens daily. Get in fiber. Only have refined sugar on Sundays.*

MY EXERCISE GOALS: Pick three forms of exercise you are committed to doing.

- Activity 1: I will (list activity) *Jujitsu* for a duration of *2 hours* on (list specific days) *Mondays, Tuesdays, Thursdays*
- Activity 2: I will (list activity) *Go for a walk* for a duration of *20 minutes* (list specific days) *every day*

- Activity 3: I will (list activity) Go to the gym for a duration of 45 minutes (list specific days) on Saturdays

MY PANIC PROOF HERBAL RECIPE: Vata Gut Anxiety Soother tincture containing 40% lemon balm (*Melissa officinalis*), 30% skullcap (*Scutellaria lateriflora*), 25% fennel (*Foeniculum vulgare*), 5% ginger. Three big squeezes in juice or water in the morning and at night.

MY PANIC PROOF SUPPLEMENTS: Anxiety-specific supplement: Happy Sleepy Powder before leaving the house.

NEXT STEPS

Matthew's journey, shaped by his unique experiences and needs, exemplifies the beauty of the principles outlined in this book. He was able to learn how to listen to his body through his symptoms, and with the help of specialized testing he created a plan that recalibrated his brain and body so that it was wired not for panic but for confidence and freedom.

And you can too.

Here are some additional next steps to consider:

1. **ASK YOURSELF:** *How does this information about the gut-brain axis relate to me? What are my symptoms trying to tell me?* Doing a deeper dive might just bring up data that would surprise you and open unexpected channels for healing.
2. **FUNCTIONAL MEDICINE TESTING:** Getting information on what is happening in your gut can indicate the best way to clear your unique symptoms.
3. **WORK WITH YOUR VAGUS NERVE:** Remember, your vagus nerve is the on-off switch for your autonomic nervous system. The more you practice, the more efficiently you will be able

to curb feelings of panic in the moment. You can read more about how to work with your vagus nerve by going to my website drnicolecain.com and typing *vagus* into the search bar.

4. **HOLISTIC SOLUTIONS:** Now that you know more about the gut-brain axis, you can take this information and jump to Part III to explore what holistic remedies might be valuable for you right now.

GUT-BRAIN TL;DR

- Anxiety that manifests in your gut is called Gut Anxiety.
- Your gut and brain communicate via the gut-brain axis.
- Your gut microbes regulate hormones, immunity, neurotransmitters, and other bodily systems.
- Psychobiotics are a group of bacteria that are beneficial for your mood.
- Your gut bacteria can stimulate the vagus nerve to stop panic and create calm.

6

NEUROTRANSMITTERS AND PANIC

"THERE ARE PEAKS AND VALLEYS, BUT THE VALLEYS HAVE BEEN COMING quicker and harder." Through the receiver, I hear David typing on his computer. He often multitasks during our calls.

"I've dealt with this my whole life. But lately it's been negatively affecting my wife and the kids. I don't sleep, then I'm irritable, anxious, and on edge. That makes me feel guilty and even more angry. I'm at my wit's end here.

"I don't want to take a drug, but clearly something's off in my brain. My therapist referred me to meet with a psychiatrist on Friday, because apparently I have a 'chemical imbalance.' "

This is the kind of thing we are told when our mental health symptoms begin to interfere in our lives: that the chemicals in our brain are out of balance, and there are medications designed to fix that.

But there is more to David's story.

Over the last five years or so, he has also been struggling with headaches, dizziness, digestive upset, and clumsiness. A primary care doctor looked at his basic blood work and gave him a clean bill of health (besides his so-called chemical imbalance), but something still wasn't right.

And so we did a little more digging.

And David discovered something that he wished he would have known 46 years sooner. More on that in Chapter 7.

IN THIS CHAPTER

In this chapter, you'll learn a lot about the chemicals in your brain: how they work, what they do, and some myths that have been circulating about them since the 1960s. You'll learn:

- How to screen for a chemical imbalance
- How your neurotransmitters play a role in your panic
- How and why your neurotransmitters go out of balance
- How to test for chemical imbalances

THE CHEMICAL IMBALANCE THEORY

In 1937 the Italian scientists Maffu Vialli and Vittorio Espamer came across something that turned out to be one of the most important discoveries in neuroscience: a signaling molecule that they named enteramine (later renamed *serotonin*), located in little cells in the gut. In the years that followed, researchers identified many other chemicals such as dopamine, adrenaline, and GABA.

More than three decades after the discovery of serotonin in 1937, a groundbreaking study emerged in 1974. This research proposed a novel treatment for mood disorders: fluoxetine (Prozac), a drug designed to elevate serotonin levels in the brain. The theory was that depression and anxiety were caused by lowered serotonin in the brain, and that increasing serotonin levels with a selective serotonin reuptake inhibitor (SSRI) would improve a person's mood. This was the birth of the chemical imbalance theory, and despite many publications that followed questioning its veracity, it has dominated the medical establishment's understanding of mental health.

Until recently.

In 2022 a giant meta-analysis and systematic review, published in the journal *Molecular Psychiatry,* took down the chemical imbalance theory. Its conclusion can be boiled down to the following quote: "There is no convincing evidence that depression is associated with, or caused by, lower serotonin concentrations or activity."

And just like that, we find ourselves back at square one.

And this is a wonderful place to be, because when we don't have answers, we look for them. Instead of assuming someone has a chemical imbalance, we have the opportunity to ask questions like:

- Why do antidepressants help some people but not others?
- Why is it that within 30 minutes of taking an SSRI like Prozac, the levels of serotonin in neural synapses rapidly increase, but it takes upward of two weeks for someone to feel better?
- What else might be going on beneath the surface?
- What do we do now?

I'm so glad you asked.

Let me start by introducing you to your neurotransmitters.

MEET YOUR NEUROTRANSMITTERS

In the remainder of this chapter, you are going to learn a *lot* about neurotransmitters: what they are, how they're made and broken down, how they relate to panic, how to test imbalances, and much more.

I've created self-administered checklists to help you identify the neurotransmitters that may be more relevant for you, but this comes with three disclaimers:

1. **YOUR NEUROTRANSMITTERS ARE AFFECTED BY MANY VARIABLES.** Your experiences, traumas, nutrient levels, gut microbes, detoxification, genetics, *other* neurotransmitters, and much more are also parts of your total experience. While I am teaching you about your neurotransmitters, I want you to keep in mind that they are only one part.

2. **MEDICATIONS AND SUPPLEMENTS CHANGE YOUR BODY CHEMISTRY.** Even if you are on medications, you can still get great information. For example, let's say you are on an antidepressant that aims to increase serotonin, and your self-assessment result reveals that you have super low serotonin. You can follow that assessment by testing serotonin metabolites, and while we cannot directly test the neurotransmitters in your brain, we can test their overall levels. So don't worry if you're taking medications. This chapter can still be very useful to and relevant for you.
3. **YOU COULD FILL BOOKS AND BOOKS WITH INFORMATION ABOUT THE HUMAN NERVOUS SYSTEM.** It's been done. While I can't cover everything in these pages, I've done my best to distill the most useful and relevant information.

Okay, now for the good stuff.

Serotonin

If there were a popularity contest for neurotransmitters, serotonin would win, hands down. SSRI-modifying antidepressants are among the top-ten most commonly prescribed medication types worldwide. There's even a Serotonin Club dedicated to research involving all things serotonin. With publicity like that, it's no wonder that serotonin has dominated the mental health market for decades.

Think of serotonin as the friend who always gets all the credit for good feelings. You feel happy and cheerful? It must be that your serotonin is working smoothly! You feel grumpy and sad? You must need more serotonin! While it is true that serotonin plays an important role in your moods, it is only one part of a complex system that regulates how you think and feel.

To get you started on your journey of learning all about your mood-regulating neurotransmitters, I have created a Serotonin Checklist. All you have to do is check the box(es) that you resonate with!

SEROTONIN SELF-ASSESSMENT CHECKLIST: SIGNS OF IMBALANCED SEROTONIN

Instructions: Check the box(es) that relate to you, and write your total score in the space provided.

- ❑ Increased appetite, with cravings for carbohydrates and sweets
- ❑ Difficulty falling asleep and/or staying asleep
- ❑ Migraine headaches
- ❑ Diarrhea, nausea, or irritable bowel syndrome
- ❑ High sensitivity to pain

TOTAL: ____/5

SCORING: If you checked more than two boxes, consider getting a workup to screen for too-low serotonin.

- ❑ High body temperature, sweating, and fever
- ❑ Dilated pupils
- ❑ Muscle spasms, tremors, and rigidity
- ❑ Extreme agitation
- ❑ Restlessness

TOTAL: ____/5

SCORING: If you checked more than two boxes, consider getting a workup to screen for too-high serotonin right away. Excess serotonin is associated with a condition called serotonin syndrome, which can be life threatening.

It is essential to note that marking checkboxes does not necessarily indicate abnormal serotonin levels but can aid in identifying areas that require further investigation.

Relationship Status Between Serotonin and Mood: It's Complicated

The chemical imbalance theory suggests that depression and anxiety are caused by low serotonin levels. However, we now know that this theory isn't entirely accurate.

There are many different theories about how and why serotonin can affect our mood. Here are a few:

- **PROMOTING THE GROWTH OF NEW BRAIN NEURONS.** Some research suggests that serotonin can promote the growth of new neurons in parts of the brain that control fear, memory, and mood. However, these effects can vary depending on which type of serotonin receptor is activated in the brain. For instance, activating certain receptors in the amygdala (the fight-or-flight part of the brain) can help reduce anxiety, while activating other receptors in this region can conversely heighten it.
- **REDUCING INFLAMMATION.** Inflammation is linked to anxiety and depression, and serotonin may help reduce inflammation and modulate the immune system. Some SSRIs, such as citalopram (Celexa), fluoxetine (Prozac), and sertraline (Zoloft), have stronger anti-inflammatory effects than others, like paroxetine (Paxil) and fluvoxamine (Luvox), making them more useful for people with panic related to inflammation. However, there are natural and holistic ways to reduce inflammation that can be even more effective without the side effects of antidepressants. Part III offers information on these strategies.
- **ACTIVATING THE STRESS RESPONSE.** Another theory is that serotonin can ease anxiety by supporting our ability to respond to stress. It does this by stimulating cortisol release via the hypothalamic-pituitary-adrenal (HPA) axis.
- **COMMUNICATING VIA THE GUT-BRAIN CONNECTION.** Serotonin isn't made only in your brain—it is also produced by cells in your immune system (such as mast cells), in your stomach, and in your small intestine. Additionally, certain microbes present in your gut produce serotonin, such as *Lactococcus, Lactobacillus, Streptococcus, Escherichia coli,* and *Klebsiella* species. The serotonin in your gut will influence your brain and vice verse. We explored this topic in more detail in Chapter 5.

Here's a fun fact: Did you know that only about 5 percent of your body's serotonin is actually made in your brain? The other 95 percent

is made in your gut. It just goes to show that the health of your gut is a pretty big deal.

Most likely, our emotional experiences are due to a blend of all the theories listed above (and more). Your mood and your predisposition to panic and anxiety are influenced by a variety of factors, such as your stress response system, gut microbes, inflammation levels, and the amount of important nutrients and minerals in your body.

As you work toward becoming Panic Proof, it is important to recognize how your diet, inflammation, and mood are interconnected. Making even the smallest changes to your health routine can have a big impact on your overall well-being.

Let's dive into the science of serotonin so that we can figure out how to tweak your Panic Proof Protocol. We'll explore:

- The science of serotonin
- Is too much serotonin too much of a good thing?
- Is serotonin right for you?
- Serotonin testing

The Science of Serotonin

Serotonin is made from tryptophan, an amino acid found in many foods such as fish, eggs, bananas, and turkey. Although tryptophan is often associated with post–turkey dinner sleepiness, the amount present in turkey is insufficient to cause drowsiness. The sensation of grogginess is more likely to result from the quantity of food consumed.

In order to make tryptophan into serotonin, the body undergoes a series of steps that requires specific vitamins and minerals, such as vitamins B1, B2, B3, B6, C and D, iron, and magnesium.

Ultimately, tryptophan is converted into a substance called 5-hydroxyindoleacetic acid (5-HIAA), which gets removed from your body through the urine. This is important to know because you can learn a little bit about your serotonin metabolism by measuring the levels of 5-HIAA in urine through a test, which I will explain later in this section.

This next part is where things can go haywire. In the presence of inflammation, serotonin metabolism changes, and tryptophan may be directed toward a different pathway known as the kynurenine pathway, which is involved in regulating inflammation. Meaning, even if you have enough of the right brain chemicals present, you can still experience symptoms of anxiety or depression if your body is not processing those chemicals properly.

The kynurenine pathway actually has *two* branches. One is helpful and the other is problematic. You can support the helpful pathway and keep inflammation in your brain down by supplementing with vitamin B3 (niacin).

Here are two important points to remember: (1) you need to keep your inflammation levels in check, and (2) you need to make sure that you are getting enough of the right vitamins and nutrients to support your body's essential pathways.

Are you wondering how to determine what is causing your inflammation, imbalances in gut microbiota, and other factors that influence serotonin levels? That's where testing comes in. But first, we need to talk about the dark side of serotonin.

Too Much of a Good Thing? Serotonin's Fall from Grace

What happens when you take too much of an antidepressant such as sertraline (Zoloft)?

Agitation. Tremors. Heart palpitations. Diarrhea. High blood pressure. Dilated eyes.

You run the risk of developing serotonin syndrome—a potentially life-threatening condition that occurs when there is an excess of serotonin in the body.

What if you swapped out the serotonin-boosting medication for excessive amounts of something natural, such as 5-hydroxytryptophan (5-HTP)?

Same thing.

Many years ago, Jenny, a patient of mine, shared her story of what happened when she took too much of a "good thing."

"I was going through a bad time. Really bad. I had just broken up with my partner, my mother was sick and moved in with me, and finances were strapped."

Jenny has always been a health advocate. After she received her diagnosis of bipolar disorder, she worked hard to change her life, starting with her health. She got a job as a fitness instructor and was a nutrition and mindfulness coach. Whenever she got sick or injured, she would turn to natural and holistic remedies, generally with good success.

But this time was different. She felt like she was drowning in overwhelm, her sleep was touch and go, and she struggled to keep her racing and anxious thoughts at bay.

"I went to my doctor, and she suggested I try an antidepressant, which I did. It was taking too long to kick in, and I was desperate. So less than a week later I went to the health food store and purchased some 5-HTP. I've read that 5-HTP can also boost serotonin, and who doesn't want more of a good thing?"

Not long afterward Jenny's symptoms changed, but not for the better. "It started with confusion. I remember lying in bed, and the walls started to shift and move. I tried to reason through how it was impossible for walls to take on a life of their own, but my thoughts were jumbled and frightening. By habit I reached for my partner, but I was alone."

Jenny got out of bed and stumbled down the hallway to her mom's room. "[Mom] tried to help. She drew me a bath and offered me tea, but for some reason I thought she was trying to hurt me instead. My thoughts were paranoid and not logical."

Soon afterward Jenny spiked a fever and began to vomit. Her mother called for an ambulance. "When the paramedics arrived, I was rocking back and forth on the floor, laughing one moment and sobbing the next. They asked me if I had taken any drugs, or new medications."

The diagnosis?

Possible serotonin syndrome—essentially, where the body and brain get flooded with excess serotonin levels.

But she had another risk factor for an adverse reaction to serotonin that her doctor did not catch. Did you notice it?

Is Serotonin Right for You?

Not only is serotonin not a one-stop shop for relieving depression, anxiety, or issues with sleep. For some, increasing serotonin can actually make matters worse.

CONTRAINDICATIONS FOR TAKING SEROTONIN BOOSTERS

- You have bipolar disorder and are not taking a mood stabilizer.
- You are already on a serotonin-enhancing protocol.
- You are taking medications that can interact with serotonin medications such as monoamine oxidase inhibitors (MAOIs), certain migraine medications, or substances like MDMA (Ecstasy).
- You have a hypersensitivity to serotonin.
- You are pregnant or breastfeeding.

The status quo solution to Jenny's symptoms of depression, insomnia, and anxiety was to work to boost her serotonin levels. Unfortunately, the results were not what Jenny had in mind. This could have been due to excess serotonin in her system, but Jenny also had a diagnosis of bipolar disorder, a condition that puts a person at risk of developing mania or hypomania when they take a serotonin-modifying medication or supplement.

I can't help but wonder how her outcome would have been different if she had been guided to interpret her symptoms as signals for healing. Jenny's story, as well as many others, are part of why I've written this book.

Serotonin Testing

Because serotonin does not cross the blood-brain barrier, any test that doesn't directly access the brain or cerebrospinal fluid will provide only approximations, at best, of what is happening with serotonin in the brain. In lieu of direct serotonin testing, we can test for the next best thing: serotonin metabolites.

My go-to test for screening for suspected serotonin imbalances is the Organic Acids Test (OAT). This test can measure serotonin metabolites that can cross the blood-brain barrier, such as 5-hydroxyindoleacetic, quinolinic, and kynurenic acids. However, the OAT measures serotonin metabolites from both the brain and gut, so it may not always be clear which source the metabolite came from.

SEROTONIN TL;DR

- Clinicians used to believe more serotonin was associated with less anxiety and depression. It turns out that it's not that simple.
- 95 percent of your serotonin is made by the microbiota in your gut.
- When you are inflamed, serotonin metabolism is shunted down the kynurenine pathway.
- Healthy serotonin metabolism requires many nutrient cofactors such as vitamins B1, B2, B3, B6, C and D, iron, and magnesium.

Dopamine

There are technically only three things you love in life: serotonin, oxytocin, and dopamine.

Allow me to introduce you to dopamine, your favorite feel-good neurotransmitter. Dopamine is part of the reward system of your brain and is involved in helping you feel pleasure. You know that feeling you get when you smell freshly baked cookies, receive a much-cherished gift, or your favorite song comes on the radio? You might want to thank your dopamine for the warm fuzzies.

All sorts of things stimulate the release of dopamine: food (especially foods high in sugar, salt, and fat), exercise (cardiovascular and weight training), novelty and excitement, positive social interactions, certain supplements, and drugs and alcohol.

And as you get flooded with dopamine, you might find yourself wondering, *Am I feeling blissed out, or is that just the chemicals in my brain?* The answer is YES.

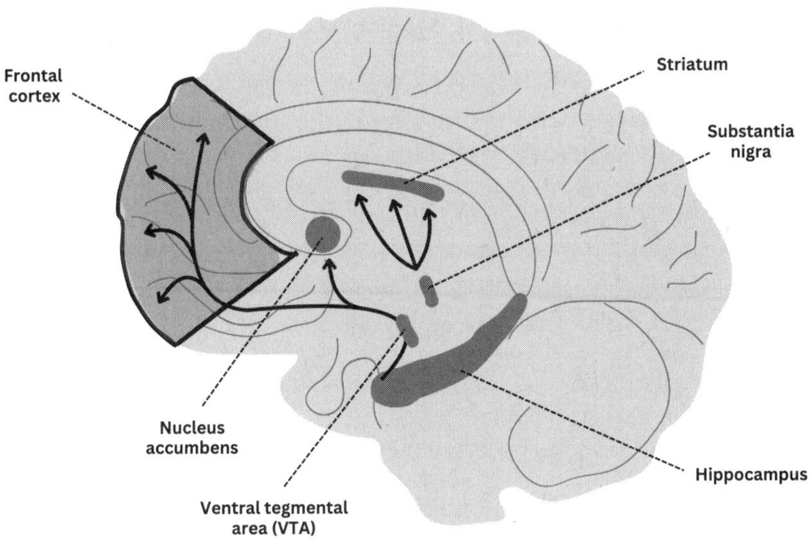

Pleasure starts with a spark deep in six key regions in the brain: the nucleus accumbens, the ventral tegmental area, the substantia nigra, the amygdala, the striatum, prefrontal cortex, and hypothalamus.

Stimulation in these regions results in activation of a certain type of neuron called a dopaminergic neuron, which releases dopamine throughout your system.

The result? You feel intensely rewarded, and you want more.

In addition to creating those feel-good feelings that we all love and rely on, dopamine plays other roles in your health.

- **REGULATION OF MOOD.** A regulated mood boils down to balance. While low dopamine is associated with depression, too much dopamine can cause anxiety and paranoia.
- **COORDINATION OF MOVEMENT.** Dopamine is involved in coordination of movement. Low levels of dopamine are associated with movement disorders such as Parkinson's disease.
- **MOTIVATION AND REWARD.** Dopamine reinforces behaviors, making you want to keep doing them. If you feel "bleh" or lack motivation, low dopamine may be (in part) to blame.
- **MEMORY.** Dopamine signaling in the hippocampus, a brain region important for memory consolidation, is essential for the long-term storage and retrieval of memories.
- **FOCUS AND ATTENTION.** Dopamine is necessary for focus. Dopamine-increasing drugs are in the spotlight for treatment of attention deficit (hyperactivity) disorder.

Here's a checklist comparing the signs of high dopamine versus the signs of low dopamine. While a checklist is not a replacement for a diagnostic tool, it can be a helpful guide for deeper digging.

SELF-ASSESSMENT CHECKLIST: TOO HIGH VS. TOO LOW DOPAMINE

Instructions: Check the box(es) that relate to you and write your total score in the space provided.

- ❑ Muscle stiffness and/or tremors
- ❑ Difficulty with focus and attention
- ❑ Apathy, lack of interest or motivation
- ❑ Anhedonia, inability to feel pleasure
- ❑ Craving sugar and/or carbohydrates

- ❑ Panic, agitation, and/or paranoia
- ❑ Excessive sweating, body temperature regulation problems
- ❑ Restlessness of mind/body
- ❑ Drug addiction, sexual addiction, screen addiction, or compulsive gambling
- ❑ Overconfidence and risk-taking behavior

TOTAL: ____/5

SCORING: If you checked more than two boxes, consider getting a workup to screen for too-low dopamine.

TOTAL: ____/5

SCORING: If you checked more than two boxes, consider getting a workup to screen for too-high dopamine.

What did you score? Do you have any signs that your dopamine levels may be out of balance? If so, let's dive into the next sections together, where you'll learn a bit about the science of dopamine and hacks for getting your dopamine levels back on track.

The Science of Dopamine

Bear with me in the next few paragraphs because we're going to wade even deeper into the science. My goal for teaching you these details is so you can identify areas where dopamine balance is breaking down. I also want to equip you with research-backed strategies to get your neurochemistry back on track.

Dopamine belongs to a group of three similar chemicals called catecholamines, which also include norepinephrine and epinephrine. These three chemicals all come from the same amino acid called tyrosine.

In brief, dopamine metabolism begins with the absorption of phenylalanine and L-tyrosine from food sources such as nuts, eggs, beans, fish, and chicken. Phenylalanine is converted into L-tyrosine, which is then transformed into L-DOPA, a precursor to dopamine. Vitamin B6 aids in the conversion of L-DOPA into dopamine, which is used by the brain and body before being broken down. Dopamine breakdown occurs through three pathways. The transformation of dopamine into norepinephrine requires the assistance of copper and vitamin C. S-adenosyl-L-methionine (SAMe or SAM-e) then converts norepinephrine into epinephrine, which is eventually broken down into vanillylmandelic acid (VMA) and removed through urine.

Now that we know the basics on how dopamine is made, let's take a look at how the process of dopamine balancing can go wrong.

Where Dopamine Balancing Breaks Down

Identifying gaps in dopamine metabolism and breakdown can be especially helpful. Here are the three most common root causes of dopamine imbalances that I see in clinical practice:

- **NUTRIENT IMBALANCES.** To maintain optimal dopamine levels, it's important to ensure that our bodies have the necessary building blocks for production and metabolism. These include amino acids, enzymes, vitamins B6 and C, and all the nutrients needed for many detoxification pathways.
- **SEROTONIN ENZYME STEAL.** Serotonin and dopamine share an enzyme called aromatic L-amino acid decarboxylase (AAAD). Taking supplements or medications that enhance serotonin levels, like 5-hydroxytryptophan or escitalopram (Lexapro), can require more AAAD, which can limit the enzyme's availability for making dopamine. Conversely, taking dopamine boosters, such as L-tyrosine or bupropion (Wellbutrin), can reduce AAAD's accessibility for producing serotonin. This is one reason why people taking SSRIs may experience depression, lack of motivation, or sugar/carbohydrate cravings. The increased serotonin demand is "stealing" the enzyme you need in order to make dopamine.
- **OXIDATIVE STRESS.** Oxidative stress occurs when the body's production of unstable molecules called free radicals overwhelms its natural antioxidant defenses. Free radicals can damage cells and tissues throughout the body. Research suggests a link between oxidative stress and various health problems, including depression, Parkinson's disease, and Alzheimer's disease.
- **JAMMED PATHWAYS.** Several environmental toxins have been shown to interfere with dopamine in the brain, including organophosphate pesticides, lead, and mercury. These toxins can disrupt the production, release, reuptake, and metabolism of dopamine, which can lead to imbalances in the brain and

potentially harmful effects on behavior, mood, and cognition. Chronic exposure to these toxins may also increase the risk of neurodegenerative disorders such as Parkinson's disease.

How to Test Dopamine Levels

We can't directly measure brain dopamine, because it doesn't cross the blood-brain barrier. Indirect methods assess dopamine activity, but these measure metabolites (breakdown products) that may come from the body, not just the brain. That being said, my favorite test is the Organic Acids Test, which tests for dopamine metabolites homovanillic acid and 3,4-dihydroxyphenylacetic acid.

DOPAMINE TL;DR

- Adrenaline, noradrenaline, and dopamine are all excitatory catecholamines, which can be anxiety-producing in excess amounts.
- L-tyrosine amino acid, found in many food sources, is a precursor to dopamine.
- Too-high levels of dopamine can worsen anxiety and panic.
- Serotonin and dopamine share an enzyme, and therefore increasing one may result in a decrease of the other.

Adrenaline and Noradrenaline

"I USED TO LOVE ADRENALINE," ARIA SAYS. "IT'S A 'HIGH' UNLIKE ANYthing else. It's when my body would feel the most alive. Everything would be brighter, sharper, and more intense. But then it turned on me, and those same sensations that used to drive me to push harder and faster morphed into sensations that were alarming, soul-crushing, and devastating.

"Since 'the event,' I now live every day worried about the adrenaline coming back. Exhilaration has transformed into dread, and now 'fear of the fear' has become my greatest motivator."

* * *

HAVE YOU EVER FELT a rush of adrenaline? Maybe it's a burst of pure excitement as your body prepares for something super thrilling, such as skydiving or getting married. Or maybe it's a flush of sheer terror that runs hot and fast through your cells.

Adrenaline, also known as epinephrine, is both a hormone and a neurotransmitter that your body uses to amp you up for whatever it is you are facing. While this can be super fun and exciting in the right context, when you're about to give a presentation, go to sleep, or drive your car, adrenaline pumping through your veins can be extremely problematic.

Keep in mind that having too little adrenaline can also have negative effects. Symptoms such as low blood sugar, fatigue, and weakness may arise when there is not enough adrenaline in your body. The key is to maintain a balance, and in this chapter, you will discover how to recognize signs that your adrenaline is imbalanced and what actions you can take to address it. Let's begin with a brief self-assessment to identify any potential indicators that your adrenaline levels may be off-kilter.

ADRENALINE SELF-ASSESSMENT CHECKLIST: TOO HIGH VS. TOO LOW ADRENALINE

Instructions: Check the box(es) that relate to you, and write your total score in the space provided.

- [ ] Rapid heart rate*
- [ ] Reduced ability to feel pain
- [ ] Heightened taste, smell, hearing, and sensitivity to light
- [ ] Increased strength and/or performance (run harder, faster, longer, lift heavier as examples)
- [ ] High blood pressure

- [ ] Slow heart rate (<60 beats per minute)
- [ ] Low blood pressure (<90/<60)
- [ ] Dizziness
- [ ] Weakness
- [ ] Joint pains

* At rest your heart rate should be somewhere between 60 and 100 beats per minute. (You can test your heart rate by locating your pulse in your wrist. Count the number of beats in 15 seconds. Then multiply this number by 4 to calculate your beats per minute.)

TOTAL: ____/5

SCORING: If you checked more than two boxes, consider getting a workup to screen for root causes of high levels of adrenaline or noradrenaline.

TOTAL: ____/5

SCORING: If you checked more than two boxes, consider getting a workup to screen for adrenal health and include other root causes of low adrenaline or noradrenaline levels.

What did you score in the above checklist? Do you have any signs that your body has too much or too little adrenaline or noradrenaline? While a checklist is not a substitute for proper testing and diagnosis, your symptoms are data points that can help point to the root cause of panic.

Understanding the underlying mechanisms of your body's response is critical in making effective changes. By identifying the root cause, you can take targeted actions to address the issue. If you relate to experiencing high adrenaline like Aria did, this section will be essential in your journey toward healing.

THE EFFECTS OF ADRENALINE AND NORADRENALINE

WHAT HAPPENS DURING FIGHT, FLIGHT, FREEZE

When faced with potential danger, your body goes through a series of physiological changes.

- **EYES.** In order to allow in more light, your pupils dilate. This enables you to better see your surroundings and assess potential threats. However, it can also lead to overstimulation and sensitivity to light. These symptoms are associated with Nervous System Anxiety.
- **HEART.** Your heart rate picks up in speed and intensity to deliver more oxygenated blood to your running-away muscles, such as the quadriceps and hamstrings in your legs.

Your blood pressure may rise, and you may feel your heart pounding, fluttering, or skipping in your chest. These sensations are common in Chest Anxiety.

- **AIRWAYS.** Your airways open wider, and your breathing becomes faster and deeper. However, this can sometimes trigger hyperventilation, a condition where you feel like you can't get enough air (air hunger). This can be a symptom of Chest Anxiety.
- **MUSCLES.** Blood flow is redirected away from small muscle groups and toward larger running-away ones. This allows you to react with greater speed and strength. As a result, some muscles will feel weak while others feel strong, a common experience during Nervous System Anxiety.
- **SKIN.** As blood gets shunted away from your skin and toward your larger muscle groups, you may notice your skin turning pale and maybe even cold. Pain, numbness, and tingling may also occur in the face, fingers, or toes. These symptoms are also associated with Nervous System Anxiety.

The Science of Adrenaline and Noradrenaline

Let's start by clearing up some confusing terminology. With terms like *adrenaline, noradrenaline, epinephrine,* and *norepinephrine,* it's easy to get lost. To simplify, know that *adrenaline* and *epinephrine* refer to the same chemical, while *noradrenaline* and *norepinephrine* also refer to the same chemical. For consistency, I will be using the terms *adrenaline* and *noradrenaline*.

Let's take a closer look at the difference between adrenaline and noradrenaline, as they have distinct effects on the body. In response to perceived danger, the sympathetic nervous system springs into action. It releases a chemical called acetylcholine, which travels down nerve fibers to reach two key targets: the bundles of nerves running alongside your spine, known as the sympathetic ganglion, and your adrenal glands.

When acetylcholine triggers the sympathetic ganglion, it releases noradrenaline to activate the fight-flight-freeze response throughout the body. For example, in "white coat syndrome," a person's blood pressure may increase at a doctor's office as opposed to other settings. Noradrenaline, which is less potent than adrenaline, mainly works to maintain blood pressure.

Your adrenal glands produce adrenaline in response to stressful or dangerous situations. As we have seen, adrenaline is made from the amino acid tyrosine, which is found in many foods, including soy, chicken, turkey, fish, peanuts, almonds, avocados, bananas, milk, cheese, yogurt, cottage cheese, lima beans, pumpkin seeds, and sesame seeds. L-tyrosine is also available as a supplement. While L-tyrosine is often used to boost dopamine, it can also increase adrenaline, potentially triggering anxiety. Be mindful of this if considering L-tyrosine supplementation.

Tyrosine is converted into dopamine, then noradrenaline, and finally adrenaline. This process requires the help of enzymes and vitamins. Any abnormalities in this pathway can affect the production of adrenaline, which can lead to panic attacks. Testing for abnormalities in this pathway may help pinpoint the underlying cause of panic.

But things can get really confusing when toxic heavy metals enter the story. We will explore this topic in more depth in Chapter 7, but for now, it's worth mentioning that your body may sometimes mistake heavy metals for beneficial minerals. This can be problematic, because at high levels, these toxins can displace minerals and disrupt essential cellular processes.

For instance, the mineral copper is necessary for converting dopamine to noradrenaline. However, heavy metals such as mercury (found in skin brightening creams), cadmium (found in talcum powder, lipsticks, and shaving creams), and lead (found in body lotions, blush, eyeshadows, and lipsticks) can substitute for copper, disrupting the metabolic process of cells.

If you suspect that your body may have been exposed to heavy metals or is holding on to them, don't worry. We will explore this topic in more detail in Part III.

ADRENALINE (EPINEPHRINE)

- Is made mostly by adrenal glands
- Is extremely excitatory and strong
- Acts on all bodily tissues to help you fight, flight, or freeze during stress/danger
- Activates alpha and beta receptors throughout your body

NORADRENALINE (NOREPINEPHRINE)

- Is made mostly by the nerves
- Is less excitatory and strong
- Maintains blood pressure, but also helps with fight-flight-freeze response
- Gets converted into adrenaline via PNMT enzyme with the help of SAM-e

Your body has a pretty sophisticated system for keeping you in balance. When it is in tip-top shape, you can enjoy feeling calm, relaxed, and in the zone, while also being able to respond quickly if danger strikes. However, even a well-tuned system can experience surges of adrenaline and noradrenaline during stressful situations, including panic attacks.

Once you have enough adrenaline to meet your needs, it's important to eliminate any excess through the process of detoxification. Two enzymes play a critical role in this process: monoamine oxidase-A (MOA) and catechol-O-methyltransferase (COMT).

These enzymes' functions can vary based on each person's genetics. Mutations in your MOA and/or COMT genes can influence how adrenaline affects you.

HOW TO TEST ADRENALINE LEVELS

- **DUTCH.** DUTCH is a urine test that not only examines sex hormones but also measures levels of epinephrine and dopamine catecholamines. Unfortunately this test is not covered by most insurance, but you might check to see if you can use your health savings account.

- **URINE TESTING.** The urine catecholamine test also measures the levels of these hormones. It requires collecting urine over 24 hours. This test is usually done to rule out a rare noncancerous adrenal gland tumor called pheochromocytoma. Ask your doctor if your insurance will cover this test.
- **BLOOD TESTING.** The catecholamine blood test measures the amount of these hormones in your body at a specific time. It is most helpful in the moment of panic or nervous system arousal to rule out pheochromocytoma. Blood tests are more likely to be covered by insurance.
- **METANEPHRINE TESTING.** Finally, the 24-hour urinary metanephrine test looks for the presence of metanephrines, chemicals made when the body breaks down catecholamines. This test is also commonly used to rule out pheochromocytoma. You'll need a doctor to justify running this through your insurance.

QUICK TIP: Interpreting these tests can be tricky and confusing, and therefore I created a place where you can ask questions and learn more about functional test results, holistic remedies, and really anything holistic-health-related. It's called the Holistic Wellness Collective, and you can join by going to my website, drnicolecain.com.

ADRENALINE AND NORADRENALINE TL;DR

- Elevated adrenaline and noradrenaline can cause panic and anxiety.
- Adrenaline and noradrenaline are responsible for many of the sensations you experience during fight, flight, or freeze (autonomic arousal).

- Copper and other heavy metals can cause paranoia and fear by interfering with pathways involved in adrenaline and noradrenaline metabolism.
- Adrenaline and noradrenaline that are causing anxiety may come from your brain or from your body.

GABA

Gamma-aminobutyric acid (GABA) is nature's tranquilizer. When GABA levels rise, you feel calm, relaxed, and sleepy, but when GABA levels drop, you may be at a greater risk of anxiety, panic, and difficulty sleeping. As the primary inhibitory neurotransmitter of the central nervous system, GABA works by reducing the activity of neurons. When released, it binds to specific receptors on the surface of neurons, known as GABA receptors, and causes the neurons to become less excitable or to stop firing altogether. As a result, the body and brain slow down, and you feel more sedated.

Signs of imbalanced GABA can tell you a lot about the overall health of your nervous system. I've made this quick GABA checklist for you to use as a part of your information gathering process.

GABA CHECKLIST: SIGNS OF IMBALANCED GABA LEVELS

Instructions: Check the box(es) that relate to you, and write your total score in the space provided.

- ❑ Fast resting heart rate (above 80 beats per minute)
- ❑ Musculoskeletal spasms, twitches, jerks, ticks, and/or seizures
- ❑ Difficulty falling asleep and/or staying asleep
- ❑ Slow heart rate (below 60 beats per minute)
- ❑ Weak muscles
- ❑ Fatigue, excessive drowsiness, and sleepiness
- ❑ Poor memory, concentration, and/or alertness

- [ ] Restless or racing thoughts (Thought Anxiety)
- [ ] Restlessness of the body (can't sit still)

TOTAL: ____/5

SCORING: If you checked more than two boxes, consider getting a workup to screen for too-low GABA.

- [ ] Respiratory depression, slow and/or shallow breathing

TOTAL: ____/5

SCORING: If you checked more than two boxes, consider getting a workup to screen for too-high GABA.

What score did you get in the checklist? Remember, checked boxes do not mean you *have* imbalanced GABA, but they can help point you toward deeper digging, which this chapter will walk you through.

So let's get to it.

The Science of GABA

The production of GABA can be broken down into two main steps, as shown in the image below.

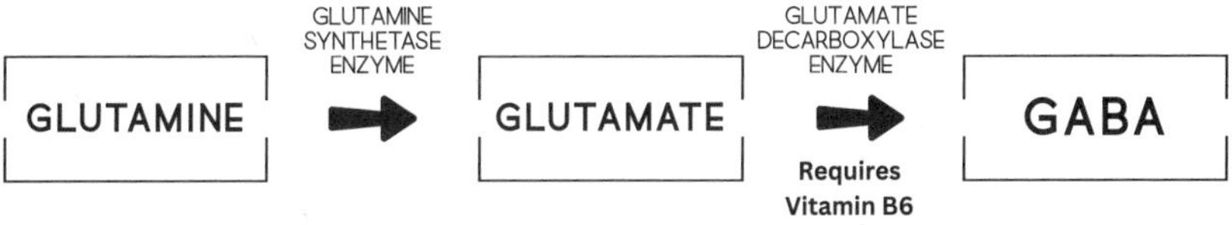

As you can see, your body needs vitamin B6 to make GABA. Since vitamin B6 is essential for GABA production, a deficiency can contribute to anxiety and panic symptoms. Luckily, many foods are rich in B6, including fish, beans, nuts, seeds, whole grains, and turkey. Additionally, you can also take a vitamin B6 supplement. My favorite form of B6 is called pyridoxal 5-phosphate (P5P), which can be found at most health food stores. I typically recommend that my clients start with a low dose of B6, between 10 and 50 mg for one week, to see how they feel before increasing the dosage.

GABA is also produced by certain gut bacteria strains, such as *Lactobacillus brevis, Lactococcus lactis,* and *Bifidobacterium dentium.*

DIET HACK. When you're planning your diet to increase GABA levels, it's important to also keep in mind the histamine content in foods. While GABA can help promote calmness and relaxation, some GABA-rich foods may also contain histamine, which can have stimulating effects and sometimes lead to feelings of anxiety. You'll learn more about histamine later in this chapter.

While the amount of GABA in foods is relatively low, you can subtly increase its levels by adding more GABA-containing foods and drinks to your diet.

HIGH-GABA FOODS AND DRINKS

- **FERMENTED FOODS.** Some fermented foods, such as kimchi, miso, and tempeh, contain GABA due to the fermentation process. Note that fermented foods tend to increase histamine.
- **TEA.** Certain types of tea, such as green tea (low histamine) and black tea (high histamine), contain GABA.
- **NUTS AND SEEDS.** Some nuts and seeds, such as almonds and sunflower seeds, contain GABA and are also low in histamine. Walnuts contain GABA but are high in histamine.
- **FRUITS AND VEGETABLES.** Some fruits and vegetables, such as tomatoes, spinach, and citrus fruits, contain GABA. These foods may also increase histamine.

Now that you have GABA, whether made by your body or taken in through your diet, medications, or supplements, you feel happy and calm and lovely.

Or do you?

Benzos: Miracle Drug or Prescriptive Nightmare?

"I STOOD IN THE DOORWAY OF MY CHILDHOOD HOME WAITING FOR the inevitable," Matthew recalled. "Sometimes it would come in a flash, an iron fist punching me directly in my gut. Other times the anticipation of the fear would be enough to make me sweat."

Matthew mimics the voice of his panic: " 'Should I strike him in five minutes, while he's still close to home, or maybe wait until he's nowhere near a toilet?' It always leads me to the same internal battle: fight the fear and risk of a mortifying episode or go back inside to safety.

"Xanax was a game changer for me. It made it possible for me to leave my house again. You'll tell me that it's just a Band-Aid, but I'm not sure it's a Band-Aid that I can live without."

IF YOU HAVE BEEN given a benzodiazepine for panic, anxiety, and/or issues sleeping, this next part is for you. If you aren't taking a benzo, feel free to skip ahead to Next Steps.

The most commonly used treatment for the relief of panic is a type of medication known as a *benzodiazepine,* including Xanax, which Matthew turned to in order to leave his house.

ARE YOU TAKING A BENZODIAZEPINE? Here are the most commonly prescribed benzodiazepines for panic and insomnia:

- Alprazolam (Xanax)
- Lorazepam (Ativan)
- Oxazepam (Serax)
- Chlordiazepoxide (Librium)
- Diazepam (Valium/Diazemuls/RecTubes)
- Clonazepam (Rivotril/Klonopin)
- Loprazolam (Triazulenone/Dormonoct)
- Temazepam (Restoril)

- Lormetazepam (Noctamid/Dormagen)
- Clorazepate (Tranxene T-Tab)
- Clobazam (Onfi)

Benzodiazepines, also known as benzos, are anti-anxiety drugs that work by binding to GABA-A receptors, which are the most common type of GABA receptor in the brain.

Stimulation of both GABA-A and GABA-B receptors can be calming, but the unique nature of GABA's calming effects will vary depending on which type of receptor it binds to.

This is especially important if you have taken, or are taking, benzodiazepine medications.

Benzodiazepines, as I mentioned, reduce anxiety by binding to GABA-A receptors. However, over time GABA-A receptors can become less sensitive to GABA, a process called receptor desensitization. This can lead to a decreased effectiveness of benzodiazepines, and more of the medication will be needed to bind to the receptors to achieve the calming effect on the brain.

We can combat some of the negative effects of benzos on the GABA receptors with trophorestorative (brain and nervous system healing) herbs and amino acids, which we'll explore in detail in Chapter 11.

Stimulating GABA-B receptors offers an additional promising alternative to benzodiazepines for anxiety relief because it targets different receptors. This creates a "GABA bridge" that can help ease anxiety as the dosage of benzodiazepines is reduced.

HERE IS A LIST of my favorite "GABA bridge" supplements for GABA-A and GABA-B receptors:

GABA-A RECEPTORS

Benzodiazepines are the most common type of medication that targets GABA receptors.

NATURAL REMEDIES THAT STIMULATE GABA-A RECEPTORS:

- Ashwagandha root (*Withania somnifera*)
- California poppy flower (*Eschscholtzia californica*)
- Ginkgo leaf (*Ginkgo biloba*)
- Jujube (*Ziziphus jujuba*)
- Kava kava (*Piper methysticum*)
- Lemon balm leaf (*Melissa officinalis*)
- Magnolia berry (*Schisandra chinensis*)
- Passionflower (*Passiflora incarnata*)
- St. John's wort flower (*Hypericum perforatum*)
- L-theanine (from Happy Sleepy Powder)
- Valerian root (*Valeriana officinalis*)

EFFECTS OF STIMULATING THESE RECEPTORS:

Decrease in anxiety, muscle tension, and seizures, as well as increased sedation and sleepiness.

GABA-B RECEPTORS

MEDICATIONS THAT TARGET THESE RECEPTORS:

- Baclofen (used to treat muscle spasms)
- Pregabalin (Lyrica) (used to treat nerve pain and anxiety)
- Phenibut (not recommended because of its high risk of dependence)

NATURAL REMEDIES THAT STIMULATE GABA-B RECEPTORS:

- Passionflower (*Passiflora incarnata*)
- Psychobiotic *Lactobacillus rhamnosus* (strain JB-1)

EFFECTS OF STIMULATING THESE RECEPTORS:

Relaxed muscles, reduced pain, feeling of calm

When GABA receptors are stimulated, GABA's effects are enhanced, nervous system activity decreases, and panic attacks subside. Benzodiazepines are very good at stimulating these receptors.

This type of powerful relief is one reason why, in the United States alone, benzodiazepine prescriptions soared to over 92 million in 2019, and the numbers keep climbing. Although benzodiazepines can have almost miraculous effects in stopping panic, they have significant drawbacks.

- **DEPENDENCE.** Dependence on benzodiazepines can develop quickly, even when they are taken as directed. Tolerance can develop within just three weeks of regular use. The American Psychiatric Association recommends not taking these drugs for more than two to four weeks.
- **SIDE EFFECTS.** Benzodiazepines can cause a range of side effects, such as depression, memory problems, confusion, and impaired coordination.
- **WITHDRAWAL.** Some experts estimate that approximately 33 percent of people taking a benzodiazepine have trouble coming off them. I would argue, based on the thousands of people I have consulted for, that this number is significantly underestimated. It is important to avoid suddenly stopping the use of benzodiazepines to prevent withdrawal symptoms, which can range from mildly disturbing to debilitating and last from days to years.

Despite these facts, benzodiazepines are routinely prescribed and taken for much longer periods, even years, leaving many people feeling like Matthew, between a rock and a hard place: on one side, suffering from anxiety, pain, insomnia, or seizures, and on the other, a prescriptive nightmare.

Winning the Benzo Battle

There is good news. You can become Panic Proof *without* benzos. I've helped thousands get there, including myself and Matthew. And you're next.

There is a wealth of information on benzodiazepines and benzo tapering that goes beyond the scope of this book. While this book will provide you with strategies to become Panic Proof if you're taking benzodiazepines, it does not contain enough information to really prepare you with all the information you need to taper off. But I've got your back! I have created a comprehensive self-paced course that covers various aspects of benzodiazepines, including tapering strategies, which you can find at my website drnicolecain.com.

Next Steps

Research in trauma-informed neuroscience teaches us exactly how to heal from panic and anxiety, and tools from holistic medicine promote long-lasting change. I know you've been dealing with anxiety for far too long. (Let's be real—even one day with panic is too long.) That's what Matthew thought, too. He had been dealing with anxiety since he was a child and thought it was too late for him. But I promise, if you diligently follow the techniques taught in this book and stay the course, you will see results.

So let's start with the next steps related to GABA.

HOW TO TEST GABA

Since GABA cannot cross the blood-brain barrier, direct blood tests don't accurately reflect GABA levels in the central nervous system (including the brain). Therefore, the most effective way to evaluate GABA levels is to indirectly assess factors involved in its production and processing.

- **TEST VITAMIN B6 LEVELS.** Remember, vitamin B6 is necessary for your body to make GABA. Without it, you would not have enough GABA, which increases your risk for panic. To get the most accurate information, you will need to do *both* a direct test and a functional test. The direct test will look at the actual B6 levels in your blood, and the functional test will measure the enzymes that need B6. Here are the tests:
    - Direct test: Plasma pyridoxal 5-phosphate (PLP)
    - Functional tests: Inflammation, comprehensive metabolic panel (CMP), which includes additional useful tests

including alkaline phosphatase, aspartate aminotransferase, serum albumin, kidney function testing, and phosphate levels

- **HISTAMINE TESTING.** If you suspect you have histamine imbalances in addition to low GABA, you can get a two-for-one by doing a *whole blood histamine test*. This test measures the response of histamine levels in the blood after a dose of histamine, with and without vitamin B6. A low response to vitamin B6 suggests a deficiency.
- **BRAIN IMAGING.** Magnetic resonance spectroscopy is a noninvasive imaging technique used to measure GABA levels in the brain. It can provide information on GABA-ergic neurotransmission, which can be helpful in understanding disorders related to GABA, such as anxiety disorders and epilepsy.
- **GABA METABOLITES.** 4-hydroxybutyric acid (GHB) and succinic semialdehyde metabolites can be tested in the urine. Just keep in mind that this test does not differentiate GABA from the periphery and GABA from your brain.

GABA TL;DR

- GABA is a calming neurochemical best known as "nature's tranquilizer."
- Vitamin B6 is needed to convert excitatory neurotransmitter glutamate into calming GABA.
- Benzodiazepine medications work by increasing GABA levels, but they are very habit-forming.
- There are no direct tests for GABA because it does not cross the blood-brain barrier.

Glutamate

What Is Glutamate?

Think of glutamate as your overexcited best friend: it wakes you up, is energizing, and can be quite stimulating. Glutamate is an excitatory neurotransmitter. This means that when glutamate levels rise, messages move more quickly from nerve cell to nerve cell. When glutamate gets released, things get done. For example, glutamate is needed for learning, memory, and wakefulness, and it is an important part of your ability to detect and feel pain. Low levels of glutamate are associated with depression, insomnia, poor concentration, and physical and mental fatigue.

However, as with most things in life, balance is key. An excess even of a good thing can lead to problems, and glutamate is no exception. Imagine that your overexcited best friend consumed too many energy drinks—she would become a little too much to handle. Similarly, an overabundance of glutamate can lead to various issues, such as anxiety, restlessness, panic, inattention, hyperactivity, amplification of pain (hyperalgesia), an increased risk of developing post-traumatic stress disorder after an aversive event, and many other problems.

If your panic attacks are linked to high levels of glutamate, it's essential to recognize this so that you can take steps to bring your glutamate levels back to normal.

GLUTAMATE CHECKLIST: SIGNS OF ELEVATED GLUTAMATE LEVELS

Instructions: Check the box(es) that relate to you, and write your total score in the space provided.

- ❑ Increased sensitivity to pain (e.g., fibromyalgia)
- ❑ Mental and emotional overstimulation: anxiety, panic, racing and/or intrusive thoughts
- ❑ Physical restlessness: excessive desire to move the body, ticks, twitches, spasms
- ❑ Difficulties with attention, attention deficit disorder (especially with hyperactivity)
- ❑ Obsessive-compulsive thinking patterns (see Chapter 3 for more on Thought Anxiety)

TOTAL: _____/5

SCORING: If you checked the first box plus at least one additional box, consider talking with your doctor about getting a workup to screen for high glutamate levels. Remember, checked boxes do not mean you *have* high glutamate, but they can help point you toward the next steps, which this chapter will walk you through.

Does this resonate? Then, let's explore glutamate together in the next section.

Glutamate 101

Glutamate comes from an amino acid called glutamine. Glutamine is created inside your body and is released by your muscles, lungs, and brain. You can also get it through your diet or from supplements. In addition to being a precursor to glutamate, glutamine has many important functions in your body; it supports your immune system, nourishes the gut, helps you build muscle, and contributes to a balanced mood.

This section may feel extra "science-y," but I promise that it offers you a better understanding of the role glutamine plays in your panic and anxiety, and what you can do about it.

Let's go back to the glutamine-glutamate connection.

Your body needs glutamine in order to make glutamate, and this requires the help of an enzyme called glutamine synthetase.

Suppose your enzyme is in tip-top shape, and now we have glutamate. What's next?

Your body uses that glutamate for all sorts of things: sending messages between the neurons in your brain, providing you with energy, making memories, making you feel inspired and get things done. Glutamate also helps your cells make proteins that keep you healthy and energized, it helps to regulate your sleep-wake cycle (circadian rhythm), and so much more.

Glutamate is also a precursor to GABA, which means glutamate gets made *into* GABA. Ah, GABA, that wonderfully calming neurotransmitter that helps us when panic or insomnia strikes! Without glutamate, you cannot make GABA.

A common treatment that I see for anxiety and panic is a low-glutamate diet. The rationale is that "less glutamate equals less excitation, which equals less anxiety." However, without glutamate you're not going to have GABA, which is your favorite relaxing neurotransmitter. So while a low-glutamate diet may be helpful for many people and absolutely necessary for others, you don't want to stop there.

Taking a small peek into the biochemistry of glutamate and GABA, we can see an important step that all too often gets overlooked. In the image below, you will see that in order for glutamate to convert into GABA you need two key things: a functioning glutamate decarboxylase enzyme and vitamin B6.

A NOTE ABOUT THE IMPORTANCE OF B VITAMINS: They are required to break down excitatory glutamate and also to get the necessary GABA. Without them, you have neither of the key elements you need. This can result in a predisposition to anxiety and/or panic attacks.

An additional critical element of the glutamate-GABA relationship is the receptors. Here's a helpful metaphor for understanding cellular receptors.

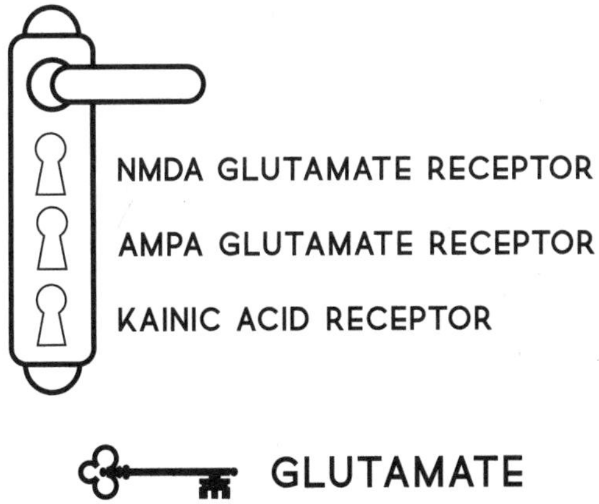

Each cell has receptors, which are like keyholes found in doors. Each keyhole corresponds to a different type of reaction. The varying molecules, such as glutamate, are the keys that are able to unlock the doors in order to carry out reactions.

Imagine that each of your cells has a door. On the door is a keyhole, which represents the cell receptor. The receptor needs to be unlocked with a key before the door can open. If a chemical, or key, approaches the cell and fits in the receptor/lock, the door will open, and a reaction can occur. If the chemical/key does not fit in the receptor/lock, the door will not open.

In this example, you want glutamate to unlock the receptor, so the door to your cell will open and enable glutamate to pass through and get transformed into GABA. Your cells have different types of keyholes that the key, glutamate, can unlock. Different reactions occur, depending on the chemical present and the receptor being stimulated.

GLUTAMATE RECEPTORS

Your body has three primary types of receptors for glutamate:

- NMDA receptors
- AMPA receptors
- Kainic acid receptors

These receptors are named after the chemicals that activate them. This is important because knowing about the actions of these different types of receptors gives us information about potential drug or supplemental therapies.

Let's dip our toe into the types of receptors and why they matter for those struggling with panic. (Note: This is not a 100 percent comprehensive analysis of glutamate but is intended to be an introduction.)

NMDA RECEPTORS

You have many NMDA receptors throughout your nervous system. When glutamate stimulates NMDA receptors, it opens the door to excitation and activation of specific areas of your brain.

The amygdala is a part of the brain that processes emotions. When there is too much glutamate in the amygdala, you may experience strong emotions, including panic and stress.

The cerebral cortex, including the prefrontal cortex (PFC), is the "brakes" of the brain. When glutamate activates receptors in the PFC, you have more control over strong emotions.

The hippocampus is part of the brain that processes memory. If you don't have enough glutamate in the hippocampus, you may have difficulty learning, remembering, or concentrating.

But what happens if glutamate stimulates too much amygdala and not enough PFC? The result is panic *plus* a feeling of being out of control.

Feeling a loss of control during panic attacks is a common experience, which is likely why you're reading this book. There are reasons why maintaining control can be difficult in these moments. While glutamate activity might play a role, it's even more about how this activity changes within the brain.

Research has found that people with post-traumatic stress disorder may have lower levels of glutamate activity in the prefrontal cortex. During emotionally charged moments, they may feel more fearful and have less logical thinking or control.

This is why it is so important to do trauma-healing work in addition to working with your neurochemicals (which you'll learn more about in Chapter 6). By addressing the underlying causes of your symptoms, your neurochemicals may naturally start to rebalance themselves.

In the meantime, let's talk about the category of anti-anxiety treatments called NMDA receptor antagonists.

NMDA receptor antagonists are a type of drug that blocks NMDA receptors. They are an emerging alternative to traditional antidepressants and benzodiazepines for treating panic and anxiety. Ketamine is one of the best-known NMDA receptor antagonists. It is a dissociative anesthetic that can make a person feel detached from their pain and surroundings. Ketamine was originally developed as an anesthetic for emergency and surgical procedures. However, it has since been found to have potential therapeutic value for conditions such as depression, anxiety, and suicidality.

HOW KETAMINE MAY BENEFIT MENTAL HEALTH:

- Ketamine may enhance brain plasticity and promote healing by increasing the brain-derived neurotrophic factor.
- It may reduce anxiety and depression by inhibiting or blocking NMDA receptors throughout the brain.

- Preliminary research suggests that ketamine can decrease reactivation of traumatic memories, allowing people to generate new feelings and associations.

Ketamine is not without risks, as it can be habit-forming and can cause side effects like hallucinations, anxiety, confusion, forgetfulness, increased blood pressure, and muscle stiffness.

AMPA RECEPTORS

Like NMDA receptors, AMPA receptors are stimulated by glutamate and pass a stimulating and excitatory signal along throughout the nervous system. Researchers have studied blocking AMPA receptors as a potential way to calm the nervous system. However, most drugs that target AMPA receptors have not been successful.

One promising AMPA blocker is cannabidiol (CBD). Preliminary research suggests that CBD may slow the activity of AMPA receptors, which could lead to reduced emotional and physical stress and anxiety.

KAINIC ACID RECEPTORS (KARs)

Kainic acid receptors (KARs) are present throughout the brain. When stimulated, they cause excitation in the nervous system, which can lead to anxiety and panic. Blocking KARs can help calm anxiety and panic.

Theanine is an amino acid that can block both KARs and AMPA receptors. It is a natural way to calm anxiety and panic. Topiramate (Topamax) is an anticonvulsant and nerve pain medication that is approved for blocking both KARs and AMPA receptors. It can help with depression and anxiety (Depressive Anxiety) by preventing excessive stimulation by glutamate. You can learn more about Depressive Anxiety in Chapter 3.

High Glutamate?

With respect to the limitations in testing, I typically hold off on testing glutamate levels unless we're hitting a lot of dead ends with treatment.

However, if you do want to look into testing, here are a few ideas to get you started.

- **URINE AMINO ANALYSIS.** This test provides an overall average of glutamate and GABA levels in your body, not specifically those from the brain.
- **BLOOD TEST.** Certain blood labs can measure blood plasma glutamate levels. But this test is also not very dependable since it only provides a snapshot of your glutamate levels at that moment instead of an overall picture.
- **MAGNETIC RESONANCE IMAGING.** Though MRIs offer valuable brain function insights, they don't definitively measure glutamate. Directly measuring live brain glutamate remains a challenge. Additionally, MRIs are expensive and have variable insurance coverage.

Regardless of whether you opt for testing or not, always explore possible root causes of neurotransmitter imbalances. We'll cover root causes in detail in Chapter 7.

GLUTAMATE TL;DR

- High levels of glutamate can cause anxiety, panic, insomnia, and high sensitivity to pain.
- You need glutamate for learning, memory, wakefulness, and motivation.
- If you do not have enough vitamin B6, you will be unable to turn glutamate into GABA.
- Lower levels of glutamate in your brain's prefrontal cortex increases your risk of developing PTSD.

Histamine

"Well damn . . . after a bad night of anxiety and watching the histamine lesson I decided to go to the store and get an anti-

histamine to try. I figured I might as well give it a shot. And I FEEL SO MUCH BETTER. I'm stunned because I really didn't think I had a histamine problem. Out of all the googling and researching I've done over the years, I would be like: "Nahhh that's not my problem. Yeah my eyes get a little watery and itchy when the pollen comes out, maybe I will sneeze for a few days. But really that's the only issue I've ever had." Who knew?"

—a Holistic Wellness Collective member, age 43

"I didn't consider that I might have a histamine issue until I listened to the histamine lesson at the Holistic Wellness Collective. I'm currently about halfway through a thirty-day histamine detox, and I'm noticing a substantial difference. It's funny 'cause I never made this connection in the past, but the only thing that helped me when my symptoms got bad was to take Benadryl, and I was magically better. Since detoxing histamine, my anxiety is better, sleep is better, energy is better. I am so amazed."

—a Holistic Wellness Collective member, age 52

Anxiety, Allergies, and Headaches

What do anxiety, allergies, and headaches have in common? They can all be triggered by the chemical *histamine*. Histamine is special because it can function as a neurotransmitter, as an endocrine cell, and as a part of the immune system. In all of these different ways, histamine communicates information between your body and your brain. Depending on where histamine is coming from and what it is doing in your body, imbalances in histamine could be a form of Nervous System Anxiety, Hormone Anxiety, or Immune System Anxiety.

You might be most familiar with the role histamine plays in allergy symptoms: itchy eyes, runny nose, or hives—you reach for a Benadryl (an antihistamine) and spend the rest of the day trying to avoid a nap. Before you grab that antihistamine or histamine blocker for your next bout of allergies, let's take a closer look at some links between panic attacks and histamine. We will also cover a variety of triggers, symptoms, and potential effects related to high histamines, as well as solutions to normalize histamine levels.

When a patient comes into my office struggling with symptoms of anxiety, allergies, and/or headaches, one of the first things I do is screen them for high levels of histamine.

HISTAMINE CHECKLIST:
SIGNS OF ELEVATED HISTAMINE LEVELS

Instructions: Check the box(es) that relate to you, and write your total score in the space provided.

- ❑ Increased mental energy: anxiety, panic, agitation, insomnia, and/or mania
- ❑ Menstrual cycle: PMS, irregular timing, cramps, heavy bleeding, spotting
- ❑ Allergies: congestion, runny, itchy, watery eyes and/or nose, and/or itchy skin, hives, or rash
- ❑ Headaches and/or migraines
- ❑ Digestive disturbances: stomach upset, nausea, vomiting, diarrhea, irritable bowel syndrome

TOTAL: _____/5

SCORING: If you checked more than two boxes, consider talking with your doctor about getting a workup to screen for high histamine levels.

Do you have these symptoms? If so, read on!

Where Does Histamine Come From?

Hista*mine* is a chemical that your body can produce, or make from the amino acid histi*dine*. Histidine is not naturally produced in the body, so it must be obtained from the diet. Some key sources include alcohol, wheat, canned foods, vinegar-containing foods, smoked foods, aged cheeses, most citrus fruits, avocados, and dried fruits. Certain foods and beverages can also trigger your body to release histamine, such as artificial preservatives and dyes, bananas, cow's milk, pineapple, shellfish, tomatoes, and wheat germ. Check out Chapter 11 for a more comprehensive list of high-histamine foods.

The pathway to convert histidine into histamine requires the enzyme histidine decarboxylase and vitamin B6, as you can see in the image below. Histamine production occurs all over the body, including gut microbiota, stomach cells, immune system cells such as mast cells and basophils, and certain neurons in your brain. Once produced or ingested, histamine gets released throughout your brain and body.

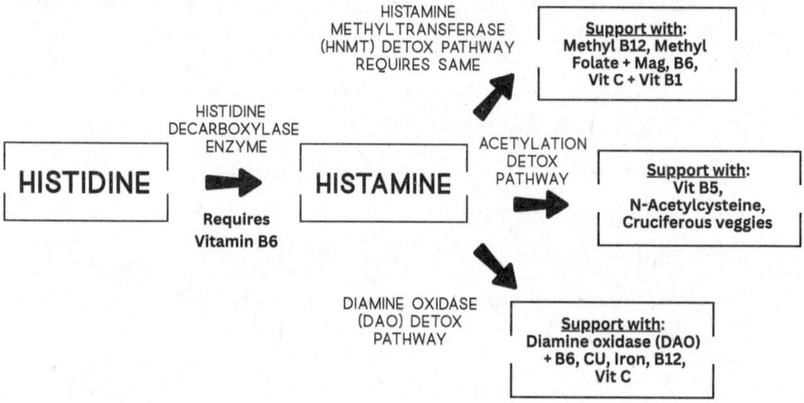

Histamine: The Hidden Cause of Your Anxiety?

But let's say you don't have allergy symptoms. You're anxious, but you don't have a stuffy nose or runny eyes, and you haven't eaten anything different or changed cleaning detergents or personal hygiene products. Nevertheless, you *feel* anxious.

It's still possible that your anxiety is caused by histamine.

Histamine is involved in a variety of functions, including:

- Controlling your mood
- Regulating your immune system
- Helping you make stomach acid, so you can digest your food
- Regulating your sleep-wake cycle
- Balancing your hormones and stimulating estrogen
- Helping you fight stress

Too much histamine, or histamine intolerance, is associated with a variety of symptoms, including:

- Allergies (sneezing, runny nose and eyes, itching, hives)
- Anxiety
- Insomnia
- Headaches
- Stomach upset (nausea, reflux, vomiting, appetite changes, stomach ulcers)
- Hormone imbalances (such as polycystic ovary syndrome, estrogen dominance, premenstrual syndrome)

Receptors for histamine are found throughout the body, in the immune system, the gut, and the brain. The effects of histamine are greatly influenced by the specific histamine receptors that are being stimulated.

Let's examine the four primary types of histamine receptors.

- **H1 RECEPTORS.** H1 receptors are involved in allergies, inflammation (seen in Immune System Anxiety), and nervous system activation (seen in Nervous System Anxiety). When H1 receptors get stimulated, you may experience allergic reactions such as asthma, atopic dermatitis, and nasal congestion. An extreme example of allergic inflammation is seen in the condition called Mast Cell Activation Syndrome. In MCAS, mast cells get triggered and can release extremely high amounts of histamine, which can masquerade as anxiety or panic disorder.

    MCAS VS. HISTAMINE INTOLERANCE. MCAS and histamine intolerance are often confused with each other. Histamine intolerance involves excessive release of histamine from mast cells. In MCAS, mast cells secrete multiple mediators in addition to histamine.

    TREATMENT. Antihistamines and other anti-allergy drugs have been developed to try to combat histamine intolerance symptoms. The first-generation medications, such as diphenhydramine (Benadryl) tend to be more sedating and can help with the restlessness, anxiety, panic, and insomnia that accompany allergic inflammation. The newer-generation H1-receptor-blocking antihistamines, such as cetirizine (Zyrtec), can combat the allergic symptoms without making you feel drowsy. To learn more about histamine and inflammation, check out the Histamine Detox Protocol in Chapter 11.

- **H2 RECEPTORS.** These histamine receptors are involved in reflux, ulcers, and anxiety. They are primarily found in the gut and brain. By way of H2 receptors in the brain, histamine can be very excitatory.

  GUT ANXIETY. If you suffer from Gut Anxiety and are taking H2-receptor-blocking medications, such as the antacid medications ranitidine (Zantac 75) or cimetidine (Tagamet HB), you may find that they help combat digestive upset but do not help your mood. That is because these medications can easily get to the gut, but they do not readily cross the blood-brain barrier to calm the brain. I've put together some excellent solutions for you that work better because they will get to the root cause of high histamine instead of just blocking it.

- **H3 RECEPTORS.** H3 receptors are the regulators of neurotransmission, or the sending of signals from one neuron to another. They are the "brakes" of the brain. They regulate the release of other neurotransmitters such as acetylcholine, glutamate, GABA, serotonin, and dopamine. It's easy to blame histamine for the effects of H1 and H2 stimulation that we just learned about, but histamine is nuanced. We don't want to throw out histamine altogether. It's all about getting the right amount of histamine to the right receptors at the right time.

- **H4 RECEPTORS.** Found in the immune cells of your brain, on your mast cells, in your bone marrow, spleen, thymus, lung, and gut, H4 receptors affect the modulation of the immune system. If histamine is elevated and stimulates the H4 receptors in your brain, you may experience the immune activation and inflammation associated with panic and anxiety.

High histamine? Here's what you need to do first.

Get your histamine tested. If you have high levels and your symptoms match up, you might consider the Histamine Detox Protocol in Chapter 11.

HOW TO TEST HISTAMINE LEVELS

- **N-METHYLHISTAMINE, 24-HOUR, URINE:** This is commonly run to test for MCAS.
- **HISTAMINE SKIN-PRICK TEST:** This test is typically run by your allergist. It involves pricking the skin with a small amount of an allergen to see if it causes a reaction.
- **HISTAMINE WHOLE-BLOOD TEST:** This test measures levels of histamine in the blood. It is not as reliable as other tests for diagnosing MCAS.
- **STOOL TEST:** Histamine is produced in the gut by the microbiota, and testing the stool can provide information about whether your gut is the source of your elevated histamine levels.
- **ELIMINATION AND REINTRODUCTION DIET:** This diet involves eliminating high-histamine foods for three to six weeks, then gradually reintroducing them to see if they cause any symptoms.

HISTAMINE TL;DR

- Histamine can be as stimulating to your nervous system as adrenaline.
- Sometimes anxiety does not come from the brain, it comes from the body in the form of histamine.

- High histamine is associated with allergy symptoms, headaches, digestive upset, anxiety, and panic.
- Detoxing histamine can help prevent and treat panic.

NEXT STEPS

You just learned so much about neurotransmitters that if any of these chemicals showed up at your next trivia night, you would be the MVP. You are now better equipped to understand some of the reasons behind the most common diagnoses and treatments for panic and anxiety.

Remember David from the beginning of this chapter? He was told that he needed medication to correct a "chemical imbalance," but as you'll learn, there was a whole lot more to his story.

In the next chapter we are going to learn all about hormones: sex, adrenal, and thyroid hormones. Are you ready?

NEUROTRANSMITTERS TL;DR

- Your neurotransmitters are in a continuous state of adaptation, changing from moment to moment.
- The nature of these adaptations gives you data on what is going on beneath the surface.
- Finding the root cause of imbalances and symptoms will direct you toward the right treatments.
- Your body is designed to self-heal, and your job is to support that process.

7

HORMONES AND PANIC

"I FINALLY DECIDED TO GET CHECKED OUT," CHARLOTTE SAID TO ME over the phone a week after our kava kava tea hang sesh. "My doctor did the basics—blood pressure, pulse—and asked me a few questions. My blood pressure and pulse rate were both high, but I've always had white coat syndrome, so we didn't pay too much attention to that." Charlotte paused, and I could imagine her shrugging.

"Anyway, I told her that I have been very jittery and anxious, losing weight, having trouble sleeping, and worrying about my kids. She agreed, saying that 'mom stress' was the real deal, and she said I was lucky that my baby weight came off so fast. She said she was still trying to get hers off two years later.

"She gave me a script for some medication [a benzodiazepine] . . . which you know I'm not going to take."

I asked if they ran any tests.

"My insurance only covers annuals." Charlotte was referring to the basic blood work she had done every year at her wellness exam. "My numbers were fine at my visit in the fall, so the doc said I didn't need to get them repeated.

"Something about that isn't sitting right with me, though," she added after a beat. "The last time I had my labs done, I felt fine. But now I don't.

So wouldn't it make sense for my doctor to want to see if anything changed?"

I agreed with Charlotte. It's important to remember that our bodies are always changing and adapting, and since Charlotte had developed symptoms since her last checkup, running current labs to determine if anything had changed made sense.

Charlotte decided to get a second opinion, and the new clinician agreed to run some basic labs. The results revealed that Charlotte's symptoms were due not just to "mom stress" but also to a problem with her endocrine system. "I didn't want to worry too much," she said. "But I'm relieved that I got my blood work done. I finally have some answers and a plan."

Stay tuned. Later in this chapter, you'll learn about the specifics of Charlotte's condition.

WELCOME TO THE WONDERFUL WORLD OF ENDOCRINOLOGY!

Endocrinology is the branch of medicine that explores the many roles hormones and the endocrine system play in our health. In this chapter, we will focus on the intriguing connection between endocrinology and anxiety, known as Hormone Anxiety (which you read about in Chapter 3).

First, the basics. The endocrine system is a group of glands and organs whose job is to produce, and release into the bloodstream, hormones that control important functions in your body.

Hormones act as messengers that transmit information throughout the body. You can think of them as the cell phones of the endocrine system. First, the gland sends a message (e.g., a hormone) directed to specific receptor(s) in the body. The targeted cells and organs receive the hormonal text message, translate it, and use this information to carry out specific functions.

In this chapter, we will delve into some of the hormones known for their potential to induce panic, including thyroid, cortisol, estrogen, testosterone, and progesterone. Then we'll explore how to optimize hormonal production, balance, and function to avoid that risk.

MEET YOUR HORMONES

Let's begin with one of my favorite hormones. It comes from a butterfly-shaped gland situated at the base of the neck that is about two inches in length.

Thyroid

The thyroid gland lies in the lower part of the front of your neck—it's just above your collarbone and below your voice box. (If you hum, you'll feel it.) It makes thyroid hormones that control many important processes in almost every cell of your body.

The production of thyroid hormone in your body is controlled by a feedback loop. When the level of thyroid hormone in your blood is low, the hypothalamus produces thyrotropin-releasing hormone (TRH). TRH travels to the pituitary gland in your brain, which releases thyroid-stimulating hormone (TSH). TSH travels to your thyroid gland, which starts producing the thyroid hormones thyroxine (T4) and triiodothyronine (T3). T4 is not very active biologically, so your liver, kidneys, and brain cells have to convert it to T3 in order for you to get the most benefit. This requires nutrients such as iodine, selenium, and zinc.

As the level of thyroid hormone in your blood increases, it sends a signal back to the hypothalamus and pituitary gland to stop producing TRH and TSH. This feedback loop helps to keep the level within a narrow range—that is, unless the loop has been impacted by various factors such as environmental burdens, viral and autoimmune disease, or an imbalance in the hypothalamic-pituitary-thyroid axis. When the thyroid hormone is out of its optimal range, you either have:

- *Hyper*thyroidism, a condition that occurs when too much thyroid hormone is made

- *Hypo*thyroidism, when your thyroid does not make enough thyroid hormone

While panic is most commonly associated with *hyper*thyroidism, *hypo*thyroidism can lead to anxiety as well. We'll get into that later.

Let's start with a thyroid self-assessment.

THYROID SELF-ASSESSMENT CHECKLIST: TOO HIGH VS. TOO LOW THYROID

Instructions: Check the box(es) that relate to you, and write your total score in the space provided.

COMMON SYMPTOMS OF HYPERTHYROIDISM

- ☐ Unintended weight loss despite healthy diet
- ☐ Heat intolerance and sweating
- ☐ High blood pressure and rapid heartbeat
- ☐ Tremors and shaking in hands and fingers
- ☐ More frequent bowel movements, diarrhea

TOTAL: ____/5

SCORING: If you checked more than two boxes, consider getting a full thyroid workup for an overactive thyroid (*hyper*thyroidism) and autoimmune thyroid.

COMMON SYMPTOMS OF HYPOTHYROIDISM

- ☐ Unintended weight gain despite healthy diet and exercise
- ☐ Cold intolerance even in a warm climate
- ☐ Dry and brittle skin, hair, and nails
- ☐ Fatigue, sluggishness, weakness even with rest
- ☐ Constipation

TOTAL: ____/5

SCORING: If you checked more than two boxes, consider getting a full thyroid workup for an underactive thyroid (*hypo*thyroidism) and autoimmune thyroid.

Checked boxes do not indicate a diagnosis. They can help guide your investigation into potential thyroid imbalances, which may be an underlying factor for your panic. Details regarding thyroid testing are discussed later in this chapter.

The best treatments for resolving endocrine-related anxiety depends on the specific causative imbalance(s). It's important to investigate the many conditions that can interfere with the thyroid hormone, such as:

- **INFLAMMATION.** An exaggerated and/or chronic inflammatory response can wreak havoc on your thyroid through oxidative stress, resulting in brain-thyroid disruption and, potentially, autoimmune disease.
- **HORMONE IMBALANCES.** As a key player in your endocrine system, sex and stress hormones can influence your thyroid function. For example, estrogen and cortisol can decrease active thyroid hormone levels, while progesterone and testosterone may increase them.
- **NEUROTRANSMITTER CHANGES.** Your neurotransmitters also influence thyroid levels. Studies suggest that low levels of serotonin and dopamine may lead to reduced thyroid activity, while high levels may increase it.
- **CHANGES IN GUT BACTERIA.** Research on the thyroid-gut axis reveals that gut bacteria play a big role in regulating thyroid function. Dysbiosis, which we explored at length in Chapter 5, is associated with poorer absorption of necessary micronutrients, exaggerated inflammatory response, and imbalanced thyroid function, while robust microbial diversity is associated with better thyroid health.
- **ENVIRONMENTAL TOXINS.** Exposure to toxic metals such as mercury, lead, and cadmium can interfere with thyroid hormone production and metabolism.

The thyroid is just one part of an intricate network in which each component can affect the others. Think of it like an orchestra: You have the violinist, bassist, harpist, and other instrumentalists. They all play their own part, and if any member is out of tune, it can throw off the entire performance. Cue Hormone Anxiety.

Three Causes of Thyroid-Related Hormone Anxiety

THYROID OVERDRIVE

Hyperthyroidism can lead to a bunch of physical symptoms, for example, a fast and/or irregular resting heartbeat, digestive upset, weight loss, high blood pressure, and emotional symptoms such as anxiety, sweating, and feeling easily annoyed or overwhelmed—all contributors to panic.

There are several causes of hyperthyroidism, such as glands in the brain sending too many signals asking the thyroid to produce more and more thyroid hormone, or the thyroid gland itself becoming overactive due to an exaggerated immune response. Graves' disease, an autoimmune disorder, is the leading cause of hyperthyroidism. In contrast, Hashimoto's thyroiditis, another autoimmune condition, primarily causes hypothyroidism, where the thyroid doesn't produce enough hormone. However, Hashimoto's can also lead to occasional spikes in hormone levels.

THYROID SLOWDOWN

Hypothyroidism causes a range of unpleasant symptoms such as depression, anxiety, constipation, weight gain, and dry skin, hair, and nails. There are various reasons why thyroid hormone output may slow down, such as a sluggish gland, external interfering variables like inadequate iodine in the diet, or reduced stimulation from the brain and/or pituitary gland resulting from endocrine imbalance.

LOW T3 SYNDROME

Low T3 syndrome—also known as nonthyroidal illness syndrome, or euthyroid sick syndrome—is a condition where the thyroid gland seems to be working properly based on basic lab testing, but you feel symptoms of low thyroid hormone levels (and there's a reason why!).

Just imagine the frustration. You check all the boxes for hypothyroidism, but you go to the doctor, they run some labs, and everything is normal. *It can't be your thyroid,* they conclude.

Don't stop your investigation here.

Here's how your thyroid can produce enough thyroid hormone but you develop symptoms of hypothyroidism: If you get really sick, are under a lot of stress, or don't have enough of certain nutrients like iodine, zinc, or selenium, your body may try to compensate by converting thyroid metabolism away from the active form of T3 thyroid into an *inactive* form of T3 called reverse T3. Reverse T3 can bind to the same receptors as T3, but it does not activate them, which is why it can cause you to experience symptoms that look like hypothyroidism: anxiety, fatigue, hair loss, and weight gain.

Unfortunately, low T3 syndrome is a commonly missed diagnosis. This is partly due to many doctors conducting *only* TSH screening tests, which usually fall within the normal range. In low T3 syndrome, you may see the pattern of test results in the Four Analyte Thyroid Panel.

> **Note:** You must have results for the entire Four Analyte Thyroid Panel to have clarity into the entire thyroid pathway.

FOUR ANALYTE THYROID PANEL

- TSH: normal
- Free* T4: normal
- Free T3: normal/low
- Reverse T3: high

Now that we have a basic understanding of how the thyroid works, let's talk about how to test its function.

* Measuring the free hormone level, as opposed to total levels, provides a more accurate assessment of thyroid hormone status than measuring total hormonal levels.

Thyroid Testing

Here are some tips for getting the most out of your thyroid testing:

- Avoid taking biotin supplements or natural thyroid remedies for 72 hours before your blood test.
- Get your blood tested in the morning, before you take any medication.
- Eat breakfast or a snack before your test, as fasting can interfere with the results of your thyroid test.
- Include a full thyroid panel, including TSH, free T3, free T4, and reverse T3, as well as thyroid peroxidase antibodies (TPOAb), thyroglobulin antibodies (TgAb), and thyroid-stimulating immunoglobulin (TSI).

INTERPRETING THYROID LABS

THYROID TEST	NORMAL RANGES*	HYPERTHYROIDISM	HYPOTHYROIDISM
TSH	0.45 to 4.5 mIU/L	Low	High
fT3	2.0 to 4.4 pg/mL	High/normal	Low/normal
fT4	0.93 to 1.6 ng/dL	High/normal	Low/normal
Reverse T3	9.2–24.1 ng/dL	Varies	Varies/high

* Reference ranges and units of measurement used can vary from lab to lab. I have included the ranges I see most commonly.

Remember, TSH can be normal, even if your thyroid isn't making proper thyroid hormone!

Charlotte's Story

LET'S CIRCLE BACK TO CHAPTER 1, WHERE WE MET CHARLOTTE FOR THE first time, and look at her symptoms: panic, difficulty sleeping, unintended weight loss, intolerance to heat, and tremors—all of which she tried to manage by drinking large amounts of calming kava kava tea. Charlotte was experiencing some of the cardinal signs and symptoms of hyperthyroidism. But in order to diagnose a thyroid condition, we need lab testing, which thankfully her second doctor was willing to order. This is what her results revealed:

THYROID PANEL

- TSH: low at 0.179 uLU/mL (the lab's reference range was 0.45–4.500 uLU/mL)
- Free T3: high at 14 (the lab's reference range was 2.0–4.4 pg/ml)
- Free T4: high at 12 ng/dL (the lab's reference range was 0.93–1.6 ng/dL)
- Reverse T3: suboptimal at 19.4 ng/dL (the lab's reference range was 9.2–24.1 ng/dL)
- Thyroid antibodies: high

Diagnosis? Autoimmune hyperthyroidism.

Next steps? Remember, effective treatment always addresses the reason behind the symptoms. Charlotte's first doctor recommended a benzodiazepine to address her anxiety, but that medication would have been only a Band-Aid. It would not have addressed the underlying autoimmunity. Instead, Charlotte dug deeper and now has information on the better next steps to take.

You'll see what happened next in Chapter 8.

THYROID TL;DR

- Imbalances in thyroid levels can be associated with panic and anxiety.
- A comprehensive thyroid test should always include TSH, free T3, free T4, and reverse T3 (consider including antibodies, too).
- Your thyroid test can look perfectly normal, and you could actually have a thyroid hormone problem.
- Your thyroid is affected by your hormones, gut, neurotransmitters, immune system, the environment, stress, and much more.

ADRENAL HORMONES

The thyroid gland and its hormones aren't the sole players that affect mood and stress/anxiety. In the next section we'll discuss your adrenals and their hormones.

Cortisol

Do you ever feel like you're on edge, ready to snap at the slightest provocation? Or do you find yourself feeling sluggish and exhausted, even after a full night's sleep? Perhaps the smallest things can provoke full-on anxiety and even panic. These symptoms could be due to imbalances in your cortisol levels. Cortisol is a hormone that helps you respond to stress. It's released by your adrenal glands when you're faced with a challenge such as a deadline at work or a fight with your partner.

Under optimal conditions, cortisol can also help you feel energized and focused so that you can deal with the stressor. But too much cortisol can lead to problems including anxiety and panic, depression, weight gain, and insomnia. If, on the other hand, your cortisol is too low, you won't be able to manage normal, daily stress, so you'll feel burned out and exhausted.

We will talk more about cortisol testing later in this chapter, but here is a simple checklist to help you set a baseline.

CORTISOL SELF-ASSESSMENT CHECKLIST: TOO HIGH VS. TOO LOW CORTISOL

Instructions: Check the box(es) that relate to you, and write your total score in the space provided.

❑ High blood pressure	❑ Rapid weight loss
❑ Easy bruising	❑ Low blood pressure (dizzy standing up)
❑ High blood sugar	
❑ Purple-ish stretch marks on skin	❑ Orange-ish pigmentation of skin and gums

- ❏ Rapid weight gain (especially face and abdomen)

TOTAL: ____/5

SCORING: If you checked more than two boxes, consider getting a full workup to screen for *high cortisol* and possible causes.

- ❏ Low blood sugar
- ❏ Recurrent infections (getting sick often)

TOTAL: ____/5

SCORING: If you checked more than two boxes, consider getting a full workup to screen for *low cortisol* and possible causes.

On the left side of the checklist, you see some of the classic symptoms associated with *high cortisol levels*. Think of high cortisol as a switch that's stuck in the "on" position, flooding your body with stress hormones even when there's no immediate danger. As mentioned, this can lead to panic, insomnia, weight gain, high blood pressure, and even acne—yikes!

On the right side of the checklist, you see the opposite problem: *low cortisol levels*. This is like a switch that's been turned off, leaving you feeling drained. You might experience muscle weakness, dizziness, or even fainting spells.

The emotional symptoms of anxiety and depression can be linked to either *high* or *low* cortisol levels, a confusing conundrum to navigate. Your body is trying to communicate, and it's up to us to decode the message and come up with a plan to get you feeling your best. To do that, we need to understand a bit of adrenal anatomy first.

Adrenal Glands: Your Body's Little Spark Plugs

Your adrenal glands are two small glands that sit on top of your kidneys, one left, one right. They are composed of two functional parts: an inner medulla and an outer cortex. Each part is responsible for producing its own set of hormones:

- The medulla produces chemicals such as adrenaline, norepinephrine, and dopamine. (Check out Chapter 6 for a deep dive into them.)

- The cortex releases a number of hormones including aldosterone, cortisol, DHEA, and testosterone.

The adrenal glands work together with the hypothalamus and pituitary gland, in the brain, to form the hypothalamic-pituitary-adrenal (HPA) axis (see page 101). When your body needs a boost of energy, like in the morning when you wake up or during times of high stress, the HPA axis jumps into action.

Here's how this magnificent biofeedback loop works:

- The hypothalamus, a pea-size gland in your brain, releases corticotropin-releasing hormone (CRH).
- CRH travels to the pituitary gland, which is located at the base of your brain, stimulating the release of adrenocorticotropic hormone (ACTH).
- ACTH travels through your bloodstream to the adrenal glands atop your kidneys.
- The adrenal glands release cortisol, which ramps up your speed, strength, and focus.
- Higher levels of cortisol cause a feedback loop that inhibits the release of cortisol-stimulating signals from the brain.

Cortisol isn't just about making you feel superhuman in the face of danger. It also suppresses noncritical bodily functions (e.g., digestion and reproduction) to make sure your body is focused on the perceived urgent task at hand. Once the danger is over, cortisol production will normally slow down, with the help of that handy feedback loop that keeps your adrenals in check (except when this feedback loop is not working correctly).

Cortisol fluctuates naturally throughout the day—and cortisol timing is one of the places where things can get wonky. As you can see in the following figure, cortisol levels should reach their peak in the morning, providing a burst of energy and motivation to start your day, and gradually decrease into the afternoon, reaching their lowest point in the evening, allowing the body to sleep, rest, and rejuvenate.

DIURNAL CORTISOL – NORMAL

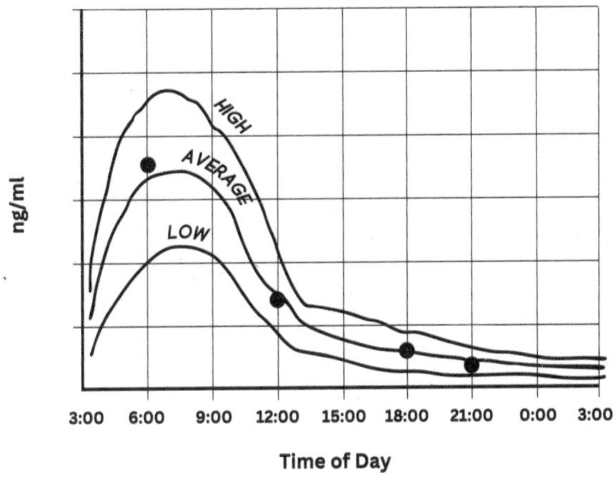

But it doesn't always work as designed. Do you ever wake with panic or feel anxious as the sun sets? Identifying the timing of your symptoms can help you zero in on their underlying cause. Stay tuned—we'll get to that soon.

Adrenal Fatigue: A Myth?

David's Story

AS YOU MIGHT REMEMBER FROM CHAPTER 6, DAVID WORKS AT A HIGH-stress job and has a long history of high anxiety and agitation. This is compounded by fatigue, brain fog, caffeine dependence, digestive upset, and unintended weight gain. "A classic case of adrenal fatigue" had been his functional doctor's conclusion. "Your adrenals are exhausted from chronic stress, which is making you tired and irritable and causing you to gain weight."

David went home with a list of supplements including adrenal glandulars—which are made from the glands, organs, or tissues of animals—adaptogenic herbs, and micronutrients. They offered minimal relief, at best because the approach was not addressing the true root cause.

HAS THIS EVER HAPPENED to you?

You may have heard the term adrenal fatigue, often used to explain a variety of symptoms like fatigue, weight gain, brain fog, and depression. However, it's not a recognized medical diagnosis, and our understanding of these symptoms and their causes has evolved significantly.

This matters for you because if you treat the symptoms without regard for the true root cause, you are not going to get the desired result: freedom from panic.

There are a few reasons why people accept the concept of a generalized adrenal fatigue. First, some websites and supplement companies claim that adrenal fatigue is a common condition that can be easily treated with supplements and herbs (commercial influence). Second, some people may experience symptoms that appear to be easily attributed to adrenal fatigue, such as fatigue, weight gain, and brain fog (generalized symptoms).

However, these symptoms can be caused by a number of things, including stress, poor diet, and underlying medical conditions (e.g., anemia, hypothyroidism, hypoglycemia, postural orthostatic tachycardia, sleep apnea, and viral infections). If you are experiencing symptoms that you think (or have been told) are caused by adrenal fatigue, it is important to take a step back and do some deeper digging.

David decided to do the deeper digging.

In order to avoid what I refer to as "spray and pray" testing, meaning expensive functional testing that may or may not elucidate the problem, we decided to be more strategic.

To get started, I had David fill out several checklists to help us zero in on which tests might be the most useful and should be prioritized, and which tests we could put on the back burner. I've sprinkled these checklists throughout this book in hopes that they will help you identify where to start and help mitigate the need for costly and potentially unnecessary testing.

DAVID'S OUT-OF-NORMAL-RANGE SCORES:

- Gut Anxiety (pitta type)
- High cortisol
- High inflammatory markers
- Low testosterone

Based on these findings, we ran these tests:

- **DRIED URINE TEST FOR COMPREHENSIVE HORMONES (DUTCH).** DUTCH evaluates cortisol levels, sex hormones, and other relevant markers. (It's not covered by most insurances.)
- **TESTS FOR INFLAMMATION.** We tested for homocysteine, erythrocyte sedimentation rate, C-reactive protein, interleukin-6, tumor necrosis factor-alpha, and complete blood count (all of which his insurance covered).
- **COMPREHENSIVE STOOL TESTING.** This test looks at gut health, which impacts inflammation, nutrient absorption, and more. (It's also not covered by most insurance plans, but be sure to check with your insurance as coverage is always evolving.)
- **ALLERGY TESTING.** A skin-prick allergy panel measures histamine reactions to specific allergens.

David's DUTCH results came back and revealed that he had:

- High cortisol throughout the day and evening. (His doctor had assumed the opposite, that David's adrenals were "fatigued" and that his cortisol would be low.)
- Low testosterone.
- High methylmalonic acid, which is a marker for vitamin B12 deficiency.
- High quinolinic acid, which is a marker for inflammation. (Remember, high inflammation markers are seen in Immune System Anxiety. Read more about this marker under "The Science of Serotonin" in Chapter 6.)

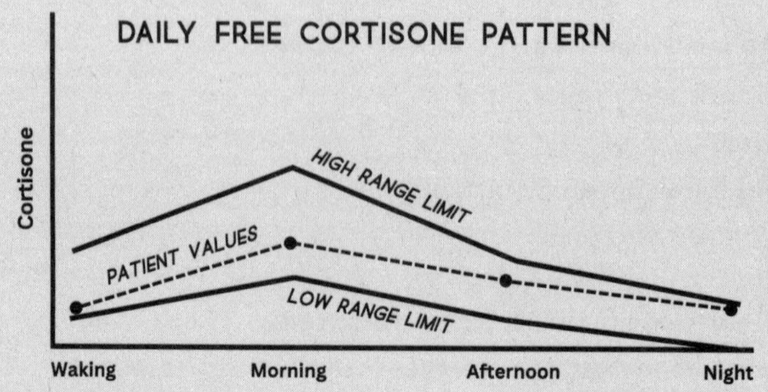

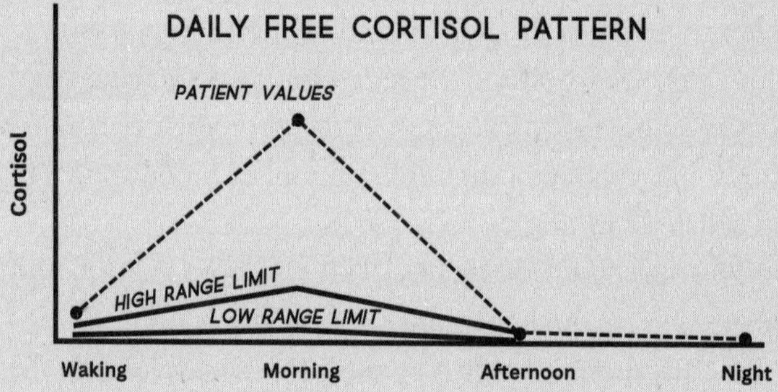

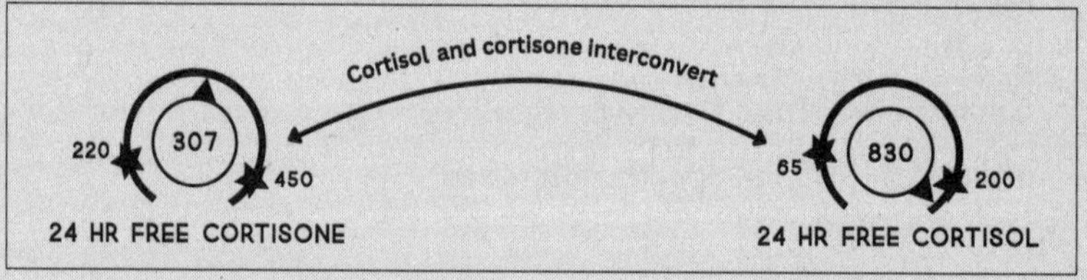

His stool testing revealed:

- Elevated levels of an inflammatory marker called fecal secretory IgA, which rises when there is inflammation and damage to the intestinal barrier, aka "leaky gut"
- Imbalances in his gut microbiome, the condition called dysbiosis that you learned about in Chapter 5

His blood tests revealed:

- High homocysteine
- Normal levels of other inflammatory markers

But why?

Our next steps included:

- **DIG DEEPER TO IDENTIFY ANY FURTHER ROOT CAUSES:** Suspecting a potential genetic link to his elevated quinolinic acid, cortisol, inflammatory markers, and low vitamin B12 (shown by MMA test), I ordered a homocysteine blood test and a genetic panel for further investigation.
- **START THE GUT HEALING PROTOCOL** from Chapter 11.

Stay tuned for what we discovered. But first, back to the adrenals.

Adrenal Gland Dysfunction

So if "adrenal fatigue" is not disrupting the adrenal feedback loop and causing unpleasant symptoms, what is the true cause?

LOW CORTISOL

Let's say you're feeling anxious and stressed all the time. You can't seem to focus, and you're always tired. You've tried everything to feel better, but nothing seems to work.

You're not alone. Millions of people suffering from anxiety and stress don't know that low cortisol could be the cause. Low cortisol can cause a variety of symptoms, including anxiety, weight loss, dizziness, and difficulty concentrating. It can even change your skin color (giving it more of an orange pigment—think John F. Kennedy). All these symptoms can compound one another, making you feel even more anxious and predisposed to panic.

HOW LOW CORTISOL CAN CAUSE ANXIETY AND PANIC:

- **LOW CORTISOL CAN LEAD TO INCREASED ADRENALINE PRODUCTION.** When your body goes into fight-or-flight mode, it needs cortisol to help cope with the stress. However, if your cortisol levels are low, your body may compensate by producing too much adrenaline. This can lead to symptoms like panic attacks, racing heart, pale skin, trembling, sweating, dizziness, nausea, and headache.

- **LOW CORTISOL CAN MAKE IT HARDER TO TOLERATE STRESS.** Cortisol helps your body cope with stress by regulating your metabolism, blood sugar levels, and immune system. Low cortisol levels can make it harder for you to handle stress, leaving you feeling drained and fatigued.
- **LOW CORTISOL CAN CAUSE HIGH LEVELS OF INFLAMMATION.** Cortisol helps keep inflammation in check, so when it's low, inflammation can go up. This can lead to changes in the brain, including neuroinflammation, that are associated with anxiety and other mental health issues.
- **LOW CORTISOL CAN CAUSE HIGH LEVELS OF ESTROGEN.** Cortisol and estrogen share a similar complex feedback loop. When cortisol levels are low, the brain thinks there's not enough hormone activity, so it sends signals to boost other hormones like corticotrophin-releasing hormone and adrenocorticotropic hormone. But these signals can also prompt the ovaries to produce more estrogen, leading to elevated overall estrogen levels. This can increase your risk of anxiety in a number of ways that you'll learn about in the "Estrogen" section of this chapter.
- **LOW CORTISOL CAN IMPAIR BLOOD SUGAR REGULATION.** Cortisol helps regulate blood sugar levels. When stress rises, cortisol helps your body break down glycogen, a storage form of sugar, and convert it into glucose to give you energy. Low cortisol levels can make it harder for your body to get sugar out of storage, which can lead to symptoms like shakiness, dizziness, and lightheadedness. These symptoms can feel a lot like a panic attack, so it's important to know the difference.

To investigate whether blood sugar issues are contributing to your anxiety, you can have your glucose and insulin levels tested while fasting and then again two hours after eating.

- When you're fasting, your glucose should be between 70 and 100 mg/dL (3.9 and 5.6 mmol/L), and your insulin should be < 25 mIU/L, or < 174 pmol/L.
- Two hours after you eat (postprandial), your glucose should be less than 140 mg/dL, and your insulin should be 16–166 mIU/L, or 111–1153 pmol/L.

Testing glucose and insulin is often a good option because these tests are typically covered by insurance. Another option that is quite a lot more thorough (but is not often covered by insurance) is continuous glucose monitoring, in which you wear a device to measure your blood glucose levels throughout the day.

OKAY, NEXT UP: WHAT'S causing your low cortisol levels? Once you have determined that your cortisol levels are low, the next step is to identify the underlying reason(s). I've included the eight most common causes of low cortisol in the figure below:

CAUSES OF LOW CORTISOL

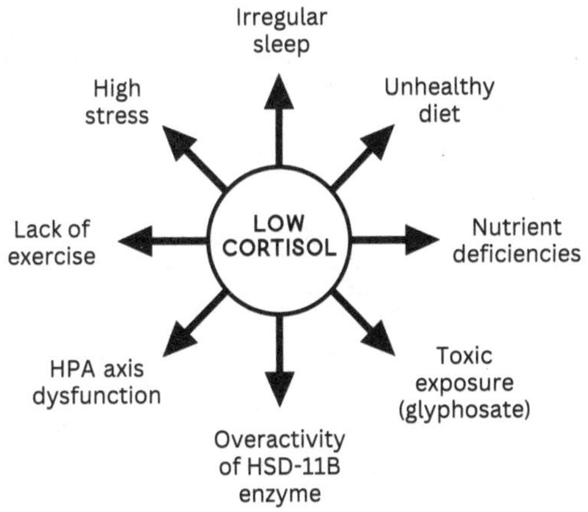

Cortisol and Panic Attacks

Now that we've learned how low cortisol can cause panic and anxiety, we're going to talk about how too-high cortisol can also cause anxiety. Remember, cortisol's main job is to jump-start your body into action. We see this in the fight-flight-freeze response. But too-high cortisol, or cortisol production at the wrong time (like when you're trying to go to sleep), can be a real nuisance.

HIGH CORTISOL

You're feeling wired and agitated, as if your head is about to pop off, but at the same time, you're feeling emotionally and physically fried. You've tried everything—supplements, herbs, meditation—but nothing seems to help. You finally get your cortisol levels tested, and your numbers are through the roof.

There are actually a lot of reasons why your cortisol levels might be high and causing panic. Here are some of the most common:

CAUSES OF HIGH CORTISOL

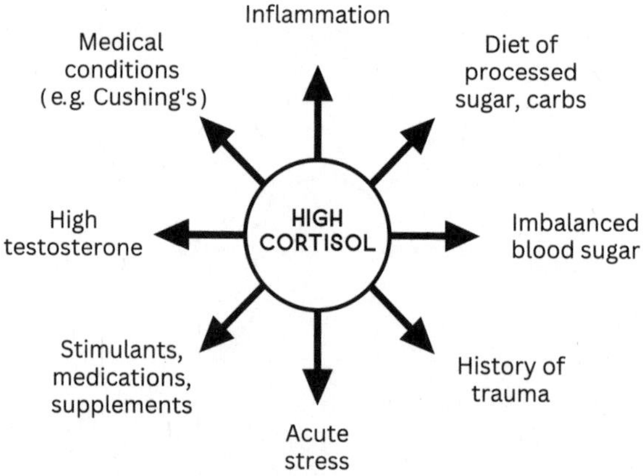

Cortisol Testing

Cortisol can be tested with blood, saliva, and urine tests. The best method for you will depend on your individual needs.

- Blood tests are the most common and can be done at a doctor's office or lab. They are typically covered by insurance.
- Saliva tests are less invasive and can be done at home, but they are less likely to be covered by insurance than blood tests.
- Urine tests can also be done at home but are also less likely to be covered by your insurance than blood tests.

> **Note:** Both saliva and urine tests can provide data on how your cortisol levels fluctuate over a 24-hour period (see page 177), which is useful if you notice that your symptoms tend to change throughout the day and night. You can get updated information about my favorite functional testing at drnicolecain.com/book-resources/.

CORTISOL TL;DR

- Both high and low levels of cortisol can cause panic and anxiety.
- Cortisol should be at its highest in the morning and reduce throughout the day and into the evening.
- Cortisol production requires vitamin C, vitamin B5, vitamin B6, magnesium, zinc, iron, and sodium.

Esme's Story

"HERE'S A FUN FACT." ESME DROPPED ONTO THE SOFA. "THE UTERUS IS a sadistic organ, whose objective is to make women's lives a living hell." Like many, Esme found menstruation to be inherently miserable, bringing wild mood swings, debilitating cramps, and a body that constantly betrays.

"I've been panicking literally every day for the last week. I'm also irritable, breaking out all over my face and shoulders, and my cramps are killing me."

In an effort to zero in on what might be leading to her panic attacks, Esme had been keeping a log of her symptoms. She retrieved her journal from her backpack.

"But here's the thing—I'm starting to wonder if there's a pattern." She read aloud what she had written a month ago.

" 'The week before my period is hell, both physically and mentally. I have more intense and frequent panic attacks with the lightning pains in my chest, claustrophobia, and terrible sleep. I'm also much more impatient and annoyed, and I've been going off on my roommates. Then there's the "bonus hair growth" on my chin. I plucked that shit out immediately. Acne is way worse; I get cysts on my T-zone and shoulders. My gut is a hot mess. It's worse with fast food—better if I just don't eat.' "

Esme looked up from her journal. "It's like clockwork," she said. "Every . . . single . . . month. My hormones are draining my will to live."

Esme's conclusion was both insightful and tragic. Insightful because she's right that our hormones can have a profound impact on our physical and mental health, and tragic because her mind and body were at war.

But here was Esme's aha! moment:

"Before, it felt like my panic was all over the place and it made no sense to me. But now that I've kept track of my symptoms for a while, I am wondering if it might not be as random as I thought. What if a lot of what I'm dealing with is related to what's going on in my hormones? What if my hormones and my uterus are actually part of why I get panic attacks?"

The weight of the question settled in the air.

Our brains don't live in a vacuum separate from our hormones, or vice versa.

Esme had just taken one step closer to understanding the messages of her symptoms.

SEX HORMONES

ESME'S EYES QUICKLY SCANNED THE PAGES OF HER LAB REPORT AS I EXplained the results.

"I think I may have an idea of what's going on," I said. "Your estrogen and progesterone are normal, but your testosterone and luteinizing hormone are elevated. Your cholesterol and insulin are also high, but your blood sugars were actually pretty good."

"So I was right." Esme didn't look up from the page. "It wasn't in my head this whole time."

"Yes, you were right. What you are dealing with—the panic attacks, acne, cramps, PMS—are all signs the body was giving you that something was out of balance. Your test results point to something called polycystic ovarian syndrome, or PCOS."

"I've heard of PCOS." Esme shook her head. "It messes with your hormones, and I know it can really affect your mood."

"Exactly." I nodded. "Now that we have a clearer idea of what we're working with, we can make a plan that is specifically tailored to you."

And then something happened that caught me off guard. Esme began to cry.

"I'm s-s-so sorry." She pressed a wad of tissue in front of her eyes. "I need a minute." As she blew her nose, I tried to hold space for what was coming up for her.

After several moments, she spoke. "You know . . . my whole life. I've been told that there was something wrong with me." Her voice trembled. "My mother called me moody. My father said I was too sensitive. Doctors even told me that if I didn't get my act together, I'd never amount to anything. I've felt so much shame and guilt."

She took a steadying breath and then her eyes met mine. "But maybe it wasn't my fault."

"Esme," I said. "You and your body were doing the best you could, but the people around you didn't understand how to interpret what was going on. You're in a different place now, you have resources you didn't have before, and that means that you now get to take your story back."

HAVE YOU BEEN THERE? Feeling judged, criticized, and condemned because the people around you didn't understand what you were going through?

I have. Growing up, I had terrible sinus congestion and asthma. My doctors gave me a prednisone inhaler, an albuterol rescue inhaler, a nasal steroid, and an allergy spray. I took a decongestant during the day, which gave me heart palpitations and anxiety, and so I was prescribed an SSRI antidepressant.

I was often criticized about my pockets full of tissues, and I was labeled "difficult" and "high-maintenance." Not until medical school did I discover I was severely allergic to dairy. After removing dairy from my diet, I was able to stop taking all my asthma and allergy medications and get rid of the Kleenex.

Just like Esme and me, you may know what it is like to be criticized for your symptoms. But you're here, right now, reading this book. And that means you're incorporating resources you didn't have before, and you're taking back your story. And that is absolutely incredible. At the end of this chapter, I'll share Esme's protocol with you, but first, let's dig into your sex hormones.

SEX HORMONES AND PANIC

Do you feel anxious during your period, or as a result of hormone treatment, or during puberty, pregnancy, menopause, or andropause? (Yes, you read that last word correctly. Cisgender males go through a form of menopause! It's called andropause and occurs as testosterone levels naturally decline with age.)

Your sex hormones are regulated by the hypothalamic-pituitary-gonadal (HPG) axis, a complex biofeedback system that controls their production and release. It's made up of the hypothalamus, the pituitary gland, and the gonads (ovaries and testes). The HPG axis works closely with other "axes" in your body such as the HPA axis (for stress response), the HPT axis (for thyroid function), and the gut-brain axis.

Hormonal imbalances can cause a variety of symptoms, including panic, depression, and irritability. These imbalances can occur during times of hormonal fluctuation, such as premenstruation, pregnancy, postpartum, perimenopause, and menopause.

Even when hormone levels are within the normal range, some people may be more vulnerable to developing symptoms during times of hormonal fluctuation. This is called *phasic vulnerability*. We'll discuss this in more detail in the Estrogen section, up next!

Estrogen

Chances are you've heard of estrogen—a hormone that's important for reproductive health. But did you know that it also plays a major role in mental and emotional well-being, especially when it comes to panic?

Estrogen is often misunderstood. While too much of it can lead to problems like painful periods, weight gain, mood swings, and hair loss, too little estrogen can also have negative effects.

For instance, did you know that low estrogen puts you at risk of panic attacks? And that having sufficient levels of estrogen will actually protect you against the effects of adverse events (traumas) and reduce your risk of depression?

Let's start with a quick self-assessment for potential estrogen imbalances.

ESTROGEN SELF-ASSESSMENT CHECKLIST: TOO HIGH VS. TOO LOW ESTROGEN

Instructions: Check the box(es) that relate to you, and write your total score in the space provided.

- ❑ Night sweats before periods
- ❑ Hot flashes
- ❑ Headaches
- ❑ Weight gain around hips and waist
- ❑ Thin and fragile skin

TOTAL: ____/5

SCORING: If you checked more than two boxes, consider getting a workup to screen for low estrogen.

- ❑ Easy startling
- ❑ Bleeding between periods
- ❑ Uterine polyps
- ❑ Fibrocystic breast tissue
- ❑ Heavy menstrual bleeding

TOTAL: ____/5

SCORING: If you checked more than two boxes, consider getting a workup to screen for estrogen dominance.

Do you have any indicators of an estrogen imbalance? The left side of the checklist lists signs that your estrogen may be too low, while signs of estrogen dominance are on the right. Alternatively, do your symptoms primarily show up during changes in hormones, such as before your period?

In the next section you're going to discover the science of estrogen, its connection to panic, and more.

Estrogen and Anxiety: What You Need to Know

Estrogen is often thought of as being produced by the ovaries (the primary source in females), but it is actually produced by many different organs in the body, including the adrenal glands, testes, fat cells, liver, bones, and brain. Estrogen is important for a number of bodily functions, including the development of sex characteristics, the regulation of the menstrual cycle, and the maintenance of bone health.

During perimenopause and menopause, estrogen levels drop as the ovaries slow down. This can lead to a number of symptoms, including hot flashes, night sweats, vaginal dryness, and mood swings.

The sources of estrogen other than the ovaries can help to buffer the effects of declining estrogen levels during perimenopause and menopause. For example, supporting the adrenal glands can help to increase the production of estrogen. This is especially important for you if your panic started during perimenopause!

There are many ways to support the adrenal glands, including eating a healthy diet, getting regular exercise, managing stress, and using herbal medicine. We will explore these methods in detail in Part III.

Estrogen and Panic

Studies have shown that an estrogen imbalance may contribute to panic attacks. This is, in part, because estrogen helps regulate the neurotransmitter GABA, which plays a role in calming the brain. When estrogen levels decline, it may lead to an imbalance in GABA, which can trigger anxiety. Additionally, estrogen helps protect the brain from stress by reducing inflammation and by increasing the production of a protein that helps sustain neurons. Low estrogen levels may make the brain more sensitive to stress and anxiety, making it harder for your brain to control your responses to fear.

Estrogen also plays a role in how the brain learns and remembers fear. Studies have shown that women with low levels of estradiol, a form of estrogen, are likely to have a stronger fear response when they are trying to forget a fearful experience. This is because estrogen helps to regulate the hippocampus and the amygdala, helping to keep the fear response in check.

Estrogen may also impact post-traumatic stress disorder symptoms. Women with PTSD may be more vulnerable to the disorder's severity due to cyclical estrogen secretion during the reproductive cycle—this is called phasic vulnerability. Estrogen replacement therapy that stimulates estrogen receptor beta has been shown to reduce PTSD symptoms. For example, one study found that women with low salivary estrogen levels were more likely to have intrusive thoughts about violent scenes after watching a film clip. This is a finding that is relevant to the re-experiencing symptoms of PTSD.

This response is evidenced by another study, published in the journal *JAMA Psychiatry,* that looked at data from more than one thousand women who had been sexually assaulted. It found that six months after the event, the women who received estrogen-based emergency contraception had significantly lower symptoms of PTSD than those who did not receive it. They reported fewer nightmares and flashbacks, less anxiety, and lower levels of depression and anxiety.

How Estrogen Metabolites Affect Anxiety: A Closer Look

There are three main types of estrogen: estrone (E1), estradiol (E2), and estriol (E3).

Estrogen is broken down into metabolites that have different effects on mood. Beneficial metabolites, such as 2-OH, can protect against anxiety, heart disease, and osteoporosis. Harmful metabolites, such as 4-OH and 16-OH, are linked to increased oxidative stress, which can put you at an increased risk of anxiety, panic, and other diseases related to inflammation (which is just about everything).

ESTROGEN TYPES AND SUBTYPES

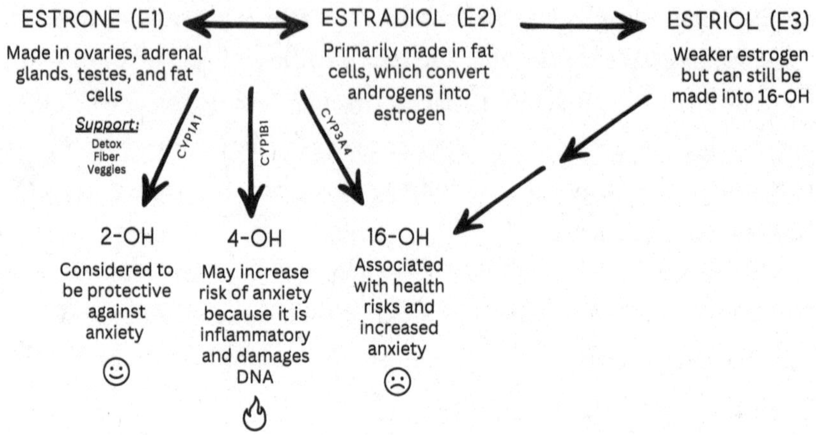

In Part III, you'll learn more about how to influence your estrogen metabolism, shifting it toward the anxiety-reducing 2-OH metabolite. Here are three steps to get you started:

- Eat more cruciferous veggies such as broccoli and Brussels sprouts. (Note: If you have hypothyroidism, your doctor may recommend avoiding cruciferous veggies.)
- Eat more foods containing resveratrol, such as cocoa and cranberries.
- Eat more polyphenol-rich foods such as brightly colored berries (e.g., blueberries and blackberries), herbs and spices (cloves and oregano), flaxseeds, and dark leafy greens (spinach and kale).

Now that we have discussed the different types of estrogen, its metabolites, and how they affect anxiety, we can focus on estrogen receptors.

The Estrogen Receptor That Could Change Your Life

Estrogen receptors are proteins that bind to estrogen. They are found in many parts of the body, including the brain. One type of estrogen receptor, called estrogen receptor beta (ERβ), is thought to be especially important for reducing anxiety.

When ERβ receptors in the amygdala bind to estradiol, it activates a signaling pathway that halts the release of stress hormones. So that means more ERβ → less stress hormones → less anxiety = Panic Proof.

Here are some suggestions to help you get started increasing your ERβ activity:

- **EAT A HEALTHY DIET.** A diet that is rich in fruits, vegetables, fiber, and whole grains can help to increase ERβ activity.
- **EXERCISE REGULARLY.** Exercise increases ERβ activity. Aim for at least 15 to 30 minutes of moderate-intensity exercise most days of the week.
- **MANAGE STRESS.** Healthy ways to manage stress, such as yoga or meditation, can help to improve ERβ activity.
- **SUPPLEMENT WITH BOTANICALS THAT BOOST ERβ.** Use herbs that contain liquiritigenin, a flavonoid found in the roots of various plant species such as licorice (*Glycyrrhiza glabra*) and skullcap (*Scutellaria baicalensis*). See Chapter 11 for specifics on herbal dosing.

While you're shifting your estrogen so that it protects you against anxiety, you're going to want to start exploring the root causes of your estrogen imbalances. Most commonly I see:

- **CORTISOL IMBALANCES.** When we are stressed, our bodies produce more cortisol. This can lead to lower estrogen levels. Cortisol can bind to estrogen receptors, blocking the effects of estrogen, and it can interfere with the production of estrogen by the ovaries.
- **GENETIC PREDISPOSITIONS.** Genetics can affect how your body

metabolizes estrogen. The catechol-O-methyltransferase (COMT) enzyme breaks down estrogen. People with a gene that codes for high COMT activity have lower estrogen levels, while people with a gene that codes for low COMT activity have higher estrogen levels. These levels are primarily genetically determined, but COMT activity can also be affected by lifestyle factors, such as diet and stress.

- **ENVIRONMENTAL TOXINS.** Some of the most common environmental toxins that can interfere with estrogen production and utilization include:

    - Heavy metals: Arsenic, cadmium, lead, mercury, and nickel are heavy metals that can mimic estrogen and interfere with the body's natural estrogen levels by damaging the ovaries, binding to estrogen receptors, and blocking estrogen from binding.
    - Endocrine disruptors: Bisphenol-A, phthalates, atrazine, and PCBs are environmental toxins that can mimic estrogen and interfere with the body's natural estrogen levels by binding to estrogen receptors.
    - Mycotoxins (molds): Aflatoxin B1, ochratoxin A, and zearalenone are mycotoxins that can interfere with estrogen by binding to estrogen receptors and disrupting their activity.

    You may consider testing your home for environmental toxins, such as getting an in-home mold inspection, or having your water tested. If you have a high risk of environmental toxins based on the self-assessment checklist on page 239, I would also recommend getting your own functional labs run, which we will explore in more detail in Chapter 11.

- **BAD BACTERIA IN THE GUT.** Pathogenic bacteria can produce toxins that bind to estrogen receptors and activate them or interfere with estrogen metabolism. These problematic organisms may include *E. coli, Salmonella, Shigella, Campylobacter,* and *Listeria* species. Stool testing can help identify the presence of pathogens.

- **IMBALANCES IN OTHER HORMONES.** Remember, changes in one hormone can cause changes in another. Polycystic ovary syndrome (PCOS) is a hormonal disorder characterized by high levels of androgens (male hormones) and insulin resistance, which can interfere with estrogen levels. PCOS can cause a variety of symptoms, including irregular periods, infertility, and weight gain. Therefore, it can be very informative if your healthcare practitioners request a complete hormone panel (covered by your insurance) when investigating the root cause. (You're going to want to remember this later when we go over one of our cases.)

Now we will delve into methods to assess estrogen metabolites and their levels.

Estrogen Testing

There are three main ways to test estrogen levels: blood, saliva, and urine.

- **BLOOD TESTS.** Blood tests are the most common method. Insurance may cover basic estrogen testing, but it may be difficult to get coverage for testing estrogen metabolites.
- **SALIVA TESTS.** Less invasive than blood tests, saliva tests can be done at home and may include estrogen metabolites.
- **URINE TESTS.** Urine tests are also less invasive, can be done at home, and may include estrogen metabolites.

WHEN SHOULD YOU INVEST in saliva or urine testing? You might really consider doing either saliva or urine testing:

- If you have had your hormones checked and they are "normal," but your lived experience is that your symptoms seem to get worse during certain hormonal cycles.
- Both saliva and urine tests can provide data on how your estrogen levels fluctuate over time, which is useful if you notice that your symptoms tend to change throughout the month.

To access my up-to-date favorite tests, go to drnicolecain.com /book-resources/.

ESTROGEN TL;DR

- Some estrogen metabolites cause more anxiety, while other types of estrogen can protect you from anxiety.
- Estrogen support can help reduce PTSD symptoms.
- Estrogen metabolite 2-OH is protective against anxiety and panic.
- Stimulating estrogen receptor beta (ERβ) may be an effective way to combat anxiety.

Progesterone

Progesterone—a hormone produced by the ovaries, testes, adrenal glands, and even the cells of the brain—promotes sleep, reduces stress, protects bones, regulates mood and menstrual cycle, and maintains a pregnancy.

Let's begin with a self-assessment checklist, then dive deeper into the panic-progesterone connection.

PROGESTERONE SELF-ASSESSMENT CHECKLIST: TOO HIGH VS. TOO LOW PROGESTERONE

Instructions: Check the box(es) that relate to you, and write your total score in the space provided.

- ❑ Premenstrual syndrome
- ❑ Bad menstrual cramps
- ❑ Insomnia
- ❑ Water retention, feeling "puffy"
- ❑ Feeling "too full" after small meals

- ❑ History of miscarriage
- ❑ Spotting between periods

TOTAL: ____/5

SCORING: If you checked more than two boxes, consider getting a workup to screen for low progesterone.

- ❑ Lack of bleeding during menstrual cycle
- ❑ Nausea
- ❑ Constipation

TOTAL: ____/5

SCORING: If you checked more than two boxes, consider getting a workup to screen for high progesterone.

On the left side of the self-assessment checklist, we see signs of low progesterone, while the right side lists signs that progesterone is too high.

Progesterone levels naturally fluctuate throughout the menstrual cycle, gradually rising throughout the first half of the cycle (follicular phase), peaking just before ovulation, and then gradually decreasing, which triggers the start of the menstrual period.

Because progesterone tends to ebb and flow, it may be valuable to circle back to this self-assessment checklist periodically to see if you notice any trends. This can give you helpful data about how progesterone is affecting your mood—for better or worse.

How Progesterone Is Made

Progesterone is made from cholesterol, a waxy substance found in all cells in the body and in some animal sources such as eggs, dairy products, and meat. Cholesterol is converted into a compound called pregnenolone, which is then converted into progesterone by a series of enzymes. Progesterone can also be converted into other hormones, such as cortisol.

See page 198 for a simplified diagram of the process.

YOUR BODY MAKES CORTISOL FROM PROGESTERONE

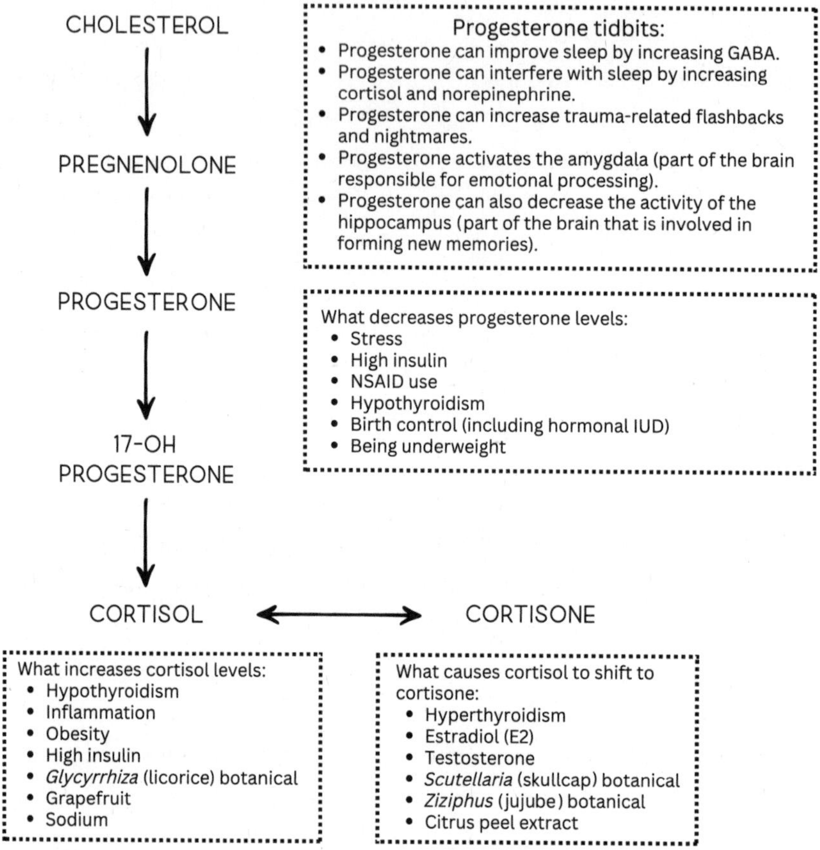

CHOLESTEROL
PREGNENOLONE
PROGESTERONE
17-OH PROGESTERONE
CORTISOL
CORTISONE
Progesterone tidbits:
• Progesterone can improve sleep by increasing GABA.
• Progesterone can interfere with sleep by increasing cortisol and norepinephrine.
• Progesterone can increase trauma-related flashbacks and nightmares.
• Progesterone activates the amygdala (part of the brain responsible for emotional processing).
• Progesterone can also decrease the activity of the hippocampus (part of the brain that is involved in forming new memories).
What decreases progesterone levels:
• Stress
• High insulin
• NSAID use
• Hypothyroidism
• Birth control (including hormonal IUD)
• Being underweight
What increases cortisol levels:
• Hypothyroidism
• Inflammation
• Obesity
• High insulin
• Glycyrrhiza (licorice) botanical
• Grapefruit
• Sodium
What causes cortisol to shift to cortisone:
• Hyperthyroidism
• Estradiol (E2)
• Testosterone
• Scutellaria (skullcap) botanical
• Ziziphus (jujube) botanical
• Citrus peel extract

Progesterone and Anxiety

The effects of progesterone on mental health vary from person to person. It has the potential to both promote and mitigate anxiety. It can have a calming effect on the brain because it stimulates the production of GABA, a neurotransmitter that helps to reduce anxiety (see Chapter 6). However, some people with PTSD report feeling more anxious after taking progesterone supplements, perhaps because progesterone can increase the production of cortisol and norepinephrine, both of which can worsen anxiety and disrupt sleep, leading to flashbacks and nightmares. Another theory is that progesterone can interfere with the production of serotonin, a neurotransmitter that plays a role in mood and anxiety.

With such different potential reactions, how do you know if progesterone will make you feel calmer or more anxious? A few factors can affect how progesterone will affect your mood.

- **STRESS.** High emotional and/or physical stress can lead to your body converting progesterone into cortisol, which can worsen anxiety. Stress-reduction strategies, such as yoga, meditation, and spending time in nature, can help protect you from these effects.
- **GENETICS.** Mutations in certain genes, such as COMT and MAO-A, can make you more sensitive to the anxiety-causing effects of progesterone. Genetic testing can help you identify genetic markers associated with progesterone imbalances, but often I do not recommend investing in genetic testing unless we are not getting results with other treatments because it can be costly and difficult to analyze without a specialist's counsel.
- **INFLAMMATION.** Immune system imbalances and high levels of inflammation can worsen the effects of progesterone supplementation. Eating a healthy, anti-inflammatory diet that is rich in fruits, vegetables, and whole grains and getting regular exercise can help reduce inflammation.

Now that we have discussed the factors that can affect how progesterone can change your mood, let's talk about the different causes of elevated versus insufficient progesterone.

Too-High Progesterone

Progesterone naturally rises and drops throughout the menstrual cycle, and it is elevated during pregnancy. Other factors such as stress and illness, ovarian cysts, certain medications such as birth control pills or hormone replacement therapies, liver disease, congenital adrenal hyperplasia, and rapid weight gain can also cause too-high progesterone.

High progesterone is associated with symptoms such as weight gain, bloating, "puffiness" or "swelling" sensations, fatigue, headaches, nausea, body pains, oily skin, and interference with the menstrual cycle. Elevations in progesterone can also lead to mental health problems, such as postpartum depression and premenstrual dysphoric disorder.

We'll learn how to lower progesterone in Chapter 11, but here are three tips you can start implementing today:

- **GET EXERCISE.** Regular exercise can balance progesterone levels.
- **AVOID ALCOHOL AND TOBACCO.** Alcohol and tobacco can disrupt hormone balance and interfere with progesterone metabolism.
- **SUPPORT ESTROGEN LEVELS.** Promote estrogen levels to bring down progesterone levels by incorporating phytoestrogens, which are plant compounds that mimic estrogen in the body. These compounds are present in soy products and flaxseeds.

Too-Low Progesterone

Low progesterone can be caused by a variety of factors, including an underactive thyroid, high cortisol levels, estrogen dominance, being underweight, deficiencies in essential nutrients, certain medications, and environmental toxins such as pesticides, heavy metals, bisphenol-A, and dioxins.

When you do not have enough progesterone, you may experience a variety of symptoms, such as irregular periods, heavy or light periods, painful periods, difficulty getting pregnant, miscarriage, fibrocystic breasts, endometriosis, weight gain, hot flashes, night sweats, vaginal dryness, and body pains that may be somewhat relieved by NSAIDs. Low levels of progesterone can also lead to conditions such as infertility and polycystic ovary syndrome.

Progesterone Replacement Therapy

Progesterone replacement is generally safe for most people, but it can cause some side effects (in addition to those we already discussed) such as weight gain, breast tenderness, nausea, vomiting, headaches, fatigue, acne, and mood swings.

While no single progesterone replacement therapy guarantees zero risk of anxiety, some options may be less likely to trigger it compared to others.

For instance, consider micronized progesterone, a bioidentical progesterone that is believed to be more easily tolerated than synthetic alternatives. Bioidentical progesterone shares the same chemical structure as progesterone and is made from plant sources, mainly yams or soybeans.

TIPS FOR INCREASING PROGESTERONE NATURALLY

- Supplement with magnesium, zinc, and vitamin B6.
- Eat a healthy diet rich in fiber, veggies, whole grains, and brightly colored fruits.
- Minimize your exposure to environmental toxins.
- Consider natural progesterone-boosting herbs such as Vitex agnus-castus, black cohosh, dong quai, and wild yam. (See Chapter 11 for more details.)

Progesterone Testing

There are three main ways to test progesterone levels: blood, saliva, and urine.

- **BLOOD TESTS.** Blood tests are the most common way to test progesterone. They are fairly accurate, can be done quickly and easily, and are generally covered by insurance.
- **SALIVA TESTS.** Saliva tests are less invasive than blood tests and can be done at home. You can order these online, but they are less likely to be covered by insurance.
- **URINE TESTS.** Urine tests are the least invasive option for measuring progesterone, and many also include progesterone metabolites. These tests can be ordered directly online and are less likely to be covered by insurance.

In women who are still menstruating, progesterone levels are checked on day 21 of the menstrual cycle. In postmenopausal women, progesterone levels are not checked on a specific day. Personally, I recommend hormone testing during peak panic and anxiety moments. Testing when your symptoms are at their worst can provide a more accurate picture of what is hormonally going on during that time.

I have compiled a list of my preferred labs on my website: drnicolecain.com/book-resources/.

PROGESTERONE TL;DR

- Progesterone supplements taken for infertility increase your likelihood of experiencing anxiety.
- Progesterone can be both good and bad for anxiety depending on the person.
- Progesterone increases GABA, cortisol, and norepinephrine.
- Progesterone supplementation can increase symptoms of nightmares and flashbacks in those with PTSD.

Testosterone

Testosterone is produced in the testes, ovaries, adrenal glands, skin, and gut. It is a type of hormone called androgens, responsible for so-called male characteristics in both men and women.

Testosterone is involved in a number of functions, including:

- Energy
- Sex drive
- Muscle growth
- Bone density
- Fat distribution
- Mood
- Cognitive function

Testosterone levels naturally decline with age, but they can be affected by a number of other factors, including stress, injury, gut health, inflammation, other hormones, and certain medical conditions (which we will explore in more detail soon).

First, take this self-assessment checklist!

TESTOSTERONE SELF-ASSESSMENT CHECKLIST: TOO HIGH VS. TOO LOW TESTOSTERONE

Instructions: Check the box(es) that relate to you, and write your total score in the space provided.

- ❏ Low sex drive
- ❏ Decreased muscle mass
- ❏ Lack of drive or motivation
- ❏ Difficulty concentrating
- ❏ Decreased bone density

TOTAL: ____/5

- ❏ Deepened voice
- ❏ Increased muscle mass
- ❏ Thinning of hair in front of scalp
- ❏ Increased body hair growth
- ❏ Anger Anxiety, short temper, irritability

TOTAL: ____/5

SCORING: If you checked more than two boxes, consider getting a workup to screen for low testosterone.

SCORING: If you checked more than two boxes, consider getting a workup to screen for high testosterone.

Testosterone imbalances can cause symptoms similar to other conditions, such as hypothyroidism, depression, sleep apnea, or medication side effects. The checklist can help you zero in on whether a testosterone imbalance is a possibility. On the left side are signs of low testosterone, and on the right are signs of high testosterone.

Let's dig into those in more detail, starting with the connection between testosterone and anxiety.

Testosterone and Anxiety

Research has shown that people with low testosterone are more likely to experience anxiety, while people with high testosterone are less likely to experience anxiety.

The exact mechanism of this link is not fully understood, but it is thought to be due to the effects of testosterone on the brain. Testosterone has been shown to alter activity in the amygdala, a part of the brain that is involved in processing fear and anxiety. When testosterone levels are low, the brain may be more sensitive to stress.

Low Testosterone

There is a growing body of evidence that exposure to environmental toxins can have a negative impact on testosterone levels. Some of those environmental toxins include:

- Heavy metals
- Organochlorines, a group of chemicals that contain chlorine and that are often used as pesticides, industrial solvents, and flame retardants, such as DDT, PCBs, and dioxins
- Pesticides

- Air pollutants
- Bisphenol-A

These toxins can interfere with the production, metabolism, and action of testosterone, leading to low testosterone levels, which may be responsible for negative health effects, potentially including:

- Reduced muscle mass and strength
- Increased body fat
- Depression
- Anxiety
- Insomnia
- Sexual dysfunction
- Cardiovascular disease
- Type 2 diabetes
- Osteoporosis
- Cancer

What's next? If you resonate with this section, your next step may be to get testosterone testing as a part of a full hormone panel. Your second step may include additional specialized root-cause testing, such as environmental toxicity testing, which you will learn more about in Chapter 11.

Gluten and Low Testosterone

A number of studies suggest that diets containing gluten, a protein found in wheat, barley, and rye, are associated with lowered testosterone levels. This may be due to inflammation, glyphosate exposure, or damage to the gut by gluten, resulting in compromised gut health and insufficient absorption of nutrients necessary for making testosterone. Gluten can also bind to the receptors for testosterone, preventing it from entering the cells.

Celiac disease is an autoimmune disorder triggered by the ingestion of gluten, but there is also a wider spectrum of gluten reactivity. Even if celiac disease has been ruled out through medical testing, you can still experience varying degrees of sensitivity to gluten. This sensitivity is notably common in the United States, where wheat is a staple food. In the United States, glyphosate is sprayed on wheat before harvest to kill weeds and to help the wheat dry down. Glyphosate can be absorbed by the body through the skin and lungs and by eating contaminated wheat. Some studies have shown that glyphosate can damage the gut microbiota, which can lead to a variety of health problems, including gluten intolerance or sensitivity.

What should you do next?

If you suspect that gluten may be negatively impacting your hormones and thus your mood, there are two main options to consider:

- **DO A SIX-WEEK GLUTEN AND WHEAT DETOX.** This means eliminating all gluten-containing foods from your diet for six weeks. After six weeks, you can reintroduce gluten-containing foods one at a time and see if you notice any negative symptoms. If you do, it is likely that this food item is negatively contributing to your overall health.
- **MINIMIZE YOUR EXPOSURE TO GLYPHOSATE BY SWITCHING TO ORGANIC SOURCES OF GLUTEN.**

For more information about gluten-free food alternatives, see Part III.

Mycotoxins and Low Testosterone

Mycotoxins are toxic chemicals produced by fungi. They can contaminate food and feed, and they can also be found in the environment. Some research has suggested that mycotoxins may be linked to low testosterone levels.

Preclinical research published in the *International Journal of Environ-*

mental Research and Public Health found that exposure to the mycotoxin aflatoxin B1 decreased testosterone levels. Another study, published in *Toxicology Letters,* found that exposure to the mycotoxin ochratoxin A was associated with low testosterone levels in men.

Here are some steps you can take to reduce your exposure to toxins:

- Remove from your home synthetic air fresheners, candles, fragrance sprays, and cleaning products containing agents that are considered environmental toxins by the Environmental Working Group.
- Consider having your home professionally tested for mycotoxins. Both My Mold Detective and Pro-Lab have at-home kits you can purchase online.
- Consider environmental toxicity and mycotoxin testing.
- Avoid high-mercury fish and Atlantic fish, such as swordfish, tuna, and shark.
- Eat organic produce to avoid pesticide exposure whenever possible.
- Use natural pesticides such as vinegar, neem oil, chili pepper spray, essential oils, and diatomaceous earth in your home and garden.
- Support gut and liver health by eating plenty of fiber, dark leafy greens, brightly colored berries, and spices like turmeric, ginger, garlic, and cinnamon.
- Avoid tobacco use and drinking alcohol.
- Exercise for 30 to 50 minutes every day.
- Aim for seven to nine hours of sleep per night.
- Manage stress with meditation, warm baths, and teas.

How to Increase Testosterone

So let's say you've been tested and your testosterone is suboptimal or low. You want to increase your testosterone and reduce your anxiety at the same time. Here are some lifestyle changes to get you started:

- **REGULAR EXERCISE.** The best form of exercise for raising testosterone is resistance-based training such as lifting weights, doing yoga, or using exercise bands.
- **HERBAL SUPPLEMENTATION.** Certain herbs such as ashwagandha (*Withania somnifera*), fenugreek (*Trigonella foenum-graecum*), D-aspartic acid, and maca (*Lepidium meyenii*) have been studied for their effectiveness at boosting testosterone.
- **TESTOSTERONE REPLACEMENT THERAPY.** TRT is a medical treatment that can increase testosterone levels. It can be given in a variety of ways, but it has risks, including mood swings, acne, heart disease, stroke, sleep apnea, prostate cancer, liver damage, and blood clots. It should be used only under the supervision of a doctor.

High Testosterone

Symptoms of high testosterone levels can vary from person to person. Some people may experience no symptoms, while others may experience a number of them, as we saw in the Testosterone Self-Assessment Checklist.

Esme's diagnosis, polycystic ovary syndrome, is a hormonal disorder that we've referred to in a few sections in this book. There is some evidence that people with PCOS are more likely to experience anxiety than people without PCOS. The exact reason behind this link is not fully understood, but it is thought that hormonal imbalances, insulin resistance, and inflammation may play a role.

There are many different causes of high testosterone, for example medications, weight gain, excess stress, and other medical conditions such as congenital adrenal hyperplasia, and androgen-producing tumors.

How to Test Testosterone

Here are the tests I often order when I suspect someone has an imbalance in testosterone:

- **TOTAL TESTOSTERONE:** This is the total amount of testosterone in the blood.
- **FREE TESTOSTERONE:** This is the amount of testosterone that is not bound to proteins in the blood.
- **SEX HORMONE-BINDING GLOBULIN:** This is a protein that binds to testosterone and other androgens.
- **DIHYDROTESTOSTERONE:** This is a more potent form of testosterone.
- **ANDROSTENEDIONE:** This is a precursor to testosterone.
- **LUTEINIZING HORMONE:** This is a hormone that stimulates the production of testosterone in the ovaries.
- **FOLLICLE-STIMULATING HORMONE:** This is a hormone that stimulates the ovaries or testicles.

Do you have high testosterone? Don't worry, the next section was written for you.

How to Reduce Testosterone Naturally

If you have anxiety caused by high testosterone, there are great options for bringing your testosterone back down to optimal levels.

- **NUTRITION.** Eat a healthy diet that includes plenty of fruits, vegetables, and whole grains.
- **HERBAL MEDICINE.** Examples of potentially useful botanicals for reducing testosterone include: EGCG from green tea, licorice (*Glycyrrhiza glabra*), and chaste tree berry (*Vitex agnus-castus*). (Read more about them in Chapter 11.)
- **SLEEP.** Aim for eight to nine hours each night.
- **STRESS MANAGEMENT TECHNIQUES.** Yoga, meditation, and deep breathing can help to reduce stress and improve overall health and well-being.

TESTOSTERONE TL;DR

- Testosterone is made in the testes, ovaries, adrenal glands, skin, and gut.
- Low testosterone is associated with a greater tendency toward anxiety.
- When testosterone is low, the brain may be more sensitive to stress.
- Dietary gluten can cause lowered testosterone levels.

Esme

ESME WAS DIAGNOSED WITH POLYCYSTIC OVARY SYNDROME, A CONDItion that may be associated with too-high androgen levels, such as testosterone. PCOS can cause mood swings, irregular periods, difficulty getting pregnant, and weight gain. It can also interfere with insulin metabolism, which can lead to higher blood sugar levels.

POLYCYSTIC OVARY SYNDROME

PCOS	DESCRIPTION	
Symptoms	Irregular menstrual cycles, excess hair growth on body, male-pattern baldness, weight gain (especially around the abdomen), infertility, acne, oily skin, deepened voice, mood swings (including depression, panic, and anxiety), and fatigue	
Test findings	**TYPICAL FINDINGS:** • Follicle-stimulating hormone: low • Luteinizing hormone: normal or high • Testosterone: high • Estrogen: normal or high • Progesterone: normal or low • Insulin: high	**ESME'S FINDINGS:** • Follicle-stimulating hormone: low • Luteinizing hormone: low • Testosterone: high • Estrogen: low • Progesterone: low • Insulin: high • Blood sugar: normal • Cholesterol: high

PCOS	DESCRIPTION	
	• Blood sugar: normal or high • Cholesterol: high • Triglycerides: high • Anti-müllerian hormone (AMH): high	• Triglycerides: high • AMH: high
Ultrasound findings	**TYPICAL FINDINGS:** Ovaries: May be enlarged and have multiple cysts. They may also be cyst-free.	**ESME'S FINDINGS:** A reported history of ruptured cysts but no cyst formation at the time of her ultrasound.
Prognosis	The prognosis is excellent! PCOS responds quite well to changes in diet and lifestyle and to herbal remedies.	

FORTUNATELY THERE ARE A lot of wonderful treatments for PCOS. Esme's treatment plan included the following:

- **GOALS:**
  - Decrease testosterone
  - Increase estrogen and progesterone
  - Support blood sugar and insulin
  - Reduce cholesterol
  - Calm Chest and Gut Anxiety (subtype kapha) and improve mood
  - Stabilize blood sugar with metformin as an option; she opted to try diet and lifestyle changes first

- **DIET:** Esme followed the Panic Proof Diet outlined in Chapter 11. The most important changes she made were to add vegetables and whole grains and to limit processed foods, sugary drinks, and unhealthy fats such as hydrogenated oils found in many prepackaged foods.
- **MOVEMENT:** Esme made a commitment to walk 10,000 steps every day and use her resistance bands three times per week.
- **BOTANICAL TINCTURE:** Following the template outlined in

Chapter 11, we made the following tincture for Esme to take during the second half of her menstrual cycle:

- 40% chaste tree berry (*Vitex agnus-castus*), which is useful in certain types of PCOS; it can increase luteinizing hormone, estrogen, and progesterone and decrease testosterone.
- 30% motherwort (*Leonurus cardiaca*), which is useful in treating PCOS. It regulates menstrual cycles and calms both Chest Anxiety and Gut Anxiety.
- 25% vervain (*Verbena officinalis*), which is great for emotional distress from hormonal imbalances. It improves mood and insight.
- 5% cinnamon (*Cinnamomum verum*), which is blood sugar balancing, warming, driving, and synergizing.

- **SUPPLEMENTS:** Esme started omega-3 fatty acids (from fish oil), N-acetylcysteine, and D-chiro-inositol, an amino acid found in Happy Sleepy Powder that balances insulin and blood sugars, lowers androgens, and relieves anxiety and depression.
- **DETOXIFICATION:** Esme incorporated 16 hours of intermittent fasting into her routine once a week. Intermittent fasting, a dietary pattern that involves alternating periods of fasting and eating, has been shown to improve insulin and glucose metabolism, cholesterol levels, and neuroplasticity.
- **COUNSELING:** Esme agreed to do trauma-informed counseling, which included Parts Work. You can read a transcript from one of her Parts Work sessions in Chapter 10.

NEXT STEPS

Let's face it: Not all of us have access to root-cause testing, whether because it's not available in your area, or your doctor is unwilling to run testing, or it's cost prohibitive. For many, this is especially true for specialty testing such as hormone metabolite tests like DUTCH, or comprehensive stool testing, which insurance does not cover.

What are our next steps if we can't run root-cause testing?

Your body is naturally designed to heal. And while some tests are necessary and lifesaving (which is why you should always have a doctor on your team who has expert training in medicine and who you trust), functional specialty tests are a relatively new thing, and people were getting better long before they came into the picture. So can you.

Here's how: we go back to the basic tenets of health and let your body do what it does best.

- **REREAD THIS BOOK AND ENGAGE WITH THE PANIC PROOF COMMUNITY.** Every time you read this book; you'll pick up new bits of information. Be sure to check out my website and Instagram to stay involved, ask questions, and become part of a like-minded and supportive community.
- **GIVE THE BODY WHAT IT NEEDS.** Give it love, movement, detoxification, nutrients, fresh air, hugs, hydration, fiber, herbs, vitamins, a good cry, and rest. What else can you think of?
- **REMOVE OBSTACLES TO CURE.** What is getting in the way of your health? There are many possibilities here, such as chronic stress, poor nutrition, lack of support, or feeling disconnected spiritually (which we'll explore in more detail in Chapter 8).
- **MOVEMENT.** Hippocrates, the father of modern medicine, advocated walking and is credited with saying, "The best medicine is movement." When in doubt, do your best to move every single day. A great goal would be 30 minutes of exercise whether that be stretching, walking, or weight training.
- **REJUVENATION.** This is so key! Rejuvenation refers to nourishing your mind, body, and spirit. It could include meditation, spending time outside, laughing, drinking a delicious golden milk tea, getting a great night of sleep, or going to

your favorite yoga class. If it makes you feel alive, fresh, healthier, and vital, take time to incorporate it into your daily life.

In the next chapter, we are going to deep dive into the obstacles to cure. Are you ready?

HORMONES TL;DR

- Imbalances in hormones can cause panic and anxiety.
- Fluctuations in hormones can also cause panic and anxiety.
- Your hormones are strongly influenced by your gut microbiota.
- Toxicity and inflammation can interfere with your hormones, causing panic and anxiety.

PART III

How to Be Panic Proof

YOU MADE IT, WE'RE FINALLY HERE, AT PART III OF *PANIC PROOF.* Now that we've gotten all that science stuff out of the way, we get to dig into the fun part: the *how* for healing panic.

I love the gift of holistic medicine. I've witnessed real-life stories of transformation, and I can't wait for you to be next.

In the rest of this book, we are going to focus on practical advice on how to overcome panic. I'll guide you through everything you need to know, from identifying the obstacles that stand in your way of having a healthy relationship with your many "parts" to retraining your nervous system so it is poised to be Panic Proof. Chapter 9 includes a ton of bottom-up strategies for combating panic, and I'll help you zero in on which ones sound like the most fun, doable, and effective for you.

And then there's the goodness about herbal medicine. Seriously, my friend, this botanical apothecary is composed of the best jewels of wisdom passed down from my teachers, decades of research, and personal and clinical experience. It is such an honor and gift to share it with you. I know that this is a lot of information to digest, and I know that overcoming panic can be a challenging journey. But you've gotten this far, and the next chapter is all about shattering glass ceilings.

You're being armed with the right tools and support so that you can reclaim your life and live free from panic. Remember, it takes 90 to 120 days to create a new habit, so be patient, keep practicing, keep digging. You can do this.

I've got you. So let's get started!

8

OBSTACLES TO PANIC FREEDOM

Aria

WHEN ARIA, WHO HAD A PANIC ATTACK DURING SEX, ANSWERED my question about what was going on right around the time the panic struck her, she mentioned taking her Happy Pill to speed up her brain. I had a pretty good idea about one of her obstacles to becoming panic-free.

"Adderall gives me the *oomph* I need to get through the day. Without it, I feel brain-dead and exhausted."

I asked, "Have you ever taken Adderall and thought, 'Hey this is over-stimulating me a little bit more than I would like'?"

Aria nodded. "Definitely. My doctor gave me an emergency prescription for Xanax for exactly that reason—it calms me back down."

"It sounds kind of like a seesaw," I observed. "Adderall gives you a boost, but too much of it can be a problem, and so you need another medication, the Xanax, to calm your nervous system back down."

"What a mess." Aria held up her hands, demonstrating a scale. "Panic, zombie, panic, zombie."

"It's a vicious circle, but one you can get out of," I said. "Having the drive to go out of your comfort zone and take risks is part of what makes you who you are, and you are amazing. However, there are risks that can accompany your current set of tools."

"And it doesn't have to be a trade-off, panic versus zombie?"

"Exactly. It doesn't have to be a trade-off."

"So . . ." The corner of Aria's lip turned up in a rare half smile. "What I hear you saying is that I can still be a vivacious and sexy beast, and that I can do it without pills that end up landing me in hotel lobby bathrooms?"

I smiled back. "You interested?"

"Hell yes."

CUPS OF MARBLES

Have you ever wondered why some people seem to be more affected by stress than others? One way to think about this is to imagine that our ability to handle stress is like a cup. The size of the cup represents our mental bandwidth, or capacity to deal with stress. The water being poured into the cup represents stressors. The marbles in the cup represent our vulnerabilities. When the cup fills up, water starts overflowing, which represents symptoms, such as panic.

Everyone's cup is different. Some people have a larger cup, which means they can tolerate more stress before they start to experience overflow. Other people have a smaller cup.

The marbles in our cup—i.e., our vulnerabilities—come from a variety of sources across five domains: lifestyle and habits, biological, psychological, social and environmental, and spiritual.

- **LIFESTYLE AND HABIT** marbles include diet, exercise, sleep, substance use, and self-care. People who use substances to cope with stress may also be more likely to experience panic attacks. On the other hand, people who engage in regular self-care activities, such as meditation, yoga, or spending time in nature, may be more resilient to stress.
- **BIOLOGICAL** marbles include genetics, health conditions, and environmental toxicities. For example, people with certain genetic predispositions may be more likely to experience panic attacks. People with chronic health conditions, such as heart disease or diabetes, may also be more vulnerable to stress.

- **PSYCHOLOGICAL** marbles include things like trauma, neglect, abuse, and a lack of coping skills. These can lead to panic attacks through learned patterns of thinking and behavior, negative beliefs, and a lack of sense of personal agency.
- **SOCIAL AND ENVIRONMENTAL** marbles include things like social support, relationships, work environment, culture, and access to resources. People who lack social support or who endure marginalization or discrimination may be more likely to experience panic attacks.
- **SPIRITUAL** marbles include things like beliefs, values, and sense of meaning in life. For example, people who have a strong spiritual foundation may be more resilient to stress. People who have lost their sense of meaning in life may be more vulnerable to panic attacks.

It is important to note that the five domains of vulnerabilities are not mutually exclusive. For example, a person's biological vulnerabilities may be exacerbated *or* mitigated by their lifestyle and habits. For example, a person with a genetic predisposition to anxiety may be more likely to experience panic attacks if they also have a poor diet, don't get enough exercise, and use substances to cope with stress.

In the sections that follow, I'm going to touch on some of the more important obstacles to cure.

LIFESTYLE AND HABITS

Here are some tips for looking at your habits and identifying what changes need to be made:

- **KEEP A JOURNAL.** Write down your daily activities and how you are feeling. This can help you to identify patterns in your behavior and emotions.
- **PAY ATTENTION TO YOUR THOUGHTS AND FEELINGS.** Notice when you are feeling stressed, anxious, or depressed. What are you doing at the time? What are you thinking about?

- **TALK TO SOMEONE YOU TRUST.** Ask them for their observations about your habits and how they are affecting you.

Personally, I find that I'm most likely to engage in unhealthy habits when I'm stressed or feeling overwhelmed. I tend to zone out on my phone, eat more carbs, and avoid exercise. When I notice that I'm starting to fall into these patterns, I try to take a step back and identify what is causing me stress. Once I know that, I can go back and recommit to healthy habits that will get me back on track.

There are plenty of resources out there for creating healthy habits, such as getting enough sleep, eating a healthy diet, exercising regularly, spending time in nature, connecting with loved ones, and practicing relaxation and mindfulness. But if you're anything like me, you need something that is a little more specific and a lot more tailored to anxiety relief.

My top recommended panic-stopping habits:

- **BODY CHECK-INS.** Make it a habit to pay attention to your body. By mindfully checking in with your body, you are strengthening the relationship between your "upper brain" and your body. This is important because it trains your brain to have more awareness, agency, and control over your physical reactions, and checking in often will give you the opportunity to identify signs that you are shifting out of balance, long before panic starts. Check out Chapter 2 to read more about this!
- **BREATHWORK.** Your breath is your most powerful and immediate road to your autonomic nervous system. Learning how to use your breath to regulate your nervous system takes time, but it works, and it's something you always have with you.
- **TALK TO YOUR PARTS.** Remember, you are made up of many different parts, each with its own unique thoughts, feelings, sensations, and behaviors. When these parts are in conflict, or if their needs are not being met, it can lead to anxiety

and even panic. Check in every day with your parts to identify signs that they are struggling long before they start to produce symptoms. Learn more in Chapter 10.

- **MOVE YOUR BLOOD AND LYMPH:** Your blood carries oxygen and nutrients to your cells, and your lymph helps remove toxins. When your blood and lymph aren't moving freely, they can become stagnant, which can lead to inflammation and anxiety. Exercise and hydrotherapy, such as alternating hot and cold showers, are great ways to move your blood and lymph, and they also have other benefits for anxiety relief, such as reducing stress and reducing your risk of panic.
- **HAVE A BOWEL MOVEMENT EVERY MORNING:** Check out the podcast I did with Hadlee Garrison called *The One About Poop* (Episode 79), and you'll learn all about how emptying your bowels daily supports gut health, detoxifies your body, and relaxes the nervous system. Learn more in the Environmental Detox Protocol in Chapter 11.

Are there any personal habits that are causing you difficulty? What about habits that you think you could incorporate into your daily routine that might be helpful? Write your ideas in the space provided below.

Panic-Producing Habits

e.g., phone use, screen time, isolation, irregular sleep, nicotine use, drinking, overworking

____

____

____

Panic-Preventing Habits

e.g., mindfulness, exercise, nutrition, counseling, hydrating, pooping, dry skin brushing

____

____

____

BIOLOGICAL OBSTACLES

Think of your body like a vehicle. (Mine is a super-cute 1960 Land Rover Series II painted moss green, but yours can be whatever you want!)

In order to get you where you need to go, your vehicle needs to be in working order: fuel in the tank, spark plugs electrified, and transmission fluid in place. If at any point one or more of these important components becomes compromised, at best the car will cough and sputter along toward its destination.

An excellent mechanic can help you identify any hiccups in your car's engine and what to do to get it in tip-top shape so you can be on your way. Let's learn how to be the best human-body mechanics and dive into some of the most common culprits getting in the way of your body running smoothly.

Nutrition

You've probably heard that what you eat can affect your mental health and well-being. And it's true!

Good nutrition is key for keeping inflammation in check, protecting your cells from damage, and promoting the growth of new brain cells. The nutrients in your food also help regulate your hormones, neurotransmitters, and gut bacteria.

As you read this section, take note of how your nutrition stacks up. If you suspect diet might be an obstacle, jot down some notes on changes you're committing to, starting today.

THREE GENERAL NUTRITION GUIDELINES

- Guideline 1: Reduce inflammation.
- Guideline 2: Load up on nutrients.
- Guideline 3: Nourish your gut microbiome.

LET'S GO THROUGH THEM one by one.

Guideline 1: Reduce Inflammation

A natural response of the body to injury or infection, inflammation is also at the root of almost all chronic diseases. Disease causes inflammation, and inflammation causes disease. It's both the chicken and the egg.

Inflammation can influence our immune system, metabolism, sleep, stress response, cognitive function, memory, mood, and more. There are a number of ways that inflammation can affect mental health, which is seen in Immune System Anxiety. For example, inflammation can damage the hippocampus, a part of the brain that is important for memory and learning. This can lead to cognitive problems and difficulty thinking clearly. Inflammation can also disrupt sleep patterns, impair the body's ability to produce serotonin and dopamine, and cause the release of other anxiety-provoking neurochemicals, such as histamine.

Inflammation can also damage the gut lining, which can lead to toxins and bacteria "leaking out" and entering the bloodstream, which can then interfere with blood sugar and hormone metabolism. It can even ultimately compromise the blood-brain barrier, resulting in toxins and pathogens entering into the brain itself.

When in doubt, bring inflammation down.

TIPS TO GET YOU STARTED:

- **IDENTIFY THE ROOT CAUSES OF YOUR INFLAMMATION.** They may include imbalances in gut flora; eating the Standard American Diet; overworking; under-resting; experiencing excess emotional, social, or environmental stress; and exposure to environmental toxicity.

- **EAT AN ANTI-INFLAMMATORY DIET.** This means eating plenty of fruits, vegetables, and whole grains; avoiding processed foods and sugary drinks; and limiting caffeine and alcohol.
- **SUPPLEMENT WITH INFLAMMATION-REDUCING NUTRIENTS AND BOTANICALS,** such as omega-3 fatty acids, vitamin D, and ginger.
- **SUPPORT YOUR BODY'S NATURAL ABILITY TO DETOXIFY.** Eat liver-boosting foods such as turmeric and Brussels sprouts, support histamine detoxification (see Chapter 6), do dry skin brushing, be sure you have a bowel movement every day, and stay hydrated.
- **GET REGULAR EXERCISE.** Exercise is a great way to reduce inflammation, promote blood flow, support sweating and detoxification, and improve mental health.
- **MANAGE STRESS.** Stress can contribute to inflammation, so it is important to retrain your nervous system so it's poised for calm and not stress (see Chapter 9).
- **GET ENOUGH SLEEP.** Getting enough sleep is important for reducing inflammation and improving mental health.

FOODS AND INFLAMMATION

FOODS THAT DECREASE INFLAMMATION	FOODS THAT INCREASE INFLAMMATION
• Brightly colored berries like blueberries • Wild Alaskan fatty fish like salmon or tuna • Green leafy veggies like kale and spinach • Nuts and seeds high in fiber and fat • Turmeric and ginger spices • 70 percent dark chocolate	• Smoked foods • Red meat like beef, pork, or lamb • Processed meat like bacon and hot dogs • Fried foods like doughnuts and french fries • Refined grains like white bread and pasta • Sugary drinks including "sugar free" drinks

FOODS THAT DECREASE INFLAMMATION	FOODS THAT INCREASE INFLAMMATION
• Cruciferous veggies like broccoli • Whole grains like quinoa and brown rice • Quercetin-rich foods like onion and cilantro	• Trans fats (hydrogenated oils) • Energy drinks (Red Bull, Monster) • Alcohol

LAB TESTING FOR INFLAMMATION

There are many tests that screen for the root causes of inflammation, such as the Organic Acids Test (OAT), stool analysis, environmental toxicity tests, and basic blood tests such as white blood cell count, C-reactive protein, erythrocyte sedimentation rate, homocysteine, ferritin, and others based on your unique needs.

Guideline 2: Load Up on Nutrients

A healthy diet rich in vitamins, minerals, oils, fats, and spices is essential for a healthy brain and body.

Sadly, due to soil depletion, nutrient density has declined over the years. This means you may be eating the right foods and still not be getting the nutrients you need. The most common nutrient deficiencies I see in my clients are deficiencies of iron, B vitamins, vitamin D, omega-3 fatty acids, and minerals.

NUTRIENT DEFICIENCIES THAT CAN CAUSE ANXIETY

You may be at an increased risk of anxiety if you're deficient in:

- **IRON.** Iron plays an important role in how your body makes serotonin, dopamine, and adrenaline. Research suggests a connection between anxiety and depression and low iron levels.
- **B VITAMINS.** B vitamins such as B6 and B12 are involved in the production of neurotransmitters like serotonin and dopamine, which play a role in mood regulation.
- **MAGNESIUM.** Magnesium is important for relaxation and the functioning of the nervous system.
- **VITAMIN D.** Vitamin D is important for overall health. Low

levels of vitamin D have been linked to increased anxiety and depression risk.

- **OMEGA-3 FATTY ACIDS.** Omega-3 fatty acids are important for brain health, and they have shown promise in reducing anxiety symptoms.
- **ZINC.** Research links low zinc with increased anxiety.
- **ANTIOXIDANTS.** Antioxidants are important for anxiety because they can help to reduce inflammation in the body.
- **SELENIUM.** Selenium's role in health goes beyond the thyroid. Studies associate low selenium levels with increased anxiety.

Let's expand on some of these nutrients in a bit more detail.

IRON: THE ESSENTIAL MINERAL FOR YOUR BODY AND MIND

"GIRL, I NEED YOUR ADVICE." JESSICA, A GOOD FRIEND OF MINE WHO was seven months pregnant, looked exhausted. "I'm a hot mess right now."

"What's going on?" I asked.

"My restless legs are making me crazy. I can't stop moving them, and so I'm panicky, not sleeping, and my skin feels like it's crawling and itches."

"What did your OB/GYN say?"

"She ordered these." Jessica handed me a piece of paper containing her lab results. "And it looks to me like my iron is low. I called her office, but it's been a week, and no one is getting back to me."

I looked at her labs and immediately identified the likely culprit. "You're in phase three of iron depletion," I said. "Which means your iron has dropped so low, you're borderline anemic. Low ferritin can cause all the symptoms you're experiencing."

"What do I do?" she asked.

"Well, for starters, you have to get your iron back up. That will help you feel better, and protect both you and your baby, especially as you prepare for delivery."

"But I've been taking a prenatal that contains iron."

"Sometimes that's not enough," I said, "which appears to be your case. You can increase your iron dose, try different forms of iron to see if one works better, and, because your levels are so low, your OB might recommend that you get an iron infusion, which is basically iron in an IV and works much more quickly."

"Honestly. I'm so tired of feeling this way, I'm game for anything that'll help," Jessica said.

YOU NEED IRON

You need iron like you need water, and sunshine, and oh yeah, oxygen.

A fun fact about iron is that even if you do not have anemia, low iron levels can contribute to panic and anxiety. This is, in part, because iron is needed for carrying oxygen throughout the body, including to your brain. Iron also helps to regulate your neurotransmitters. When iron levels are low, your brain does not get enough nourishing oxygen, and your neurotransmitter function may go out of balance, both of which can result in greater feelings of anxiety and panic.

The European Society of Cardiology guidelines define iron deficiency as a serum ferritin level below 100 ng/mL. If you're like many of my clients, you'll find that your ferritin is below that number in your most recent blood test.

If iron levels are not replenished, iron insufficiency can then develop into iron deficiency anemia, which the World Health Organization defines as blood hemoglobin levels below 12–13 g/dL.

SIGNS OF LOW IRON

- Anxiety, panic, insomnia, depression, irritability
- Fatigue
- Shortness of breath
- Pale skin
- Dark circles under the eyes
- Cold hands and feet
- Hair loss
- Brittle nails
- Heart palpitations
- Headaches
- Itching and crawling of skin
- Joint pain
- Pica (craving nonfood substances like ice, dirt, or paper)

BE PROACTIVE!

The unfortunate part, however, is that many doctors do not do iron testing unless something abnormal shows up on someone's CBC basic blood test. Typically, a CBC is run first, and when the results do not show anemia, doctors often won't order the extra iron panel. This is sort of akin to "wait until it gets really bad and then we'll do something about it." In the meantime, you're struggling unnecessarily with symptoms, as Jessica was.

The take-home here is that even if your doctor has reviewed your basic blood work and assured you that you are not anemic, yet you are experiencing anxiety, it is important to look at an entire iron panel, especially ferritin.

So let's explore what is included in an iron panel and what each test means.

IRON TESTING 101

A full iron panel should include serum iron, total iron-binding capacity (TIBC), transferrin, %Sat, and serum ferritin.

DECODING YOUR IRON PANEL

TEST	DESCRIPTION	NORMAL RANGE	LOW	HIGH
Serum Iron	Unbound iron in the serum (blood)	38–169 mcg/dL	<38 mcg/dL	>169 mcg/dL
Total Iron Binding Capacity (TIBC)	The body's ability to bind iron	250–450 mcg/dL	<250 mcg/dL	>450 mcg/dL
Transferrin	The protein that transfers iron throughout the body	215–380 mg/dL	<215 mg/dL	<380 mg/dL

TEST	DESCRIP-TION	NORMAL RANGE	LOW	HIGH
Transferrin Saturation (%Sat)	Percentage of serum iron that is bound to transferrin	15–55%	<15%	>55%
Serum Ferritin	Storage Iron	30–300 mg/L	Many labs still say: <30 mg/L Updated value: <100 mg/L	>299 mg/L

Note: Having too much iron can also be problematic. If you have high ferritin levels, it is important to determine the cause, such as high inflammation or high stored iron. Once the root cause is identified, you can begin treatment to lower your ferritin levels while addressing the underlying condition.

IRON SUPPLEMENTATION: A GAME-CHANGER FOR MANY

There are a number of ways to treat iron deficiency, including eating iron-rich foods such as red meat, poultry, fish, beans, and lentils, and taking iron supplements.

Iron supplements come in both heme and nonheme forms. Heme iron is the more easily absorbable form of iron, but it is found only in animal products such as oysters, beef liver, and sardines. Nonheme iron is found in plant foods like whole grains, nuts, legumes, leafy greens, and dark chocolate, but it is less bioavailable and should be taken with vitamin C for absorption.

HOW TO CALCULATE YOUR IRON DOSAGE

The amount of iron you should take will depend on your individual needs. You can use this formula to calculate your iron dosage:

- Nonheme iron: 5 mg/kg of body weight
- Heme iron: 2 mg/kg of body weight

To convert your weight from pounds to kilograms, divide your weight by 2.2. For example, if you weigh 128 pounds, your weight in kilograms would be 58.18.

To calculate your nonheme iron dosage, multiply your weight in kilograms by 5. For example, if you weigh 58.18 kg, your nonheme iron dosage would be 290.9 mg.

To calculate your heme iron dosage, multiply your weight in kilograms by 2. For example, if you weigh 58.18 kg, your heme iron dosage would be 116.36 mg.

TIPS FOR TAKING IRON SUPPLEMENTS

- Take iron supplements with vitamin-C-rich foods. This will help to improve absorption.
- Avoid taking iron supplements with calcium, tea, coffee, or dairy products. These all can interfere with absorption.
- Start with a low dose of iron supplements and gradually increase as needed.
- Monitor your iron levels regularly to make sure they are increasing safely. Stop all iron supplements 48 to 72 hours before your blood test, and consider testing every three to six months to ensure that your levels are increasing.

B VITAMINS

B vitamins are essential for a healthy nervous system and balanced mood.

B VITAMINS FOR PREVENTING ANXIETY AND PANIC:

- **B9.** Folate is important for serotonin production. The best form of folate for most is methylfolate, but people with MTHFR mutations may do better with folinic acid. Try to avoid folic acid.
- **B6.** Pyridoxine is also important for serotonin production and can help reduce anxiety symptoms. The best form of B6 is pyridoxal 5-phosphate.
- **B12.** Cobalamin is needed for homocysteine metabolism,

DNA production, and nervous system health. For those with MTHFR mutations, talk with your doctor; that being said, when in doubt, I start with hydroxocobalamin.

- **B1.** Thiamine is important for histamine detoxification. The best form of thiamine is benfotiamine.
- **B3.** Niacin is important for energy production, skin health, and brain function. The best form of niacin for most individuals is niacinamide, but some people may prefer inositol hexaniacinate to avoid the flushing sensation.

VITAMIN D

Vitamin D is a superhero nutrient that keeps your bones strong, your immune system in peak condition, and your mental well-being on point. Often called the "sunshine vitamin," we get most of our vitamin D when our skin is exposed to the sunlight. We can also get vitamin D from certain foods, such as fatty fish, egg yolks, and fortified milk.

If you are experiencing panic attacks, it is important to get your vitamin D levels checked. The blood test for vitamin D is called 25-hydroxyvitamin D total, or vitamin D 25-OH total. A level of 80 to 100 nmol/L is considered optimal for most people.

If your vitamin D levels are low, you may need to take a supplement. The most common vitamin D supplement is cholecalciferol. A dosage of 1500 to 2000 IU per day is a good place to start.

For best results, vitamin D should be taken with other nutrients, such as vitamins A and K, calcium, magnesium, and a fatty food such as an avocado. These nutrients help the body absorb and use vitamin D.

OMEGA-3 FATTY ACIDS

Omega-3 fatty acids are essential fats that can help reduce anxiety. Studies have shown that people with anxiety often have low levels of omega-3 fatty acids in their blood. Eating wild Alaskan fatty fish regularly and supplementing with omega-3s can help reduce anxiety symptoms, such as restlessness, racing thoughts, and panic attacks.

Two types of omega-3 fatty acids are particularly important for mental health: eicosapentaenoic acid (EPA) and docosahexaenoic acid (DHA). Both EPA and DHA are found in fatty fish, such as salmon, tuna, and mackerel, or plant-based spirulina or algae oil (from algae). I typically recommend at least 500 mg of EPA and 500 mg of DHA (combined total of 1000 mg or 1 g).

When it comes to adding fish or fish oil supplements to your protocol, be mindful about the source of the fish. Watch out for fish oils that are rancid or come from sources that are not screening for mercury, polychlorinated biphenyls (PCBs), or dioxins, the latter two of which are industrial chemical by-products.

FISH OIL VS. COD LIVER OIL VS. KRILL OIL

Fish oil, cod liver oil, and krill oil all have their own advantages and disadvantages. Fish oil is the most common type of omega-3 supplement, but it may contain mercury and other pollutants. Cod liver oil is a good source of vitamins A and D, but it may also contain high levels of mercury, PCBs, and dioxins. Krill oil tends to have fewer toxicants, but there are concerns about overharvesting threatening the species that consume it for food, including whales.

The best type of omega-3 supplement for you will depend on your individual needs and preferences.

MINERALS

Some of the most important minerals for mental health include magnesium, calcium, zinc, and potassium. These minerals can help to prevent panic attacks by regulating mood, reducing inflammation, and protecting the brain from damage.

Unfortunately, due to conventional farming practices, the soil our food grows in is often depleted of minerals. Additionally, many water filtration systems remove essential minerals naturally present in water. Therefore, it's especially important to ensure you get enough nutrients, either through your diet or supplements.

FOODS THAT ARE HIGH IN MINERALS:

- Dark leafy greens, such as spinach and kale, pumpkin seeds, sunflower seeds, and chia seeds are all great sources of magnesium.
- Yogurt, cheeses, and leafy green vegetables, such as broccoli and bok choy, are excellent sources of calcium.
- Oysters are the best source of zinc, but if you can't get down with the slime factor, consider kidney beans and lentils for their zinc-boosting abilities.
- Bananas, leafy greens, and sweet potatoes are good sources of potassium.

My favorite mineral hack is to put a pinch of pink Himalayan sea salt in my drinking water. Pink Himalayan sea salt contains a variety of minerals including magnesium, calcium, potassium, iron, zinc, selenium, and copper, as well as some lesser-known minerals such as lithium orotate, strontium, and molybdenum.

HOW CAN I TEST MY VITAMIN AND MINERAL LEVELS?

Blood micronutrient testing can be a useful tool for measuring the levels of vitamins, minerals, and other nutrients in your blood. However, it is important to note that not all micronutrient tests are created equal. For example, many nutrients, such as vitamin C and the B vitamins, are metabolized very quickly by the body. This means that a blood test may give you a snapshot of your nutrient levels only at a specific point in time. Additionally, the results of a blood test can be affected by a number of factors, such as diet, medications, and underlying health conditions.

LAB TESTS FOR MICRONUTRIENTS

Micronutrient tests to consider:

- Complete blood count (CBC): can indirectly screen for deficiencies in iron, vitamin B12, and folate

- Total 25-hydroxyvitamin D: measures vitamin D levels
- Methylmalonic acid (MMA): screens for vitamin B12
- Iron panel: screens for serum iron, TIBC, ferritin, and %Transferrin
- Omega-3 fatty acids: measures levels of omega-3 fatty acids in the blood
- Red blood cell (RBC) magnesium: measures magnesium levels in the body. It is considered to be more accurate than plasma magnesium because RBC magnesium is less affected by short-term changes in magnesium intake or status.

Guideline 3: Nourish Your Gut Microbiome

We talk a lot about nourishing the gut microbiome—the collection of microbes, including bacteria, fungi, viruses, and their genes, that naturally live on and in our bodies—and supporting the growth of health-boosting microbes (the microbiota) in Chapter 5. Here are the three most important ways you can do so:

- Eat more fiber, such as whole grains and leafy greens.
- Eat probiotic-rich foods, such as yogurt and kimchi.
- Evacuate your bowels daily.

Genetics and Panic

Knowing about our genes can help us understand our risks for developing certain mental health symptoms. If you have a long family history of panic and anxiety, you can take proactive steps to reduce your risks. And epigenetics, the study of how our genes are turned on and off, can help you to zero in on the precise steps that will likely work the best for you.

Two of the biggest influencers of our epigenetics are trauma and stress. Identifying a genetic predisposition to panic through epigenetic testing can enable us to develop targeted treatments, in addition to trauma work, that can effectively address anxiety and panic at their root.

While there are an estimated 100,000 genes in the human body, I typically zero in on genes that appear to specifically influence histamine, dopamine, serotonin, folate, glutathione, and S-Adenosylmethionine (SAM).

GENETICS AND MENTAL HEALTH

CHEMICAL	GENES I LOOK FOR	MORE ABOUT THESE GENES
Histamine	DAO NAT2 MAO-A and B	Histamine is as stimulating as adrenaline and can be a factor in panic. Learn more in Chapter 7.
Dopamine	DRD2 COMT MAO-A and MAO-B	Too much dopamine is associated with anxiety and paranoia. Learn more in Chapter 6.
Serotonin	TPH HTR MAO-A and MAO-B	Serotonin plays a role in anxiety. Learn more in Chapter 6.
Folate	MTHFR SLC19A1 DHFR	Folate (B9) is important for neurotransmitter production. Low levels and certain genetic mutations may increase anxiety risk.
Glutathione	CBS SOD2 and SOD3 GSTP	Glutathione is an antioxidant that protects the body from free radicals and regulates neurotransmitters. Low glutathione levels are associated with anxiety.
SAM	MTR and MTRR PEMT PON1 and PON2	SAM is important for neurotransmitters. Low SAM levels and genetic mutations may increase anxiety risk.

The world of genetics is like Mary Poppins's bag: endlessly fascinating and endlessly complex. If you'd like to know more about genetics and health, including testing, check out the resources I have included in Appendix B.

David

DAVID STARED AT HIS TEST RESULTS. "SO I HAVE A GENE MUTATION that makes it hard for my body to process folate," he said. "Which could explain why I've been having problems with my mood and headaches."

"Yes, that's right," I said. "The C677T MTHFR gene mutation can also have a negative impact on your gut health if you don't get the support your body needs."

"What kind of support are we talking about?" David asked.

"There are a lot of different combinations of mutations and types of mutations that require different treatments," I explained. "But for the most part, your other genes look pretty good. We're going to focus on supporting this C677T mutation. As you said, this type of mutation makes it difficult for your body to convert folate into its active form, methylfolate. Our next steps will involve a trial of methylated B vitamins and seeing how you feel. We can also assess how your body is responding in real time by measuring your blood levels of homocysteine."

"We ran homocysteine before," David remembered, "and mine was high."

"That's possibly a factor behind why your body is releasing excessive amounts of cortisol," I said. "Homocysteine is inflammatory, and one of cortisol's jobs is to reduce inflammation."

David nodded thoughtfully. "And high cortisol causes anxiety and anger."

"In some people, yes," I said.

"So . . . this genetic thing may have been causing my symptoms this whole time," David said. "I wish I had known forty-six years ago."

"I hear you," I said. "The good news is that we have more information about what might possibly be contributing to your symptoms now, and we can start to address them."

THIS IS EXACTLY WHY it's important to look for obstacles to cure. If you, like David, have been struggling with what feels like a moving target of symptoms and ever-shifting treatments, it likely means that you're missing some data. Maybe you and your trusted clinical team haven't found it yet, maybe you haven't run the right testing, or maybe the right testing hasn't been developed yet. Or perhaps you have the right tests but the solutions are all wrong.

Medications That Can Cause or Amplify Anxiety

It is important to know about your medications, including the potential side effects, so that you can be aware of any problems that may arise. Some medications, or medication interactions, can cause anxiety. In that case, it is important to identify this obstacle so that you can talk with your prescriber about changing the medication or dosage or finding other treatment options.

COMMON MEDICATIONS THAT CAN CAUSE ANXIETY:

- Antidepressants, such as selective serotonin reuptake inhibitors (SSRIs) and tricyclic antidepressants (TCAs)
- Stimulants or medications for AD(H)D, such as Adderall and Ritalin
- Corticosteroids, such as prednisone and hydrocortisone
- Thyroid medications, such as levothyroxine and desiccated thyroid
- Asthma medications, such as albuterol and budesonide
- Decongestants, such as pseudoephedrine and phenylephrine
- Caffeine, found in some over-the-counter pain relievers such as Excedrin

My favorite resource for medications and medication interactions is Drugs.com.

Toxicity and Panic

Environmental toxins are chemicals and other substances that are present in the air, water, food, and other parts of our environment. When these toxins enter the body, they can disrupt the normal functioning of the nervous system and other bodily systems, leading to a range of health problems, including panic.

We are all exposed to toxins, but the key is how efficiently our body is able to detoxify. Recall the marble analogy from Chapter 8. Marbles represent our vulnerabilities to symptoms, which can include exposure to toxins. Below is a quick self-assessment checklist for generally screening the likelihood that your symptoms may be associated with environmental toxicity.

ENVIRONMENTAL TOXICITY CHECKLIST

Instructions: Check the box(es) that relate to you, and write your total score in the space provided.

- ❑ You use nicotine or are exposed to secondhand smoke (cigarette, vape, chew, gum, patch, etc.).
- ❑ You use candles, perfumes, dryer sheets, or other scented fresheners.
- ❑ You live in a new home or have remodeled in the last five years.
- ❑ You or your neighbors use pesticides, herbicides, and other pest control chemicals.
- ❑ You have been exposed to mold, water damage, or musty buildings.
- ❑ You eat food from plastic containers (takeout, storage containers).
- ❑ You eat farmed fish (as opposed to wild Alaskan freshwater fish).
- ❑ You regularly consume (nonorganic) animal products.
- ❑ You get your nails done, wear cosmetics, go to the salon, and/or use nonnatural products.
- ❑ You have silver fillings in your teeth (or have had them removed recently).

TOTAL: ____/10

SCORING:

1–3: Low likelihood that environmental toxicity may be worth exploring.

4–6: Moderate likelihood that environmental toxicity may be worth exploring.
7–10: High likelihood that environmental toxicity may be worth exploring.

While a score on a checklist is not a diagnostic alternative to a full workup and testing, it can help you to zero in on where you might want to search for obstacles to your healing. If you scored >4 in the table above, you would likely benefit from further exploration in environmental toxicity and your health.

Here are the five most common categories of toxins associated with panic and anxiety:

TOXINS AND ANXIETY

TOXIN	EFFECTS ON ANXIETY
Heavy metals	Lead, mercury, arsenic, cadmium, and other heavy metals can cause anxiety, panic, and autonomic arousal.
Solvents	Benzene, toluene, and xylene can cause anxiety, panic, and autonomic arousal.
Mycotoxins	Mycotoxins (which are produced by mold) like aflatoxins, ochratoxin A, and fumonisins can cause anxiety.
Organophosphates	Organophosphates, which are used in certain types of pesticides and herbicides like Roundup, can cause anxiety.
Phosphonates	The phosphonate known as glyphosate is the most widely used herbicide in the world. It can cause anxiety by triggering inflammation in the brain, and it interferes with the neurotransmitters dopamine, noradrenaline, and serotonin.

Charlotte

WHEN CHARLOTTE'S THYROID TESTING CAME BACK REVEALING THAT she had autoimmune hyperthyroidism, we did deeper digging to find out why. The immune system doesn't attack the thyroid just for the fun of it. Whenever I see autoimmunity show up on a test result, the following root causes come to mind:

- **UNHEALTHY DIET.** Looking into someone's diet for foods and beverages that contain preservatives, artificial ingredients, dyes, hydrogenated oils, chemicals, caking agents, metals, organophosphates, glyphosates, and other harmful substances
- **FOOD REACTIVITIES.** Testing for celiac disease, IgG, and IgE antibodies
- **TOXIN OVERLOAD.** Testing for metals and nonmetals
- **GUT IMBALANCES.** Testing for imbalances or diseases in the gut, such as dysbiosis of yeast, bacteria, or other pathogens
- **NUTRIENT DEFICIENCIES.** Screening for deficiencies in nutrients that are involved in the immune system and, in Charlotte's case, in thyroid health, such as vitamin D, iron, iodine, and zinc

Because Charlotte was so mindful about her health, she was one of the last people I would have imagined developing environmental toxicity. But even if we make healthy choices, we live in a toxic world. And depending on our body's ability to effectively detoxify, some of us are at higher risk of accumulating toxins than others.

Keeping this in mind, I gave Charlotte my Environmental Toxicity Checklist. She checked boxes associated with the following:

- She had her silver amalgams removed recently.
- She was living in a home built within the last five years.
- She used soy candles. (Just because it's soy, doesn't mean it's better for you.)
- Her family sometimes took out food to go in plastic or Styrofoam containers.
- She grew up in a home with a parent who smoked cigarettes (even though they smoked outside and not indoors).

Based on the checklist results, Charlotte decided to do environmental toxicity screening in addition to a few other tests. It's a good thing she did.

Her results revealed high levels of many environmental toxins, but the most concerning was that she was in the 95th percentile for a chemical metabolite called perchlorate, which is found in fireworks, fertilizers, and some nonorganic contaminated foods such as eggs, milk products, and some fruits. Research has shown this chemical to be associated with autoimmune thyroid disease.

Here's what Charlotte did:

- She installed a reverse osmosis water treatment system in her house to remove perchlorate and other contaminants.
- She did the Panic Proof Environmental Detox Protocol (in Chapter 11).
- She purchased minerals to remineralize her water and aid in detoxification.
- She started taking a botanical tincture that contained herbs that aid in the treatment of hyperthyroidism, such as lemon balm (*Melissa officinalis*), bugleweed (*Lycopus europaeus*), and motherwort (*Leonurus cardiaca*). Her protocol also included immunomodulating herbs to support and balance the immune system (which, depending on the particular substance, works by increasing or decreasing activity of immune cells as needed), including cordyceps (*Cordyceps sinensis*). Her tincture also contained relaxing nervines passionflower (*Passiflora incarnata*) and lavender (*Lavandula officinalis*).

Charlotte's endocrinologist gave her four days to try her holistic protocol before recommending a more aggressive treatment. Charlotte, true to her two-feet-forward nature, dove into her holistic protocol with gusto.

Within three days she was feeling significantly better. At the end of the week, she retested her thyroid numbers and antibodies, and they were dropping.

Her endocrinologist agreed to watch and wait and gave her another week. When she called for a follow-up, feeling even better than before, her doctor agreed to retest her numbers in six weeks but advised her to call sooner if she needed anything from her.

Charlotte never needed to call her endocrinologist back. The last time I talked with her, she was living her best life.

What's Next?

It would be amazing if we could live in a world with clean air, water, and food, but unfortunately, we are all exposed to toxins in our daily lives. The good news is that our bodies can detoxify more effectively when we're healthy and resilient.

Getting your body tested for toxic substances like organophosphates, glyphosate, mycotoxins, solvents, and heavy metals can be a helpful way to assess your body's overall toxic burden. By retesting periodically, you can also see if any detox protocols you're following are working effectively.

You can learn more about each of these toxins and gain access to testing education in my Holistic Wellness Collective. I also recommend checking out the resources listed in Appendix B.

BIOLOGICAL OBSTACLES TL;DR

- Certain medications and supplements can be obstacles to anxiety healing.
- People with certain genes may be more predisposed to experience panic.
- Imbalances in neurotransmitters, such as serotonin and norepinephrine, may also cause anxiety and panic.
- Medical conditions, such as thyroid problems and heart disease, can trigger anxiety and panic attacks.

PSYCHOLOGICAL OBSTACLES

Feeling stuck in your fight against anxiety? Hidden internal obstacles might be holding you back, both mentally and emotionally. Here are ten of the most common ways these obstacles may manifest:

- **AVOIDANCE BEHAVIOR.** When you're feeling overwhelmed, do you feel the urge to avoid situations or triggers that make you more anxious? Remember Matthew, who had the traumatic bowel incident during childhood? This is what he did.

But the more he avoided the situation, the worse his anxiety got and the smaller his world became. Avoidance might provide temporary relief, but it also prevents you from reclaiming your agency and having experiences that challenge anxiety's messages.

- **MIND-BODY DISCONNECT.** Many anxiety sufferers are highly intelligent and thoughtful people. But these same people tend to be dissociated from their bodies. Do you ever feel like you're ignoring physical sensations of stress or anxiety? Remember, what we resist will persist, and what we deny will amplify.
- **LACK OF SELF-CARE.** What is your self-care regimen like? Do you take enough time to tend to your own needs? Poor self-care habits, such as neglecting exercise, sleep, and nutrition, can exacerbate anxiety symptoms.
- **LACK OF COPING SKILLS.** When panic strikes, do you feel equipped with skills to help you be in the feeling? Without effective coping skills, we often resort to quick fixes, which may help in the short term but hold us back in the long term.
- **NEGATIVE THOUGHT PATTERNS.** Do you believe that you can't get well? Do you feel helpless in your ability to feel strong and confident? Negative thought patterns, such as catastrophizing (imagining the worst possible outcome), overgeneralizing (drawing broad negative conclusions from specific events), and self-criticism strip away our power and exacerbate anxiety.
- **PERFECTIONISM.** Has anyone ever accused you of being a perfectionist? Perfectionism might tempt you to push yourself harder, but aiming for unrealistic standards can leave you feeling inadequate and anxious.
- **RUMINATION.** You get caught up in thoughts about things you've said, past events, or future worries. This pulls your attention away from the present moment and can send your nervous system into overdrive. Ruminating is a sign that

your default mode network (DMN) is running the show. Onboarding your executive control network (ECN) is one big step toward achieving anxiety freedom.

- **RESISTANCE TO CHANGE.** Have you ever stopped and wondered, *Who would I be if I weren't anxious?* Sometimes fear of the unknown is more terrifying than our current reality, even if our reality is fraught with panic and anxiety. How do you respond to change? Do you embrace it wholeheartedly or are you resistant? Overcoming anxiety often requires stepping out of one's comfort zone, which can be difficult and scary. However, doing it can be incredibly powerful.
- **NEGATIVE SELF-IMAGE.** I've worked with many anxiety sufferers who had such a poor self-image that they struggled even to look in the mirror. What is your self-image? Do you feel worthy of anxiety freedom? Do you feel like you deserve to live a joyful life? Sometimes struggling with our self-esteem can show up as an obstacle to healing, and therefore it is an important place to start.
- **UNREALISTIC BELIEFS.** Remember, healing comes one step at a time. While suppressive medications can make us feel like we're back on track, in all reality, the healing process takes time. Do you ever get impatient with your healing process? Do you feel like you may jump from one solution to the other, never giving any solution time to work? Unrealistic expectations about yourself, your healing process, and the treatments themselves can contribute to anxiety. Challenging and changing these beliefs is crucial for making lasting progress.

PSYCHOLOGICAL OBSTACLES TL;DR

- Psychological obstacles are the emotions, thoughts, and beliefs that block us from healing.
- Your thoughts and beliefs about yourself and the world can contribute to anxiety and panic.
- It is important to identify and challenge these obstacles.

SOCIAL AND ENVIRONMENTAL OBSTACLES

The social and environmental experiences we had in childhood can have a lasting impact on our emotional well-being. Our environment is like the foundation of our house. A solid foundation provides stability and support, while a shaky foundation can make us feel insecure and unsteady.

JENNY GREW UP IN A HOUSEHOLD THAT WAS UNSTABLE AND UNPREdictable. Her father was absent, and she lived with her mother, who never stayed in one place for long.

"As soon as I felt settled into my new school, she would uproot us again," Jenny remembered. "One day I came home from school to find that my entire bedroom was packed up and some of my toys and belongings were in the trash at the end of the driveway.

"I asked my mom where we were going, and all she said was, 'You'll find out when we get there, Chickadee.' She always called me Chickadee back then."

Jenny's mother was emotionally abusive. She would often make negative comments about Jenny, which made her feel insecure and unworthy.

"She would always find a way to get under my skin," Jenny said. "She would often make little remarks like 'Oh, Jenny. You do try so hard. It's just a shame that you're not smart.' Maybe she really believed the things she said. Or maybe it was her way of keeping me down, so that I wouldn't leave her. Which worked for a long time."

For many years, Jenny believed her mother's criticisms. She wasn't as good at school as the other kids, she struggled with math, and the teachers said she was emotionally delayed.

"It took me a long time to be willing to consider that maybe my struggles weren't because there was something wrong with me but because I was constantly on edge, waiting for my mother's next mood swing, or because the next day I'd come home and learn that we were moving again."

Jenny lived with her mother until she was in her late twenties. It wasn't until she had the terrifying manic episode that she finally started counseling. At that time she began to understand the impact of her childhood and her relationship with her mother on her mental health.

She learned about attachment theory and codependency, and she began the process of working through how traumas had wired her brain, body, and nervous system to be poised for danger.

"For the first time in my life I've started asking questions like . . . who was I before the world told me who I was? Who do I want to be? What types of relationships help me see who I truly am and nourish my soul?"

JENNY'S STORY REMINDS US that many of us carry the weight of difficult childhood experiences that can impact our emotional well-being even today. If you're struggling with the lasting effects of a challenging past, you're not alone. There's immense strength in acknowledging that, and there's also immense hope for healing.

This book, along with resources like therapy, support groups, and other self-help options, can be powerful tools on your journey. Remember, you have the strength to overcome the challenges of your past and build a healthier, happier present. Let's explore ways to find that healing together.

Here's a list of common social and environmental obstacles that I see impeding the anxiety healing process in my clients:

- **LACK OF SUPPORTIVE RELATIONSHIPS.** Building strong, supportive relationships is key to healing anxiety, but it can be tough to put yourself out there and connect with new people. The good news is that there are steps you can take to start building a more fulfilling social circle while also addressing the dynamics of your current relationships.
- **MENTAL ILLNESS STIGMA.** The stigma around mental illness can prevent us from getting the help we need and deserve. We may feel hesitant to open up about our anxiety for fear of being judged. Remember that anxiety affects millions of people around the world. Seeking help is wise and brave.

- **INEQUALITY AND SYSTEMIC DISCRIMINATION.** Inequality and systemic discrimination can also be major obstacles. These experiences can lead to feelings of fear, helplessness, and hopelessness, which can exacerbate anxiety. In addition, inequality and systemic discrimination may obstruct access to resources such as mental health care.
- **ECONOMIC BARRIERS TO TREATMENT.** The high costs of mental health care can be a major barrier to healing. Therapy and medication can be expensive, and many people don't have health insurance that covers mental health services. However, many resources are available to help people afford mental health care, such as sliding-scale therapy and free clinics. (See Appendix B for resources.)
- **LIMITED ACCESS TO SUPPORTIVE COMMUNITIES.** Marginalized individuals may face challenges in finding supportive communities that understand their experiences. They may find it difficult to find people who can relate to their experiences and offer support. For example, LGBTQ+ people of color might feel isolated and misunderstood by their families and communities. Fortunately, there are many wonderful online and in-person support groups available for people from all walks of life.
- **LACK OF ACCESS TO TREATMENT.** People who live in rural areas or in communities with limited mental health resources may have difficulty accessing the care they need, especially if they have specific needs. The good news is that telehealth options are expanding access to care, making it possible for people in rural areas to connect with providers more easily.
- **LANGUAGE BARRIERS.** People who have limited proficiency in the dominant language of their country may have difficulty accessing mental health services. But many mental health services are becoming more inclusive by hiring multilingual providers and offering interpretation services, making it easier for everyone to access care.

IMPORTANT RESOURCES

- 988 Suicide and Crisis Hotline: call or text 988 or chat 988lifeline.org
- LGBTQ+ National Hotline: call 1-888-843-4564
- Black Emotional and Mental Health Collective: visit BEAM.community
- National Domestic Violence Hotline: call 1-800-799-7233 or text LOVEIS to 22522
- Veterans Crisis Line: call 988, then select 1, or text 838255
- To find a treatment facility in your local area, visit findtreatment.gov
- To find a therapist that takes your insurance: psychologytoday.com

SOCIAL AND ENVIRONMENTAL OBSTACLES TL;DR

- Your past and present social relationships can be anxiety healing or anxiety provoking.
- Stressful and chaotic environments can contribute to anxiety and panic.
- A strong network of friends, family, and community members can buffer you against the effects of panic and anxiety.
- Culture and economics play a role in many people's anxiety and panic.

SPIRITUAL OBSTACLES

You are more than the sum of your parts.

Have you ever *known* something that your brain didn't actually really *know*?

Some people refer to this experience of *knowing* as tapping into our sixth sense or intuition. Others chalk up these seemingly mystical experiences to imagination or wishful thinking.

Maybe you are versed in the art of manifestation, or in listening to your inner voice, or perhaps your idea of getting what you want comes from a well-thought-out strategic plan.

Wherever you are on the spectrum of materialist to mystic, ask yourself the following question:

Am I more than a trillion little chemical synapses, experiences, and adaptations? If so, what does that mean?

Traditional Chinese Medicine, Ayurveda, Indigenous practices, and vitalism all teach that the mind, body, and spirit are interconnected. They teach that true healing must address all three aspects of your being.

For example, Traditional Chinese Medicine healers use the Eight Extraordinary Meridians to balance the flow of energy in the body. Ayurveda uses the doshas to understand each person's unique constitution and how they can create balance in their lives. Vitalist healers believe that health is a matter of honoring the universal principles of nature.

Modern medicine also recognizes the importance of the mind-body connection. *Soul sickness* is a term some clinicians are using to describe a vague, unexplained sense of loss of purpose and hope. It is thought to be caused by a disconnection from one's spiritual self.

Teachers like Eckhart Tolle teach that we are all interconnected by a great unifying force and that symptoms emerge when we are disconnected from that force and get stuck within our ego's protective armor.

All of these mythologies rest on one foundational belief: *You are more than just the sum of your parts.*

The Hero's Journey

Writer, teacher, and philosopher Joseph Campbell was famous for a monomyth that he called the Hero's Journey. It is a template of how stories have been created and told through time:

> A hero is invited on a journey. They say yes, meet a mentor, go through a series of challenges, find themselves in the abyss. There they are transformed and unified with a greater sense of purpose and connectedness. And then they bring their gift to others. Rinse. Repeat. Rinse. Repeat.

You can see these heroic journeys every day. The single mom beaming at her child's graduation. The now-sober young adult leading a support group. The thrice failed entrepreneur making it big. The kindness of a stranger.

There can be a purpose to everyday suffering, and that purpose lies at the foundation of spiritual awareness and integration.

Anxiety Healing Through Spiritual Alignment

You are more than just your physical body. Mind, body, and spirit are all intricately connected. When one aspect feels off-balance, it can ripple through the others. Feelings of being stuck, lost, or isolated might be a signal that your spirit needs some attention.

Being spiritually unaligned can create a state of disharmony that manifests in emotional and physical problems. An imbalanced mind, body, and spirit can get locked in a cycle that impacts the others. Healing can begin by opening your spirit and rewiring the patterns that keep you feeling stuck.

A spiritual quest can be a powerful journey of self-discovery. It's a chance to delve into your purpose, beliefs, values, and what truly matters to you in life. The focus shifts from being in the individual ego to recognizing that we are part of a larger whole. This journey of discovery is unique for everyone. Some embark on literal quests while others find solace in meditation. Some explore altered states of consciousness with psychedelic substances while others seek connection within their spiritual communities.

Regardless of your beliefs, finding your soul or spirit often involves a process of introspection, self-discovery, and personal growth. This may include exploring your values, passions, strengths, and weaknesses, as well as engaging in practices that promote mindfulness, meditation, or self-reflection. It may also involve seeking guidance from mentors, counselors, or spiritual leaders who can provide support and insight.

A FEW IDEAS TO GET YOU STARTED:

- **SET AN INTENTION.** Before beginning your spiritual quest, it can be helpful to set an intention or a goal for what you hope to gain from the experience. It could be something like anxiety-freedom, relief from physical pain, inner peace, exploration of your purpose, or a deeper understanding of yourself.
- **EXPLORE DIFFERENT SPIRITUAL PRACTICES.** Many spiritual practices can help you connect with your inner self, your soul, and the great beyond. Some common ones include meditation, prayer, retreats, yoga, journaling, listening, and spending time in nature. Try experimenting with different practices to see what resonates with you.
- **SEEK GUIDANCE.** Consider finding a spiritual mentor or teacher who can guide you on your journey. This could be a religious leader, an intuitive, a meditation teacher, a spiritual coach, or simply a compassionate friend.
- **PRACTICE SELF-REFLECTION.** Spend time reflecting on your thoughts, feelings, and experiences. Journaling can be a helpful tool. Take time to explore your beliefs and values, and consider how they shape your understanding of the world and your place in it.
- **CONNECT WITH A COMMUNITY.** Connecting with a spiritual community can provide support, encouragement, and opportunities for breaking barriers. Consider joining a local religious or spiritual group, attending a retreat or workshop, or connecting with others online.
- **EMBRACE THE JOURNEY.** Remember that a spiritual quest is a journey, not a destination. Embrace the process of self-

discovery, and be open to the insights and experiences that come your way.

Ultimately, the search for meaning and purpose is a lifelong adventure, unique to each of us. It calls for openness, honesty, and self-exploration, guiding us toward a life that feels authentic and fulfilling.

SPIRITUAL OBSTACLES TL;DR

- Spirituality is a journey of self-discovery that explores the concept of something beyond ourselves.
- Healing the soul involves reconnecting with your inner self and discovering a sense of purpose and belonging that transcends the individual.
- A spiritual journey is a lifelong process, not a destination.

9

RETRAIN YOUR NERVOUS SYSTEM

Jenny

JENNY WAS INCREDULOUS. "YOU'RE SUGGESTING THAT MY BRAIN IS stuck in a time warp from the car accident?"

"In a sense, yes." I nodded. "We have a part of our brain that is sometimes referred to as the Time Keeper. It helps us differentiate between the past and the present. But when we go through something traumatic, the Time Keeper doesn't work as well, and our brain can sometimes have difficulty distinguishing between what's occurring now and what happened in the past."

"So that's why it can feel like it's happening all over," Jenny said.

"Yes. It's very common for people who have had a traumatic experience like a car accident to have panic attacks in cars later in life. And it's totally treatable."

"So they say." Jenny looked dejected. "I've been at this therapy thing literally for over a decade."

I understood Jenny's doubts. She had tried many different therapies with limited results. But she had never tried nervous system repatterning practices before.

"I hear you," I said. "You've put a lot of time into healing, and I know you're discouraged. But I'm glad you're here, and I really believe you can get better. Are you willing to give it ninety days?"

"After ten years, what's ninety more days?" Jenny joked.

"Piece of cake." I grinned.

She took a big breath. "I'm ready. How do we start?"

WE START WITH BOTTOM-UP processing.

BOTTOM-UP PROCESSING

Bottom-up processing is a type of healing that gathers information from the body's sensations, nervous system, and other bodily systems to understand how they have adapted to stressors.

It also gathers information, through careful observation or functional testing, about the feedback loops that are maintaining a traumatized panicky state.

Doing bottom-up work helps us to understand our reactions to stress and trauma by paying attention to physical sensations and emotions. This gives us access to information from the parts of our brain, body, and nervous system that lie beyond our conscious awareness.

When we develop new coping mechanisms and lay the foundation for reintegrating our higher and logical brain centers with our lower brain centers, we become more resilient and learn to change the way our body reacts to stress and anxiety, including those bodily reactions that are often seen as involuntary (such as heart rate and breathing). Bottom-up approaches can also lead to positive changes in our gut, neurotransmitters, immune system, hormones, and organ systems.

When you learn how to repattern your body, you can start to experience the benefits of living in a body that feels fundamentally safe and in the present moment. No more panic out of the blue, no more fear of the fear, and no more attacks of anxiety that control your life. Instead, you'll have more energy, get better sleep, and enjoy a greater sense of well-being. You'll also be better able to cope with stress and adversity.

THE PANIC RESET

The Panic Reset is a 90-day program designed to teach you how to rewire your brain and body so that you can experience panic-free living. The program is based on the latest research in neuroscience and psychology, and it uses strategies that have been shown to be effective in helping people to overcome panic disorder.

The Panic Reset is a four-step process:

Step 1: Calm the nervous system.
Step 2: Onboard your wise and analytical mind.
Step 3: Reintegrate mind and body.
Step 4: Restructure panic-producing patterns.

Research suggests that it takes 90 to 120 days for your brain to create a new habit. So while you should start to see results at around the 30-day mark, I want to encourage you to give yourself 90 days of consistent effort in practicing the skills from the Panic Reset. If you do, I am confident that you will see results.

Also note that there are many ways to do bottom-up work, beyond what we will be able to cover in this book. So I encourage you to get creative with what works best for you!

Step 1: Calm the Nervous System

When you're feeling anxious, your brain may go into autopilot mode. In this mode, the logical part of your brain shuts down, and the emotional part of your brain takes over. (Refer back to Chapter 4.)

In this first step, we are going to learn how to turn your logical brain back on via activation of your brain stem.

When your autonomic nervous system (ANS) is in a state of sympathetic arousal, it sends danger signals throughout your body. Activating the brain stem can transition you into the present moment, and a more parasympathetic state. This shift decreases the amygdala's emotional activity, so that the prefrontal cortex can come back online and give you some logical input.

TOOLS FOR ACTIVATING THE BRAIN STEM:

- **USE YOUR PANIC PACK.** The Panic Pack is a small bag or container that you can make and keep with you at all times. Fill it with items that stimulate your brain stem to help you relax.
- **PRACTICE TIPPSSSS.** This acronym stands for Tip the temperature, Intense exercise, Paced breathing, Paired muscle relaxation, and the four *S*'s: Scene, Scent, Sip, Stimuli.

Exercise 1: Make a Panic Pack

A Panic Pack is a small, portable bag that you can bring with you everywhere you go. It contains tools that can help you stop a panic attack in its tracks. The items in the Panic Pack target the brain stem in different ways, such as touch, temperature, texture, scent, taste, breath, sound, and movement.

ITEMS FOR A PANIC PACK:

- **A PORTABLE BAG.** Choose a bag that's small enough to fit in your purse, backpack, or even your pocket. A fanny pack, a crossbody bag, or a small pencil case would all work well.
- **DISPOSABLE INSTANT COLD PACKS.** Applying a cold pack to your face for 30 seconds on and 30 seconds off can be one of the quickest ways to stop a panic attack. It triggers a response called the mammalian dive reflex, which is associated with a slower heart rate, lowered body temperature, and less anxiety.
- **PLASTIC REUSABLE STRAW THAT HAS BEEN CUT IN HALF.** Inhaling and exhaling slowly through a cut straw can activate your body's relaxation response (parasympathetic nervous system). This helps prevent hyperventilation and promotes a sense of calm.

- **TWO ESSENTIAL OILS OF YOUR CHOICE.** Scent is one of the most powerful ways to change your nervous system's state. Therapeutic-grade essential oils such as lavender and rose can be very effective at reducing panic and anxiety. You can apply the oils topically or orally or even inhale them.
- **REUSABLE EARPLUGS.** If you find yourself feeling overstimulated, using earplugs or noise-canceling headphones can help reduce sensory input and calm your nervous system.
- **PAIR OF SMALL PORTABLE HEADPHONES.** Listening to music can also be helpful for calming the nervous system. Choose your favorite music or try listening to alpha wave music, binaural beats, or nature sounds. Check out my soundtrack on Spotify, which can be found at https://open.spotify.com/user/nicole.a.cain.
- **A ROUGH STONE AND A SMOOTH STONE.** Grounding techniques like touch can help to calm your nervous system by activating your brain stem. Different textures can help to ground you in the present moment and reduce anxiety.
- **A PACK OF GINGER CHEWS.** Salty, sour, and bitter flavors are all known to have calming effects on the autonomic nervous system. Ginger is a particularly good choice because it can also help to soothe nausea that can be caused by anxiety.
- **A BUBBLE WAND.** Blowing bubbles can help to stop anxiety in two ways. First, it forces you to slow your exhale, which stimulates your vagus nerve and promotes relaxation.
- **YOUR FAVORITE SUPPLEMENT OR BOTANICAL FOR ANXIETY.** Many different natural remedies can help to reduce anxiety. Some popular options include chamomile (*Matricaria chamomilla*), valerian root (*Valeriana officinalis*), and magnesium.

WHEN TO USE YOUR PANIC PACK

Your Panic Pack is a great tool to have on hand when you're feeling overwhelmed, whether you're in the Yellow Light Zone or the Red Light Zone. It can also be helpful to use as a preventive measure if you know you're going to be in a situation that triggers your anxiety.

TIPS FOR USING YOUR PANIC PACK:

- **ITEMS.** Choose the items that you think will be most helpful for you. For example, if you're feeling overstimulated by noise, you might want to use the earplugs or noise-canceling headphones.
- **SENSATIONS.** Focus on the sensations that you're experiencing as you use your Panic Pack. This will help you stay present and grounded.
- **EXPERIMENT.** Don't be afraid to experiment with different items and techniques. What works for one time might not have the same effect later.

Exercise 2: TIPPSSSS

One of the best tips for stopping a runaway train that's headed straight into panic is to leverage the powers of temperature, intense exercise, paced breathing, and paired muscle relaxation. If you've ever studied Dialectical Behavior Therapy, you've heard these strategies summarized as TIPP Skills. But I've refreshed them just a bit and expanded the name to TIPPSSSS.

TIPPSSSS STANDS FOR:

- **T**ip the temperature
- **I**ntense exercise
- **P**aced breathing
- **P**aired muscle relaxation
- **S**cene
- **S**cent
- **S**ip
- **S**timuli

TIPPSSSS is an amazing strategy that can be used during any and all of your stoplight phases, and it is one of your best assets if and when you go into the Red Light Zone.

Let's go through these one at a time.

TIP THE TEMPERATURE

This technique can work quickly to calm the nervous system as it evokes what is called the "mammalian dive reflex," which causes your heart rate to slow down, interrupting panic. Here are some ideas for tipping the temperature:

- **COLD WATER BOWL.** Hold your breath and place your face in a bowl of cold water for 15 to 30 seconds.
- **COLD WATER PACK.** Apply a freezer pack, or a cold chemical pack, or a Ziploc bag of cold water to your eyes and cheeks. Hold it there for 15 to 30 seconds.
- **SHOWER.** Get in the shower and turn the temperature to cold, and then hot. Alternate every 30 to 60 seconds, three times in a row.
- **POOL.** Jump in a cold pool and then a hot tub. Alternate every 30 to 60 seconds, three times in a row.

INTENSE EXERCISE

When the nervous system is firing on all cylinders, it can be helpful to channel that energy into something productive. Otherwise, your body is going to get creative with ways to release the endorphins, and you will experience all sorts of not-fun symptoms. Here are my three favorite outlets to direct panicked energy:

- **RUNNING.** You can run outside (if you feel safe in your neighborhood), in the local gym (some gyms are open 24/7), in a public park, or on a treadmill or elliptical. Run as hard as you can for 15 seconds, then walk and let your heart rate return to normal. Repeat several times.
- **BIKE RIDING.** When I was in a record groove of panic, I would ride my bike all around town. I'd pedal vigorously up hills, then slowly through the park, listening to the sounds of the gears on the bike and the sounds around me or my music of choice.

- **SWIMMING.** With swimming, you get the benefit of a nice cold-water and energy-channeling exertion. It's also easy on the joints. Feel the coldness of the water on your skin, and experience the bubbles and splashing water.
- **YOGA.** There are many types of yoga practices. Some are more intense, and others are more about de-escalation and calming. Try out a few different types of classes and see what works for you.

PACED BREATHING

According to research out of Harvard Medical School, paced breathing is one of the most effective ways to calm the stress response.

The Four-Square Breath, also known as Box Breathing, is a specific type of paced breathing that involves counting to four as you breathe. We are going to super-charge this process by adding an alternating nostril component, which is referred to as Nadi Shodhana breathing.

Imagine that as you are breathing, you are drawing the lines of a square or a box.

- Close your right nostril and inhale deeply through the left nostril for four counts. As you inhale slowly, imagine drawing the first line of your box.
- Hold at the top of the breath for four counts. As you count, imagine drawing the second line of your box.
- Close your left nostril, open your right nostril, and exhale for four to six counts. Draw the third line of your box.
- Hold at the bottom of the exhale for four counts. Draw the last line and complete your box.
- Repeat as many times as needed.

PAIRED MUSCLE RELAXATION

Paired muscle relaxation can help especially if your body becomes tense and trembles with extreme emotion. Start at your head and work your way down your body. While doing your Four-Square Breath, clench each muscle group for four seconds, then release and move to the next muscle group.

- As you inhale, clench your muscles in your head and face. Hold for four counts.
- As you release the muscles, exhale on the word *relax*. Release for four counts.
- Then inhale and clench the muscles in your shoulders and upper back. Hold for four counts.
- As you release the muscles, exhale on the word *relax*. Release for four counts.
- Continue to work your way down your body. Remember to count to four with each muscle group and each breath.
- Repeat as necessary.

SCENE

Our senses are powerful tools for calming the mind. The brain forms strong associations between sensory details and emotions. Think about the warm and comforting feeling you get from the smell of freshly baked cookies. A "scene" is all about these sensory details—sights, sounds, smells, tastes, and touches—that combine to create a complete picture in our minds. When we encounter specific sights, sounds, or smells, it can trigger memories and emotions linked to those experiences.

When I was dealing with extreme anxiety, I found that being in my apartment made it worse. So I would leave and go to a park or visit a friend and hang out at their house. Changing the scene may also help your brain let go of associations feeding into your current state.

SCENE-SHIFTING SUGGESTIONS:

- Physically relocate yourself. If you are inside, go outside, and vice versa. If you're in your office, get up and go to the bathroom.

- If you're in a dark room, go into a light room, or vice versa.
- Go for a run, walk, bike ride, or jump on your longboard.
- Change your bedspread, or rearrange your furniture. Move the things on your desk.

SCENT

Scents can be powerful cues for the brain stem, and they can be activating or calming.

Here's an example of how scent can trigger anxiety. Dental visits weren't exactly a walk in the park for me growing up. Throughout elementary school and adolescence, I had many teeth pulled, some without adult replacements waiting. Needless to say, the experience wasn't pleasant. Even today, the telltale scent of a dentist's office—a potent cocktail of antiseptic and novocaine—triggers a surge of memories so acute, it's as if those childhood visits were yesterday.

Many years later, as an adult, I took my cavapoo, Sheva, to a daycare so that she could romp around with her dog friends. When I picked her up, I pulled her into my arms. The first thing I noticed was a surge of anxiety in my chest. The second thing I noticed was the smell. It reminded me of the numbing gel the dentist had used on my gums before my surgeries.

SCENT SUGGESTIONS:

- Make sure your environment is clean, smells fresh, and is clutter-free.
- Consider inhaling essential oils. You can use a diffuser, a candle, or whatever you like. Some of my favorite scents for anti-anxiety are citrus (especially lemon), lavender, chamomilla, vetiver, rose, and ylang ylang.
- Apply essential oils to the insides of your wrists, the bottoms of your big toes, your temples, or beneath your nose on your upper lip.
- Smell a perfume or a candle scent that you love.

SIP

The vagus nerve is a major nerve that runs through the body, including the root of the tongue, and can be activated during activities like sipping and swallowing, aiding in anxiety reduction.

SIPPING SUGGESTIONS:

- Sip a calming herbal tea. Chamomile, lavender, and lemon balm have all been shown to have calming effects.
- Suck on ice or eat a frozen-fruit Popsicle. The cold temperature can help to soothe the body and mind.
- Apply a pinch of sea salt to the back of your tongue. It can help to stimulate the vagus nerve.
- Suck on sour candy such as a lemon drop or ginger chew. The sour taste can also help to stimulate the vagus nerve. Research suggests that sour flavors can be particularly effective at calming anxiety.

STIMULI

Sometimes feelings of anxiety may be due to the wrong type or amount of stimulation in your environment. Try different things, notice how your body reacts, and jot down some notes so you can remember what works for next time.

STIMULUS SUGGESTIONS:

- **CHANGE YOUR BODY TEMPERATURE.** Take a hot or cold shower, apply a cold compress to your face, or wear different clothing.
- **CHANGE YOUR ENVIRONMENT.** Open a window, change the lights, use a HappyLight, turn on some music, use white noise, or go for a walk.
- **CHANGE YOUR FOCUS.** Watch a funny movie, read a book, or talk to a friend.
- **ENGAGE IN PHYSICAL ACTIVITY.** This can help release endorphins, which have mood-boosting effects.

- **PRACTICE RELAXATION TECHNIQUES.** Do deep breathing, meditation, or yoga.

ADDITIONAL SUGGESTIONS:

- Choose stimuli that are strong enough to distract you from your anxiety but not so strong that they overwhelm you.
- Focus on the positive aspects of the stimulus. For example, if you are listening to music, focus on the lyrics or the melody.
- Allow yourself to enjoy the stimulus without judgment. Don't worry if you don't feel instantly relaxed. Just keep practicing, and you will eventually find what works for you.

The next time you're feeling anxious, try to pay attention to the scene around you. What are you seeing, hearing, smelling, tasting, and feeling? These sensory cues can be helpful in grounding you in the present moment and distracting you from your anxious thoughts.

CALM THE NERVOUS SYSTEM TL;DR

- Mindfully activating your brain stem helps to shift the autonomic nervous system out of arousal and into a state of calm.
- Body-based interventions work quickly and effectively to calm your nervous system.
- A Panic Pack is a small, portable bag that contains tools to activate your brain stem.
- TIPPSSSS are eight steps that you can take to stop a panic attack in its tracks.

Next, I am going to walk you through the process of keeping your mindful brain on board while noticing your body.

Step 2: Onboard your wise and analytical mind

Now that you've calmed your nervous system and your amygdala, you're ready for the next step. The goal of Step 2 is to balance your two brain states: the default mode network (DMN) (autopilot) and the executive control network (ECN) (your wise and analytical mind). While they are both important in mood regulation and cognitive function, your ECN is going to be your best asset at giving you a sense of agency over panic and anxiety.

In this step, you will learn how to strengthen your logical brain's ability to quickly engage, so that you have more power to decide if something is actually dangerous and can choose how you want to react. This will help to bring your system out of the past, with its time warp, and the future, with its worries, and allow your self-awareness and executive function to return to the present moment and take back the reins.

The more you practice Step 2, the more automatic it will become. In other words, "the way you wire it is the way you'll fire it."

Here's how to recruit your wise and analytical mind:

Exercise 1: Focused Attention Meditation

This type of meditation is unique because with it you sustain focus on a single thought, mantra, or object to help yourself stay in the present moment. It shifts you out of autopilot and activates your thoughtful and logical brain networks, the ECN. For best results, practice the Focused Attention Meditation for five minutes every day.

FOCUSED ATTENTION MEDITATION

- Sit upright in a comfortable position. Allow your body to relax, and keep your spine tall.
- Choose a target for your attention. Either focus your eyes on a fixed spot at a comfortable height and distance, or close your eyes and focus on your breath.

- As you inhale, imagine breathing in a mantra, word, sound, or phrase.
- As you exhale, imagine exhaling a mantra, word, sound, or phrase.
- For example, you may inhale the word *It's* and exhale the word *Okay*. Or you may choose the phrase *I am safe,* or a sound such as *ohm,* or a mantra given to you by a mentor or teacher.

Exercise 2: Do things that challenge your brain.

When you learn a new skill, do a puzzle, read a complex book, or otherwise challenge your brain, you're activating the ECN and helping it to stay strong. Try to challenge your brain for 30 minutes every day. Here are some ideas:

- Jigsaw puzzles
- Sudoku
- *New York Times* crossword puzzle
- Chess
- Strategy board games
- Brain-boosting apps. Tons of them are popping up every month!

You've calmed your nervous system and onboarded your wise and analytical mind. Now it's time to reintegrate your wise mind with your body.

WISE MIND TL;DR

- Parts of your brain associated with the ECN are activated when you are in your wise, logical, analytical mind.
- Strengthening your ECN will help you have more say about how you react to your experiences.
- You will have greater control over your bodily responses to stress by strengthening your ECN.

- Practices that increase the amount of gray matter in your brain will help you have more emotional control and better cognitive performance.

Step 3:
Reintegrate mind and body

Your amygdala is calm, and your analytical brain is onboarded. Now you can start to synchronize or reintegrate your analytical brain with your body. But you may be wondering, *How do I know if my analytical brain and my body are not in sync?*

SIGNS THAT YOUR ANALYTICAL BRAIN AND YOUR BODY ARE NOT IN SYNC:

- **HYPERAROUSAL HIJACK.** Hyperarousal can show up as symptoms like increased heart rate, sweating, muscle tension, and anxiety.
- **REDUCED ACTIVITY IN THE PREFRONTAL CORTEX.** You may notice that it's difficult to think logically, regulate your emotions, or make decisions. These symptoms are hallmarks of Thought Anxiety.
- **INCREASED ACTIVITY IN THE AMYGDALA.** You may notice exaggerated startle responses or even big mood swings.
- **DEFAULT MODE NETWORK TAKEOVER.** You may find yourself zoning out, forgetting things, or noticing symptoms of dissociation, derealization, or depersonalization. These symptoms are seen in Nervous System Anxiety.

If, despite using your logic and coping skills, your body continues to produce panic and anxiety, it's time to learn how to synchronize your body and your logical brain. This will help your central nervous system to be calm and in control when you need it to be.

Notice Your Body's Communications

Sensory processing is the way the brain interprets and responds to sensory information from the environment. This includes information from the five senses (sight, hearing, taste, smell, and touch), proprioception (the sense of body position and movement), and interoception (the sense of body signals such as heart rate, muscle tension, and body temperature). The brain receives this information through sensory receptors located throughout the body, interprets the signals, and generates a response.

If you have a history of adversity or trauma, it may have affected your sensory processing in ways that make it difficult for you to feel comfortable in your own body and that may even cause symptoms of anxiety about your health. This is a normal response to trauma. You may be extra sensitive to every little sensation, or you may not notice anything until it's really strong. These symptoms are not a sign of weakness or failure.

The good news is that you can learn to honor your symptoms and see them as messages from your body about what needs healing. Self-compassion is key to this process. When you notice a symptom, remind yourself that it's a normal reaction to high stress, unpredictability, and/or chaos and that you're not alone. You can also try body awareness techniques, such as paying attention to your breath and the sensations in your body. These techniques can help you to calm down and connect with your body in a healthy way.

TIPS FOR PRACTICING BODY AWARENESS:

- **BE PRESENT.** Take some time each day to sit quietly and focus on your body. Notice the sensations you're feeling, both inside and out. Do this for 5 to 20 minutes, whatever works for you.
- **PAY ATTENTION TO YOUR BREATHING.** Notice how your chest rises and falls. Observe the motion of your belly. Is your breath shallow or deep? Is it fast or slow?
- **NOTICE THE TENSION IN YOUR MUSCLES.** Are there any areas that

are particularly tense? As you notice them, continue breathing gently.

- **BE PATIENT WITH YOURSELF.** It's normal for thoughts to come up when you're trying to focus on your body. Just acknowledge them and let them go. Don't judge yourself for having them.
- **BE CURIOUS.** When you notice your body, what comes up for you? Where are the sensations? Are they moving or still? Are they large or small? Heavy or light? Soft or rough? What else do you notice?

I know that when you are feeling anxious and experiencing unpleasant physical sensations, it can feel counterintuitive to focus on those sensations. But as the saying goes, "What you resist persists." When you try to push away your anxiety, it only gets stronger. Instead, you can learn to acknowledge your anxiety without judgment. You can do this by creating a safe space for yourself where you can practice paying attention to your thoughts, feelings, and sensations in a way that is predictable, moderate, and controllable. This means choosing when, how much, and how you want to focus on your anxiety.

Notice Your Reactions to Your Observations

Once you're aware of your sensations, you can be aware of your feelings about your sensations, which is meta-awareness. In essence, meta-awareness enables you to step back and observe your own thoughts, feelings, and sensations from a distance, enabling you to observe them without becoming anxious about them. Just practice noticing.

Here's an example:

> Suzie is gathering berries in a field to take home to her family. Well aware that tigers live nearby, Suzie's senses are attuned to any signs of danger in the brush. A hungry tiger growls in the distance, and before Suzie logically realizes it, a fear signal starts

> in her limbic system that causes a cascade of changes in both her brain and body that results in autonomic arousal.
>
> Her heart is beating faster so that her cells and muscles can receive the energy they need in order for her to run. Her breathing speeds up so that she can keep up with the increased demand for oxygen. Her blood pressure rises with her faster heart rate. Her body deprioritizes sending blood to the fingertips in favor of sending blood to the heart and large muscle groups, causing numbness and tingling on her cheeks and fingertips. Her body temperature rises with all the metabolic activity. Her muscles are clenched and are pumping as she zigzags around trees and jumps over fallen branches and stones and safely escapes.

Thankfully, Suzie's quick responses enabled her to escape. If she was to stop and reflect, she might feel appreciation for her body's response.

But what if Suzie were to experience these sensations later that night, while trying to go to sleep? Heart throbbing, muscles twitching, rapid breathing, numbness and tingling, body temperature rising, and thoughts racing?

In this context, these sensations may feel very frightening. Meta-awareness can help Suzie calm down during a panic attack. By taking a few deep breaths and focusing on her body, she can start to observe her thoughts and feelings from a distance. This can help her to realize that she is no longer in danger and that her body's reaction is just a normal response to stress.

Meta-awareness can also help Suzie to prevent panic attacks from happening in the future. By learning to recognize the early signs of a panic attack, she can take steps to calm down before it gets worse.

Befriend the Body

Some time ago I read a very moving quote by author and poet Nayyirah Waheed that read, "and i said to my body. softly. 'i want to be your friend.' it took a long breath. and replied 'i have been waiting my whole life for this.' "

What comes up for you as you read her words? If you're a panic sufferer, you might relate to the feeling of being at odds with your body.

Many of us who deal with panic attacks don't want to go anywhere near the body, let alone befriend it. If your origin story is anything like mine, you were brought up believing that your body was flawed and that you needed doctors to fix it. However, there is another perspective: that our bodies, in their infinite wisdom and love, are inherently designed to heal. If you cut your finger, your body will jump into action, and before you know it, that cut will be healed. Why wouldn't it be the same with other parts of our bodies and minds?

The important thing is to understand what your symptoms are doing for you: how your symptoms are adaptations to what has and has not happened to you, and what they are telling you that you need in order to be healed, and how to accomplish that.

By changing our perspective from being at war with our bodies toward having self-compassion and love, miraculous things will happen.

Exercise 1: How to Befriend Your Body

In this exercise, we're going to explore the idea of befriending your body. We'll look at how you can start to see your body as a source of wisdom and strength, and how you can use this new perspective to attune to the wisdom from your panic symptoms.

STEPS TO BEFRIEND THE BODY:

- **CONVERSE WITH YOUR BODY WITH KINDNESS AND COMPASSION.** Talk with your body as if it were a friend. Acknowledge the ways it has been there for you. Let it know that you're committed to working together.
- **LISTEN TO YOUR BODY AND ACKNOWLEDGE ITS VOICE.** Let's say you're having a conversation with your body, and you notice your legs, and a thought comes to mind such as, "You don't give me gratitude for carrying you where you need to

go. You just judge me for how I look." You could listen with compassion, acknowledge the message, and respond with something honorable such as, "I hear you. I'm sorry for the judgment. I'll try to do better. Thank you for carrying me every day of my life."

- **DO THINGS THAT MAKE YOUR BODY FEEL GOOD.** Spend time in nature, listen to music, get a massage, or do self-massage. For self-massage, try placing the palm of your hand on your opposite shoulder and allowing its weight to gently pull your shoulder down. Find a lotion or oil with a scent that you love, and massage it on your feet. Take time to brush your hair, and notice the feeling of the bristles on your scalp.
- **FILL YOUR HEART.** Place your hand on your heart and close your eyes. Imagine being surrounded by a white light, and as you inhale, draw that light in through your nose or mouth and direct it to your heart. As you exhale, imagine breathing out stress, tension, and any other unwanted symptoms.
- **DANCE.** Put on a song that represents your relationship with your body or maybe how you *want* your relationship with your body to be. Allow whatever comes up to come up through the movements with love and acceptance. Feel the movement in your body, and notice thoughts, feelings, and sensations that emerge. Movement can remind you of positive strength, or of fear and sadness, or it can trigger past things that need to be dealt with.
- **PRACTICE TRAUMA-INFORMED YOGA.** Have a conversation with the stressed parts of your body during movement. Breathe into that area of the body, asking, "What is it you need me to know? I'm listening."

Befriending your body is not a destination, it's a journey. It takes time and practice to learn how to listen to your body and to develop a greater compassion and stronger alliance.

As you do these things, you'll start to see your body in a new light. You'll come to see it as a powerful ally rather than an enemy. And you'll start to experience the benefits of befriending your body, including reduced anxiety and panic symptoms.

Exercise 2: Mindfulness

Mindfulness is the practice of cultivating explicit awareness of one's thoughts, feelings, and sensations by focusing on the present moment without judgment. When you are mindful, you are aware of your thoughts, feelings, and sensations, without getting caught up in them.

POPULAR MINDFULNESS TECHNIQUES

- **MEDITATION.** Meditation is a great way to focus your attention on the present moment and let go of distracting thoughts. There are many different types of meditation, so find one that works for you.
- **BODY SCAN.** A body scan is a type of meditation where you focus your attention on different parts of your body, one at a time. This can help you to become more aware of your physical sensations and how they are connected to your thoughts and feelings.
- **SELF-MASSAGE.** Massage your feet, rub your neck, do dry skin brushing, or give yourself a butterfly hug.
- **YOGA.** Yoga is a mind-body practice that combines physical postures, breathing exercises, and meditation.
- **QIGONG.** Qigong is a Chinese practice that combines gentle movements, breathing exercises, and meditation. It can help to improve your circulation, reduce stress, and boost your mood.
- **TAI CHI.** Tai chi is a Chinese martial art that combines slow, graceful movements with deep breathing. It can help to improve your balance, flexibility, and focus.

Spending at least five minutes each day doing one or more of these practices will enable you to stay in the present moment instead of getting hijacked by events from the past or getting lost in worries about the future.

Mindfulness activates your ECN, and it strengthens the salience network, reinforcing the connection between your filtering thalamus and your analytical prefrontal cortex. This means that you'll be able to respond to stressful situations from a place of personal power instead of your amygdala sending a danger signal straight to your body. Mindfulness practices have been studied as effective strategies for increasing the amount of gray matter in the brain, which gives you more control over your emotions, movements, and reactions.

Exercise 3: Interoception

Practicing interoception can help you reduce anxiety about the sensations you notice in your body. With greater understanding, you will experience fewer misunderstandings about your body's messages. Interoception can help you better receive information from your body as you move through the different stress response stages (the Green, Yellow, and Red Light Zones) and make changes so that your body can shift back to a calm state.

INTEROCEPTIVE BODY SCAN

- Body-scan from your toes to your head. Each time you identify a sensation, stop, and then practice simply observing the sensation. You do not have to change anything about the sensation, just observe it without judgment and breathe.
- Notice subtle reactions, changes, sensations, and signals inside your body, like warmth, change in heartbeat, tightening of your throat, stiffness of your tongue.
- Breathe into each sensation, inhaling and drawing the breath to that sensation for four counts. Hold at the top for four counts, then exhale any tension, stress, or other sensa-

tions for six counts. Hold at the bottom of the exhale for four counts. Repeat.

- Notice reactions on the outside of your body such as a hunching posture, furrowing of your brows, reddening of your skin, or breaking a sweat.
- Breathe into each sensation, inhaling and drawing the breath to that sensation for four counts. Hold at the top for four counts, then exhale any tension, stress, or other sensations for six counts. Hold at the bottom of the exhale for four counts. Repeat.

INTEROCEPTIVE CHANNEL-CHANGING

CHANNEL-CHANGE EXERCISE

- Get comfortable in a quiet place where you won't be disturbed. Close your eyes and take a few deep breaths.
- Slowly scan your body from your toes to your head, noticing any sensations you feel. Don't judge the sensations, just observe them.
- Imagine yourself in a calm place. This could be a place you've been or a place you've created in your imagination. Spend a few minutes in your calm place, noticing the sights, sounds, smells, and sensations.
- Bring to mind a stressful thought, image, or memory. Notice the thoughts, feelings, and sensations that come up for you.
- Take a deep breath and shift your attention back to your calm place. Spend a few minutes in your calm place, noticing how it feels to be there.
- Visualize a protective box at your feet. As you inhale, draw

the breath to any areas where you feel tension or discomfort, and as you exhale, imagine breathing out that tension and discomfort and putting it in your protective box. Once you feel complete, close the lid of the box and set it aside for safe keeping.

Experiment with different techniques we've explored in this section, and find what works best for you. Once you know which ones are your favorites, pick two and practice them every day for the duration of this 90-day program.

BEFRIEND THE BODY TL;DR

- The goal of reintegrating is to keep your logical brain active while you observe sensations and symptoms in your body.
- Explicit awareness is the ability to be consciously aware of your thoughts, feelings, and sensations.
- Interoception is the ability to feel your body's internal sensations.
- Meta-awareness enables you to step back and observe your thoughts, feelings, and sensations from a distance.

Now that you have been practicing observing with unattachment, you are ready to do the work of unpacking and reprocessing panic patterns that are stored in your body and your nervous system.

Step 4: Repattern your defense posture

The latest research in neuroscience teaches us that our brains and nervous systems are incredibly "plastic." This means they can change and adapt, and that we can repattern our inner maps. We can change the programming of our brains and restructure our nervous systems to respond to our internal and external environments in a more helpful way.

There are many tried-and-true techniques that we can use to do this. As you read through the techniques below, circle the ones that you are willing to experiment with throughout the 90-day program.

EXPOSURE. This technique involves gradually exposing yourself to the things that you fear in a controlled, predictable, and moderately intense way. Practicing exposure techniques can help to repattern your nervous system, as they can teach your brain and body that the experiences and sensations it dreads are not actually dangerous.

Exposure is used in a variety of therapeutic approaches such as Eye Movement Desensitization and Reprocessing Therapy (EMDR) and trauma-focused Cognitive Behavioral Therapy, as well as in martial arts, wall climbing, high-ropes courses, and other activities that activate autonomic arousal in a safe setting.

CHANGE YOUR BODILY POSITIONING, CHANGE YOUR MIND. When we are in autonomic arousal, our bodies move into a defense posture. The lower body is in extension, the legs straightened and tense, ready to run, while the upper body is in flexion, with the arms pulled in, either to block or protect the core or to throw a punch. Research, especially from the field of orthopedic medicine, suggests you can change your mental and emotional state and regulate your physiological arousal by changing your panic defense postures.

In essence, the technique involves getting into the defense posture, then breaking the posture by going into the opposite state. We see this done in yoga, qigong, tai chi, martial arts, and even in games we used to play when we were kids. For example, did you ever play the "popcorn parachute" game? My whole class would sit on the floor in a great big circle, each of us grasping the edge of a parachute. The teacher would toss in fluffy balls, and we would work together to lift and drop the parachute in order to cause the balls to pop into the air. It was great fun, and we didn't realize that we were patterning our nervous systems to be fluid and flexible.

REPATTERNING TECHNIQUES

- **FIRECRACKER.** Exhale and crouch down, with your feet flat, back bent forward, knees bent, and your arms tucked in, like a squatted fetal position. Then as you inhale, stand and lift your arms up and out, arch your back slightly, and spread your fingers like "jazz hands." Repeat two or three times.
- **SUN SALUTATION.** Begin in mountain pose, standing tall with your arms extended downward to your sides. Inhale, and bring your arms out to the sides and up to the ceiling. At the top, either bring your palms together over your head or point your fingers straight toward the sky. Lift your gaze and look upward. As you exhale, release your arms to either side and continue bending forward so that you are reaching down toward your toes. (It's okay if you can't reach them—I can't reach mine.) Inhale again, lift your head, and allow your hands to travel up and rest on your shins as you come to a flat back. You can start over by returning to mountain pose, or you can do what is called a yoga vinyasa flow, which you can learn more about online. My favorite free online resource is "Yoga with Adriene," which you can find on YouTube.

YOGA. Yoga can be a powerful tool to retrain your nervous system and positively repattern the structure of your brain. A great deal of evidence suggests that trauma-informed yoga practices can help people feel greater self-compassion, groundedness, and sense of control.

During a yoga process, you may have thoughts like:

Wow, I didn't expect that thought to come up.

Oh my gosh, I'm not going to be able to hold this pose any longer.

Your teacher may direct you to focus on your breath. You inhale and exhale, counting each breath. *One,* you say to yourself. You breathe again. *Two.* You have two more breaths to go. *I don't know if I'm going to make it,* you think.

Sometimes you do make it, and sometimes you don't. But the process is transformative and healing, even if you don't hold the entire pose.

THINGS TO KEEP IN MIND DURING A DIFFICULT POSE:

- **THE DISCOMFORT ALWAYS ENDS.** You hold a pose, you feel discomfort, and it can be intense. But then you shift out of that pose and enjoy the delicious relief as your muscles relax. And then you mindfully move into the next.

  Yoga teaches us important messages such as: *This too shall pass, we can get through hard things, we are often stronger than we realize,* and *breath is powerful.*
- **YOU HAVE AGENCY.** Yoga retrains your nervous system to reclaim agency. You can choose when to go into a pose and when to come out of it. You can choose to go to a class, or you can choose to skip it. You can make adaptations to poses and make the practice yours. There is no right or wrong way to do yoga. Which, I think, is a beautiful metaphor for living life.
- **YOU HAVE LOTS OF OPTIONS.** If you find that you tend to feel more anxious or activated from yoga, you may want to consider a type of yoga called trauma-informed yoga. It's designed to be gentler and more supportive than traditional vinyasa flow yoga. It includes self-awareness, grounding, and techniques designed to help you process difficult emotions and sensations in a safe and supportive environment.

EGO STATE THERAPY, INTERNAL FAMILY SYSTEMS THERAPY, AND PARTS WORK. Chapter 10 is dedicated to these therapies, so I won't expand on them here. I have included them as a reminder that using them can help heal panic-producing patterns.

SOMATOGRAPHIC IMAGERY. Somatographic Imagery is a process I created that merges mindfulness and bodily awareness. The four goals of Somatographic Imagery are:

- **AWAKEN.** Gain awareness and clarification about the physical sensations associated with your emotional state.
- **INSIGHT.** Learn about emotions and memories associated with your physical sensations.
- **EMPOWER.** Promote the breaking of old patterns and build new, desired patterns.
- **RENEW.** Create new patterns and use techniques from hypnosis and mindfulness to "install" new images, sensations, emotions, and thoughts about memories.

You can access the guided meditation at drnicolecain.com/book-resources/.

EYE MOVEMENT DESENSITIZATION AND REPROCESSING THERAPY. EMDR can help you process traumatic memories in a safe and controlled way. It combines eye movements, taps, or tones with talk therapy to help you feel less distressed by your memories. This can help you feel more present, in control, and able to build new, positive associations with the memories.

HOW IT WORKS:

- You'll focus on a specific memory or thought that's causing you distress.
- The therapist will use eye movements, taps, or tones to help you process the memory.
- As you focus on the memory, you'll notice that your thoughts and feelings about it change.
- You can repeat the process until you feel less distressed by the memory.

BREATHWORK. Your breath is your quickest and most effective strategy for modulating your central nervous system. If you are in autonomic arousal with your heart racing and muscles tensing, you can use your breath to slow down your heart and relax your muscles. The most powerful part of the breath is the exhale. As you exhale, your parasympathetic nervous system is activated, and so if you are feeling stressed, the first thing you should do is to simply elongate your exhale.

My favorite breathwork practices:

- **FOUR-SQUARE BREATH/BOX BREATHING.** Refer back to page 261 for instructions.
- **ALTERNATE NOSTRIL BREATHING.** Research suggests that alternate nostril breathing can activate your parasympathetic nervous system, with left-nostril breathing being more relaxing. My favorite approach is to inhale through the left nostril, then exhale through the right. Repeat three times several times throughout the day.

SOMATIC EXPERIENCING. Somatic Experiencing is a therapeutic approach developed by Peter Levine, PhD. It is based on the understanding that traumatic experiences can get trapped in the body's nervous system, causing a range of physical, emotional, and psychological symptoms.

This is what happened to Jenny. Many years after the frightening car accident, her body held on to the memory of the event and kept reliving the trauma as though it were still happening.

Somatic Experiencing techniques are based on the belief that the body has the natural ability to heal itself. Practitioners help clients rest in a safe place where they can process and release their traumatic experiences.

BIOFEEDBACK/HEART RATE VARIABILITY. It's common to think the heart keeps a consistent rhythm like a metronome, picking up speed when stressed and slowing down to its normal rhythm when relaxed. But a healthy heartbeat is actually not like a metronome; in fact, its rhythm should be somewhat variable.

Heart rate variability is the variation in time between heartbeats. A healthy and relaxed nervous system will have high variability, meaning that the rate of your heartbeat is constantly changing. This allows your system to rapidly adjust to sudden emotional or physical changes.

A stressed nervous system and heart will have low variability. This means that the time between heartbeats is more consistent, which can make it difficult for your body to adapt to change.

Biofeedback is a technique that uses sensors to track your body's responses to stress, including heart rate variability. My favorite program is HeartMath, which gives you real-time feedback on your heart rate so you can practice relaxation techniques and see the results immediately. This information can be used to help you learn how to control your body's response to stress.

NEUROFEEDBACK. Neurofeedback is a type of biofeedback that uses electrodes to measure brain waves. The idea is that once you can see or hear your brain waves, you can learn how to control them and improve your overall mental and emotional health. Not all neurofeedback is the same, however, so be sure to do your research before signing up with a practitioner. My personal favorite approach is to start with an at-home wearable device such as the Muse or Mendi.

I typically recommend practicing biofeedback or neurofeedback for 30 to 45 minutes at least three times weekly for best results.

EXPRESSIVE ARTS THERAPY. This type of therapy uses art, singing, music, dance, movement, and writing to help people express their emotions, process difficult experiences, and develop a sense of personal control and mastery. Acting can be a helpful way to heal from trauma by providing a safe and supportive space to explore and express painful emotions and act out what it feels like to be in different roles, thus rewiring your brain.

If this sounds like something that could be helpful for you, I encourage you to check out the International Expressive Arts Therapy Association at IEATA.org. IEATA is a professional organization that promotes the use of Expressive Arts Therapy and provides resources for therapists and clients.

VAGUS NERVE STIMULATION. We talked a lot about the vagus nerve in Chapter 5, so we won't repeat it here. Be sure to check out the Vagus Nerve Hack at drnicolecain.com. Search for the word *vagus* if you want more information.

REPATTERNING TL;DR

- If your brain and body are stuck in feedback loops that are designed to keep you hypervigilant of stress and danger, you will need to retrain these systems to heal.
- Neuroscience shows that our brains can change. By practicing bottom-up techniques, we can reprogram our bodies and minds, building resilience in the face of stress and overwhelm.
- Healing from panic requires consistently engaging in bottom-up strategies to provide your brain, body, and nervous system with new and corrective experiences.
- Stick with it for 90 to 120 days, and you will see results.

NEXT STEP

The next step is to add some of this goodness to your Panic Proof Protocol. The template is in Appendix A.

Remember, being regulated is not about being calm all the time. It's about being able to manage your emotions and behaviors in a mindful and embodied way.

This means being aware of your current state of being and having the ability to choose how you want to respond to it. When you're feeling activated or dysregulated, take a few moments to pause and check in and ask yourself: *What emotions am I experiencing right now? What thoughts are running through my head? How does my body feel?*

Once you have a better understanding of your current state, you can start to choose how you want to respond. Do you need to take some deep breaths and ground yourself in the present moment? Do you need to talk to someone you trust? Do you need to do a coping mechanism that works for you?

There is no right or wrong way to regulate your emotions. The important thing is to find what works for you and to be patient with yourself. It takes time and practice to develop the skills of emotional regulation.

Refer to each of the four steps outlined in this chapter and then turn to Appendix A, where you will find your Panic Proof Protocol template. Fill in the blanks on the template based on what you are willing to commit to practicing for the next 90 to 120 days.

10

RELATING TO YOUR MANY PARTS

Esme

"TELL ME WHAT YOU'RE NOTICING."

Esme was seated across from me, her eyes closed. She was holding an EMDR tactile device in each hand, and they were buzzing bilaterally between her left and right hand. We were doing a guided visualization exercise to explore what her body had to say about her Gut Anxiety.

"I see my little self. She's crouching beneath a coffee table in the living room."

"What's going on?" I asked.

"She's hiding from Dad," Esme answered.

"Is she open to talking with us?"

Esme nodded. "But she only knows Vietnamese. She doesn't understand you."

"Okay. Can you translate for her?"

"Yes, I can do that."

"I'm glad to hear that. So let's make sure that Little Esme knows that you are here for her, that you hear and understand her, and that you can help her and I understand each other."

Esme translated my words to her inner self and then said, "She feels better hearing that."

"Good," I replied. "Is there anything that Little Esme wants to talk about?"

Esme nodded. "She wants to talk about something, but she doesn't know if she's allowed."

"How do you want to respond to her?"

Esme opened one eye and looked at me. "Can I talk about violence here?"

"Yes, as long as you both feel comfortable and safe."

"We do. We both feel safe." Esme was silent for several minutes, then said: "She's telling me now."

Esme's breathing slowed, her eyes moving beneath her now closed eyelids. "When I was four or five, my mom moved us from San Francisco back to where she had grown up in Vietnam. We were getting away from my father, who was dealing with pretty bad rage at that time. He followed us back. We tried to hide, moving from place to place, but he eventually found us."

Esme's cheeks were flushing, and her posture stiffened. "One day there was a loud banging at the door. My mom opened it and he was standing right there. I don't know why, but I started to scream at the top of my lungs. My mom tried to shush me, but I wouldn't. I don't know why I was screaming."

"It sounds like your little self was experiencing some really big feelings and expressing them in the best way she knew how."

A single tear dripped down her cheek. "Yes. That's exactly right. But they didn't see it that way. My dad came at me and kicked me right in the gut. No one helped me. My mom and younger brother sat right there, saying nothing. I can feel it now, the pain in my gut." Esme placed a hand on her lower abdomen.

"You're safe," I said gently. "You're no longer in that house. You're grown up, you have power and resources now. Show your little self that she doesn't have to stay in that time or in that place if she doesn't want to."

Esme inhaled through her nose, then exhaled through her mouth slowly.

After several moments she said, "She climbed out from under the table, and I brought her to Calm Place. She's feeling better there."

Another moment or two passed, and then Esme tilted her head to the side, curious. She placed a hand on her abdomen, and after a breath she opened her eyes, looking into mine. "The pain in my abdomen is gone," she said.

YOU HAVE MANY PARTS

Have you ever felt like you were divided, as if one part of you was totally freaking out while another part was trying to stay calm? It can be really confusing and frustrating to feel completely different about the same thing. As you'll learn, feeling divided happens because we are all made up of many varying parts, each with its own psychological and physical differences.

WHAT IS A PART?

Our minds are made up of many parts, each with its own thoughts, feelings, sensations, and behaviors. These parts are often formed in response to stress and adversity. For example, if you were bullied as a child, you might have developed a part of yourself that is afraid of conflict. This part might cause you to feel anxious and afraid when you need to speak up, such as in a meeting at work.

TWO PARTS THERAPIES

Therapeutic approaches, Internal Family Systems (IFS) and Ego State Therapy (EST), share a fundamental concept: Our minds can be understood as a collection of different parts, each with its own role and function.

- **INTERNAL FAMILY SYSTEMS (IFS):** This therapy views the mind as having a core "Self"—a wise, compassionate, and healthy center. IFS believes we also have various "sub-personalities" or "parts" that can hold on to negative emotions or coping mechanisms from past experiences. The goal of IFS is to help us heal by strengthening our connection to the Self and achieving harmony among our parts.

- **EGO STATE THERAPY (EST):** EST also views the mind as composed of different "parts" or "ego states," formed in response to life experiences, especially challenging situations. For example, a part might be created to help you avoid conflict or to feel in control.

While the language used in IFS and EST are different, the foundations of these two therapies are similar. Both believe that our parts are formed in response to stress and adversity. Both therapies also believe that our parts can help us to cope with difficult situations.

PARTS AS PROTECTORS

When you encounter a trauma or stressor, your mind, body, and nervous system automatically adapt. This adaptation recruits cooperation from your gut, hormones, immune system, and other bodily systems. (It can later show up in the form of symptoms from head to toe, including and especially panic—but we'll get to that in a moment.)

Additionally, your nervous system will memorize and store each unique state of being, creating a part that is better able to cope with similar situations in the future.

Esme had to cope with abuse from her father and feeling unprotected by her mother and brother. Her brain, body, and nervous system adapted by creating a part that was sensitive to and avoidant of conflict. As a result, she may have been better able to avoid being targeted later in life, but it also prevented her from taking risks and pursuing her goals. It also showed up in her body.

When Esme became an adult, she found herself needing to speak up. But the child-part of her didn't feel safe. She was anxious and afraid and remembered the physical experiences of being in danger. Esme's five-year-old self may have contributed to Esme's physical symptoms.

Despite the powerful messages of her anxiety, Esme was also excited about the opportunity to live life on her own terms, to contribute to society and share her ideas. That part helped her be tenacious, knowing that she had something valuable to contribute. You have that part in you too; that's why you're reading this book.

That part is called the Self.

The Self is the part of you that is intuitive, self-aware, compassionate, and resourceful. In Dialectical Behavior Therapy, the Self is referred to as the Wise Mind. In Eye Movement Desensitization and Reprocessing Therapy (EMDR), it is called the Ego. When you are in Self, you are able to see the big picture, make wise decisions, feel compassion for yourself and others, take care of your needs, and make plans for the future.

While your anxious parts are trying to keep you safe, the Self is excited about the opportunity to adapt and learn. This is the root of internal conflict.

You need all your parts, because they protect you and carry your burdens so that other parts of you, including the Self, don't have to. This is a beautifully adaptive gift. It's like being able to put on a warm jacket in the winter and take it off in the summer.

However, a problem arises if the zipper on the jacket gets stuck. If the jacket won't close in the winter, a cold draft can chill you. If the jacket won't open in the summer, you can't cool down. This is what happens when your mind or body gets stuck in a memorized state that is no longer adaptive. The jacket has become rigid. It is no longer serving you in a positive way. In fact, it may be interfering with your life and causing symptoms.

At a very young age, Esme developed a protective part that became wired throughout her mind, body, and nervous system. This part "remembered" the physical pain long after the event and the danger of it recurring had passed.

Even if you have done therapy on your past traumas, if your body and nervous system haven't received the all-clear message, they are going to continue behaving as though you are still back in the past, which can make it difficult for you to access your Self.

This is where Parts Work comes into play.

THE GOALS OF PARTS WORK

There are many ways to work with your parts, but the method I am going to teach you is an amalgamation of the most useful strategies from the different schools of thought about Parts Work. (See Appendix B for more Parts Work resources.)

THE GOALS OF PARTS WORK:

- **UNCOVER THE ROOT CAUSE(S).** By understanding the root causes of your symptoms, you can create solutions that help you heal and move forward.
- **FREE YOUR PARTS.** A time warp has trapped them into repeating old and no longer necessary patterns. You can free the parts by helping them to understand that the present moment is safe.
- **HELP YOUR PARTS RELEASE THEIR BURDENS.** You can do this by listening to the parts and validating their experiences.
- **TEACH YOUR MIND AND BODY TO SETTLE INTO THE PRESENT MOMENT.** Teach them to observe and accept reality without judgment or the need to change it. You can do this through mindfulness practices such as meditation and yoga.
- **DISENTANGLE YOUR TRUE AND MOST PURE SELF FROM YOUR OTHER PARTS.** Once you do this, they can collaborate toward your higher purpose and bring joy into your life. This is the ultimate goal of Parts Work.

The good news is that your parts are not fixed. They can be changed and transformed.

HOW TO WORK WITH YOUR PARTS

You are going to learn my favorite protocol for doing Parts Work at home. It's called the Meeting Place.

I have also created a second protocol, which is particularly useful for when symptoms start in the body, called Somatographic Imagery.

You can find free recordings to walk you through both of these exercises by going to drnicolecain.com/book-resources/.

First, we'll walk through the eleven steps of the Meeting Place exercise. Then I'll share with you a transcript from a session with Jenny.

Before you start, get a pen and some paper so that you can take notes. I personally like to draw my meeting place, who goes where, and add little notes to remind me what comes up for each part.

Meeting Place

THE ELEVEN STEPS FOR THE MEETING PLACE

1. Create your meeting place.
2. Establish boundaries and rules.
3. Invite your parts.
4. Make introductions.
5. Gather stories and learn about behaviors, thoughts, and sensations.
6. Identify goals and strategies.
7. Express respect and gratitude.
8. Time-stamp the time warp.
9. Determine resources.
10. Set down backpacks.
11. Meet unmet needs.

Find a quiet place where you can relax and won't be disturbed. After you read this paragraph, close your eyes and take a few deep breaths. As you breathe in, imagine that you are filling up with a golden light and calming energy. As you breathe out, imagine that you are releasing your stress and tension. When you are ready, move on to Step 1.

Step 1: Create your meeting place.

In your mind's eye, imagine a comfortable space where you can meet with the different parts of yourself. Imagine that space has some sort of door that you can open or close whenever you want. This will give you control of who you allow to enter your space. This space can be anything you like, such as:

- An office with soft lighting and comfortable furniture
- A cozy room with a fireplace
- A big beautiful garden with a big ivy-covered wall

As you look around your meeting place, notice what you see, smell, hear, and feel. What colors do you see? What textures do you feel? What sounds do you hear? What smells do you detect?

Then allow your imagination to make any and all changes that you would like in order to ensure the space feels comfortable for you.

TIPS FOR CREATING A COMFORTABLE MEETING SPACE:

- Make sure the space is quiet and peaceful.
- Choose colors and textures that you find relaxing.
- Add some personal touches, such as photos or objects that make you feel happy.
- If you have any favorite scents, you can diffuse them in the air.

Stop reading and take a moment to make notes on your piece of paper. Be sure to include as much detail as you can about this space so that you can more easily return the next time you do this exercise.

Step 2: Establish boundaries and rules.

Rules for the meeting place:

- Rule 1: You are in charge of this space—no one else is.
- Rule 2: Parts can enter and exit only when you give them permission.
- Rule 3: Parts must be respectful of you and each other.

Take a moment to write each of these rules on your piece of paper, including anything you feel needs to be added.

Step 3: Invite your parts.

In this step, you are going to invite your parts to come to your meeting place. Open the door, and as each part arrives, introduce yourself and get to know them. Some parts may be easy to identify, while others may be more hidden. Be mindful of how your parts interact with you, how you feel when you meet them, what they say, where they orient themselves in the meeting place, and any other details you notice. There is no right or wrong way to do this. Just allow yourself to be open to meeting all your parts.

Take a few moments to write down what comes up for you in each of the steps that follow.

Step 4: Make introductions.

Once you have met each of your parts, introduce your parts to each other. You can name them whatever feels right for you. Some you may name based on their age or their role, or maybe they'll tell you what they want to be called. For example, in the transcript at the beginning of this chapter, you met Esme's very young part who had stomach pain and hid under the table. Esme named her Little Esme. In Internal Family Systems, they have preexisting names such as Protectors, Firefighters, Exiles, Managers, Seekers, and Wise Self. Jenny named two of her strongest protector parts Caretaker and Strength. There are no right or wrong names. Pick whatever ones resonate best.

You may be surprised to find that some of your parts are aware of other parts, while others may have no idea of certain ones existing. This step is very important in helping you and your parts to realize they are not alone. It allows them to connect, build understanding, and establish trust with one another.

Some parts may be very open to meeting each other, while others may not. Again, there is no right or wrong way to do this step. Allow yourself to be guided by your intuition.

Step 5: Gather stories and learn about behaviors, thoughts, and sensations.

Remember, every single one of your parts has an origin story. That story is the reason they are with you today. One at a time, ask each part if they are willing to tell you what was going on in your life when they showed up. How old are they? How are they affecting your life today? What are their insecurities, fears, hopes, and dreams? What are their unmet needs?

As you listen to your parts' stories, be compassionate and understanding. Remember that they are all trying to do their best to protect you.

As you get to know your parts, you will be able to identify them more easily when they show up in your day-to-day life. In this step, take some time to learn about the behaviors, thoughts, sensations, and general mannerisms of your parts. For example, I always know when my husband's twelve-year-old self comes out, because he's a lot quirkier and louder than his adult clinical director self, who is calmer and more focused.

What behaviors do your parts exhibit? What thoughts do they have? What sensations do you feel in your body when they are present? You may ask them to tell you stories and share memories, and you can learn a lot by simply observing what they reveal. As you observe your parts, be curious and nonjudgmental. Just allow yourself to see them as they are.

Step 6: Identify goals and strategies.

Now take some time to learn about your parts' goals. What are they trying to achieve? What are they doing to try to reach their goals? Parts can do all sorts of creative things to accomplish their goals such as causing different physical sensations in your body, giving you urges and impulses, changing your thinking patterns or cravings, or doing other amazing things. Remember, parts show up as *states* of being, which may involve every single cell in your body, from head to toe.

As you listen to your parts' goals, continue to be supportive and encouraging—even if some of their strategies are those same ones that you'd label as problematic symptoms that you are trying to get rid of.

Step 7: Express respect and gratitude.

This next step is very important. By giving your parts the benefit of the doubt, respecting that they were doing the best they could with the resources they had, you will be able to see how your parts have shown up to try to protect you and how they have held on to the grief and stress so that you didn't have to. What amazing parts you have!

Now take some time to honor and thank your parts for their contributions in your life. Sincerely acknowledge what they have done to help you and the ways they have made your life better.

Step 8: Time-stamp the time warp.

Trauma can sometimes get stored in nontemporal parts of the brain, which means that your parts can get stuck in a sort of time warp, not realizing that time has passed. Like leaving your winter coat on even when summer has arrived.

To help your parts reorient to the present moment, you can use a technique called Time-stamp the Time Warp. Ask your part what year they think it is, then share with them the current time and date, and update them on your current life. Show them how far you have come and how much you have learned.

By asking these questions, you can help your part to understand that time has passed, that they are no longer in danger, and that they can let go of the past.

Step 9: Determine resources.

Your parts need assurance that they can rely on you to take care of them, your other parts, and yourself, if they are to step down from their role in protecting you. So this next step is about sharing with your parts your skills, knowledge, support, and love. Be generous and openhearted as you share these things with your parts. Remember that just as you need your part, your part also needs you.

As you share this information with your parts, you might also add it to your Panic Proof Protocol.

Step 10: Set down backpacks.

Trauma can sometimes feel like a heavy backpack that we carry around with us. It weighs us down with the burdens of the past, causes us to continue to reenact our safety-seeking strategies, and makes it difficult to enjoy life in the present. In this step, we ask our parts if they are willing to set down their burdens and allow us to care for them.

Some parts may be overjoyed by the invitation to be free from their backpacks, while others may negotiate and set them down as an experiment to see how you do. Still others may need more time and support first.

Let them know that you are here for them and that you will do everything you can to help them heal. Be patient and understanding. Remember that this may take time.

Step 11: Meet unmet needs.

Sometimes trauma is not what happened to us, it's what *didn't* happen to us. Ask your parts what desires they have that are unfulfilled that you can safely fulfill. What do they need, long for, and crave? Let them know that you are here to help them make their dreams come true. Be creative and resourceful. Remember that anything is possible.

Session Example: Jenny

"LATELY, MAKING EVEN THE SMALLEST DECISION FEELS LIKE A MONUmental task." Jenny was sitting across from me, shoes off, a pillow in her lap. "Part of me wants to dopamine-dress and throw on the red pantsuit.

But an even stronger part wants to lie on the floor of my closet and cry. Since the latter isn't an option, I typically wind up putting on the same black athleisure wear pants, gray top, and blazer."

"It sounds like your parts have a lot of differing opinions right now," I said.

Jenny nodded. "It's mayhem. Reminds me of my life growing up. It was constant indecision."

"Okay. Let's see what your parts have to say. Is there a place you'd like to start?"

"The self-doubt. Maybe. I think." She smirked at her own joke.

We both got settled, taking a few moments to get comfortable and bring our attention to the present.

"Okay, Jenny. Let's go to your meeting place. Tell me when you get there."

"I'm there. I opened the garden door, and the fire pit is lit, and there are pillows and chairs, twinkle lights, and cups of tea are already set out for everyone."

"Wonderful. Remember, this is your space, you are in charge, and we can stop at any time."

"Yes."

"Okay, are you ready to invite your parts?"

"Yes." Jenny nodded, eyes closed. "I already asked them to come. I see ages four, ten, and thirteen. Anger is also here. She's standing in the corner. And here comes the Caretaker and Strength."

"Is there anyone else that you want to invite?" I asked.

Jenny paused. "There is someone, but she's standing outside the door."

"What do you want to do?" I asked.

"I want to invite her in, but she's—she's hesitant. I feel it in my throat, a constriction."

"Ask her what she needs in order to feel comfortable coming in."

"She needs to know that I'm not going to punish her."

"Tell her that this place is safe, that you will protect her, and that you and your other parts want to hear what she has to say."

"She feels more comfortable," Jenny said. "She came in but wants to stay near the door."

"That's fine. I'm glad she trusted you to come in. Would she be willing to share a little bit about her worry of being punished?"

"Mom was big into punishing. She'd read my emails and text messages. She said that I was her best friend, but if I said or wrote something wrong, she'd get very upset. She'd lock herself in her bedroom and cry very loudly, or she'd blame me for making her depressed."

"How did your younger self respond to all that?"

Jenny's voice changed—she sounded younger. "I tried to keep quiet. I was always waiting to make another mistake that hurt my mom."

"Adult Jenny, what are you noticing right now?"

"My throat hurts a lot. It's making me feel panicky, and my heart is beating faster. I feel like I'm that little girl again. I can't trust myself, and so I feel like hiding."

"Tell Little Jenny that she is so brave, and that we are grateful for her trying to protect you, and that we appreciate her sharing her feelings with us," I said.

Jenny was silent for several moments as she relayed the message to her younger self.

"Ask her if she knows that the year is 2019," I said. This was the year we did this session.

Jenny paused. "She . . . she is surprised."

"Tell her that it's 2019 and she doesn't have to carry this heavy burden anymore. She's not responsible for Mom's feelings. Explain that you have grown up, you're strong, and you have resources now that she didn't have then."

"She wants proof," Jenny said.

"Show her proof. What would you like her to see?"

Jenny hesitated as she thought, then said, "My degree. My apartment. My job, helping people. My best friend. You. Sophie [the cat]."

"What does she think of all that?"

"She's impressed." Jenny smiled.

"She also has all your other parts," I reminded her.

"Caretaker and the four-year-old both want to hug her."

"How does she feel about that?"

"She likes it." Jenny's voice sounded a bit stronger. "It helps her believe we're not mad at her."

"Good. It's important for her to know she matters and that she's loved."

"And that she doesn't have to be perfect," Jenny added.

"Exactly." I paused. "Next, let's ask your younger part to imagine that all her worries and stressors are inside a backpack. Ask her if she would be willing to set that backpack down."

"She wants to throw it into the firepit," Jenny quickly answered. "She doesn't want to carry it anymore."

"Then let's throw it into the firepit."

Jenny nodded slowly, then took a deep breath. "Wow."

"What do you notice?"

"My throat feels completely normal."

"That's wonderful to hear. It sounds like your younger part is feeling a little better?"

"Yes," Jenny said, "much better. The anxiety has . . . lifted."

"Okay, before we finish up, ask your younger part what else she needs from you today."

"She wants me to know she likes the red jumpsuit. She thinks it's pretty."

"For the record, I happen to agree," I said.

"Yeah, she's in my closet." Jenny's smile was radiant. "She said she wants me to wear the red jumpsuit tomorrow."

JENNY AND I WENT on to finish her session, including an assignment for Jenny to journal what her part shared with her today, and to pay attention to any other messages she got from her parts over the coming weeks.

NEXT STEPS

By learning to understand and work with our parts, we can begin to heal from panic and live more peaceful and fulfilling lives. Your next steps are to dive into this exercise yourself.

PARTS WORK TL;DR

- Your mind, body, and nervous system automatically adapt to stress and adversity by forming parts.
- We are all made up of many varying parts, each with its own state of body and mind.
- Parts can get stuck in a time warp where they continue to react as though you are stuck in the past.
- Parts Work can help repattern your mind, body, and nervous system, creating healing in both the mind and the body.

11

THE PANIC PROOF PROTOCOL

YOU DID IT! YOU DOVE INTO THE DETAILS, LEARNED THE NITTY-gritty science, and completed the self-reflection exercises. Now it's time to put it all together!

The Panic Proof Protocol will walk you through the process of creating your trauma-informed and holistic protocol based on the results of the self-assessment checklists you have filled out. As you follow your protocol, be sure to track your progress and refer to the checklists regularly. This will help you evaluate what's working and what's not and make any necessary adjustments. Think of it as a cross-country road trip. There will be zigs and zags, detours, ups and downs. But frequent check-ins will help you navigate this journey like a pro.

Throughout this chapter, you're going to learn about holistic solutions from a wide variety of traditions, such as naturopathic medicine, trauma-informed neuroscience, and Ayurveda. We'll talk about your specific obstacles to healing from anxiety, and the foundations of Panic Proof living, including lifestyle and healthy habits. Once those pieces are in place, we'll zero in on the nine types of anxiety and how to create a protocol that is as specific as possible for your unique experience.

You'll notice the protocols mix of all sorts of holistic solutions: nutrition, botanical remedies (including mushrooms), supplements, psychobiotics, essential oils, flower essences, and a ton more. I've given you recipes under each protocol, but at the end of this chapter I've also included a bit more information on different kinds of herbs and supplements in case you're the more independent type and want to learn how to create your own protocol.

The best part is that you get to make it yours. So have fun with this process! Dig in! And get ready to see some amazing results.

STEP 1: MY OBSTACLES TO CURE

No matter what you do, if you haven't addressed the obstacles to your healing, your solutions will be palliative and temporary at best. This book is not called *Panic Palliation,* it's called *Panic Proof.* So let's zero in on how to start.

Begin by referring to Chapter 8, where you learned about different types of obstacles to cure. In each of the spaces provided below, write down all the potential obstacles that stuck out to you as potentially relevant in your life.

My Lifestyle and Habit Obstacles

My Biological Obstacles

My Psychological Obstacles

My Social and Environmental Obstacles

My Spiritual Obstacles

What next steps can you take to address these obstacles? Is there a change you can make, a test you can order, more research you'd like to do? Write down your ideas here:

Zeroing In

Look at your list and identify the top three most prominent obstacles. List them here:

Based on Chapter 8, do the types of obstacles you resonate with indicate any testing? If so, write some notes in the space provided below.

ESME EXAMPLE:

Biological obstacle suspected because symptoms ebb and flow with menstrual cycles. This suggests a hormonal component. Root-cause testing: sex-hormone testing. Esme researched hormone testing options and opted to do a DUTCH.

STEP 2: MY FOUNDATIONS

Just as healthy soil is essential for a bountiful fruit and vegetable garden, healthy habits are the foundation of healing your mind, body, and spirit.

Throughout this book, I've shared quick tips on diet, lifestyle, and habit changes that can help you create a Panic Proof lifestyle. Here they are:

Panic Proof Diet

The best diet for healing the brain and body will be rich in antioxidants (which help eliminate tissue-damaging free radicals), anti-inflammatory foods, gut-nourishing fermented foods and fiber, and brain-health-boosting nutrients. It is also low in saturated fat, trans fat (hydrogenated fat), and processed foods. My go-to protocols are the Mediterranean diet and intermittent fasting.

FOODS FOR HEALING THE BRAIN AND BODY:

- **ANTIOXIDANT-RICH FOODS.** Fruits, vegetables, whole grains, legumes, nuts, seeds, and spices
- **ANTI-INFLAMMATORY FOODS.** Leafy green vegetables, berries, fatty fish, olive oil, and turmeric
- **GUT-NOURISHING FOODS.** Fermented foods such as yogurt, kimchi, and sauerkraut, and fiber-rich foods such as fruits, vegetables, and whole grains
- **BRAIN-HEALTH-BOOSTING FOODS.** Fatty fish, leafy green vegetables, berries, nuts, and seeds

In addition to eating a diet that is rich in the foods listed above, it is also important to avoid foods, ingredients, drinks, and additives that may increase anxiety. These include:

- **CAFFEINE.** It's found in energy drinks, coffee, and some teas.
- **SUGAR.** It can cause spikes in blood sugar levels, which can lead to anxiety.
- **ALCOHOL.** In your liver, alcohol breaks down into a chemical called acetaldehyde, which damages your DNA, is a neurotoxin, and can cause anxiety and panic.
- **PROCESSED FOODS.** They are often high in sugar, unhealthy fats, and artificial ingredients such as food coloring, all of which can contribute to anxiety.
- **ARTIFICIAL SWEETENERS.** If a package says "no sugar," be sure to check the ingredient label for the presence of artificial

sweeteners. These sneaky chemicals can trigger anxiety, inflammation, and all sorts of other problems.

We've talked a little bit about the relationship between panic and genes, which adds a lot of nuance to nutrition. For example, eating leafy greens is generally a safe go-to, but certain gene mutations or medical conditions may require specific dietary adjustments. While this is out of the scope of this book, I do have a great resource for you in Appendix B.

Lifestyle

Your lifestyle consists of the broader patterns of how you live your life: your daily work routine, leisure activities, social interactions, and dietary choices. Do your patterns promote stress or calm?

Sometimes the stress-provoking variables in our lives are out of our control, but in certain areas we do have some control.

FOUNDATIONS OF A HEALTHY LIFESTYLE

- **EXERCISE REGULARLY.** Exercise is a great way to reduce stress, improve sleep, and boost mood. Aim for at least 30 minutes of moderate-intensity exercise most days of the week.
- **GET ENOUGH SLEEP.** Most adults need seven to nine hours of sleep per night. Getting enough sleep helps to regulate mood and reduce anxiety.
- **SET HEALTHY BOUNDARIES.** For example:

    - Set limits on your time and energy. Don't be afraid to say no to requests that you don't have time for or that will drain you.
    - Learn to say no to unhealthy relationships. If someone is making you feel stressed, anxious, or unhappy, it's okay to end or put limits on the relationship.
    - Take care of yourself first. Make sure you're getting enough sleep, eating healthy foods, and exercising regu-

larly. When you take care of yourself, you're better able to take care of others.

- Be assertive. Learn to express your needs and wants in a clear and direct way.
- Avoid people-pleasing. Don't try to make everyone happy all the time. It's impossible, and it will only make you feel worse.

- **SPEND TIME IN NATURE.** Being in nature has been shown to reduce stress and improve mood. Take some time each day to go for a walk in the park, hike in the woods, or simply sit in your backyard and enjoy the fresh air and sunshine.
- **CONNECT WITH LOVED ONES.** Social support is important for everyone, but it's especially important for people with anxiety. Make time for friends and family who make you feel good.

Habits

Habits are activities, actions, or behaviors that you repeatedly perform that become ingrained in your routine. Habits can produce panic, or they can protect you from panic. For example, nicotine is a habit that some people use to try to combat stress, yet numerous studies reveal that nicotine does the opposite—it makes you anxious. On the other hand, brushing your teeth every morning and night can actually help you have better mental and emotional health.

There are many habits you can start practicing to help prime your body, mind, and nervous system to be able to shift between being appropriately aroused and relaxed, which we explored in Chapter 9.

Identify three bottom-up activities from Chapter 9 that you are committed to incorporating into your daily life and making into habits. Write them in the space provided:

____

____

____

I know that making changes to your lifestyle can be challenging, but it's worth it for your health and well-being. I'm here to support you every step of the way.

Okay, now that we have foundations in place. Let's zoom in and get a bit more specific.

STEP 3: YOUR TYPE(S) OF ANXIETY

Next, refer back to the Nine Types of Anxiety Quiz that you filled out in Chapter 3, and write your results in the table below:

YOUR NINE TYPES OF ANXIETY QUIZ RESULTS

ANXIETY TYPE	SCORE AND SUBTYPES
Chest Anxiety	Score: __/20
Nervous System Anxiety	Score: __/20
Immune System Anxiety	Score: __/20
Gut Anxiety	Score: __/20
Thought Anxiety	Score: __/20
Anger Anxiety	Score: __/20
Depressive Anxiety	Score: __/20
Hormone Anxiety	Score: __/20
Trauma Anxiety	Score: __/20

Write down your top-three highest anxiety type scores, starting with the highest score or the most bothersome one in the space below:

____

____

____

Now we've identified your three starting points. Start with the first one you listed and flip to the page with the associated protocol. This will be your first protocol. With your foundations in place, add to your lifestyle elements from the first protocol that you resonate with. Give it about a week and a half to see shifts in your symptoms. Sometimes the protocol you start with will create a domino effect resulting in relief in other areas. Other times you will need to move on and add strategies from the next protocol.

Write your plan in the Panic Proof Protocol in Appendix A. Be sure to remember your "obstacles to cure" goals, and include any testing that you need to get ordered, and tips from the Ayurveda section about your dosha, in your protocols.

Ayurvedic Medicine

Ayurveda practitioners believe that each person is born with a unique combination of the five elements: ether (space), air, fire, water, and earth. Your particular combination is called your dosha. Your dosha determines your physical and mental constitution, your natural tendencies, and it gives you direction on how to restore your health and promote remission of symptoms. There are three doshas, which are vata, pitta, and kapha.

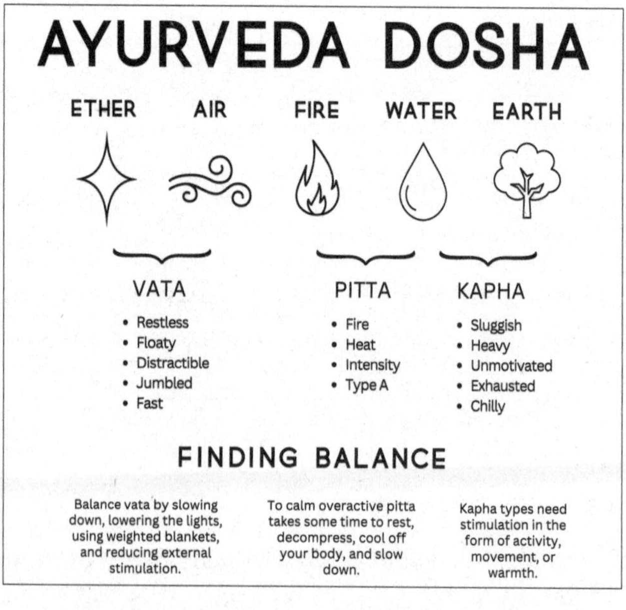

CHEST ANXIETY

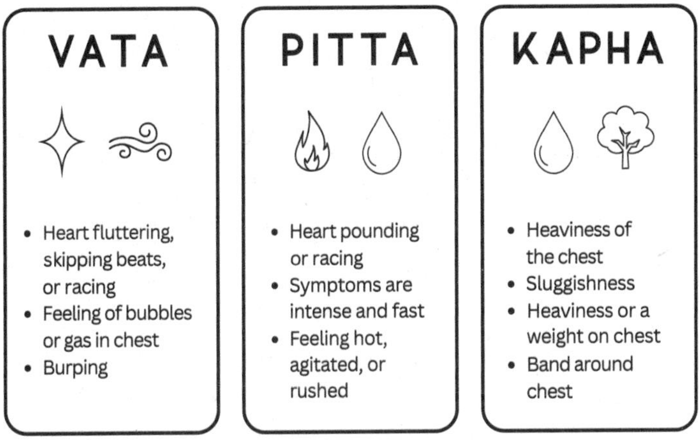
VATA
• Heart fluttering, skipping beats, or racing
• Feeling of bubbles or gas in chest
• Burping
PITTA
• Heart pounding or racing
• Symptoms are intense and fast
• Feeling hot, agitated, or rushed
KAPHA
• Heaviness of the chest
• Sluggishness
• Heaviness or a weight on chest
• Band around chest

So let's say you have anxiety. We do a little digging and learn that much of your anxiety is centered in your chest: Chest Anxiety. Ayurveda takes us a step deeper, showing us how Chest Anxiety can take on different forms.

As you can see, each of these dosha types can have symptoms of anxiety in the chest, but the symptoms are quite different. An Ayurveda practitioner would treat your vata Chest Anxiety differently from a pitta or kapha Chest Anxiety.

Adding dosha-balancing specific strategies to your anxiety protocols will get you better results. Here's how:

FIRST: IDENTIFY YOUR PARTICULAR dosha imbalance. Below are general indicators of each imbalance, and for even more detail, you can take my free dosha quiz by going to my website and typing the words *dosha quiz* into the search bar.

SYMPTOMS OF IMBALANCE IN EACH DOSHA

VATA	PITTA	KAPHA
Think: Light, dry, moving, cold Symptoms: Changeable, distractible, irregular, fluttering, and floaty	Think: Fiery, hot, intense Symptoms: Coming on with a vengeance, tend toward tenacity, with lots of inflammation	Think: Heavy, soft, chilly Symptoms: Sluggish, slow-moving, weighed down, depressive, lethargic

NEXT: INCORPORATE DOSHA BALANCING, foods, habits, and spices into your Panic Proof Protocol. Here are some starting points. I have a ton more free resources on my podcast *Holistic Inner Balance,* too!

- **BALANCING VATA.** Do regulating and grounding exercises such as yoga or qigong or midstrength weight training. Walk outside on the grass in your bare feet. Eat foods that are warm, cooked, and oily such as ghee, cooked root vegetables, and wild Alaskan salmon. Use vata-balancing herbs such as ginger (*Zingiber officinale*) and gotu kola (*Centella asiatica*).
- **BALANCING PITTA.** Do soothing exercises like swimming or yin yoga. Be still in nature. Eat foods that are cooling and nourishing such as mint, cucumbers, and watermelon. Use pitta-balancing herbs such as peppermint (*Mentha piperita*), cilantro (*Coriandrum sativum*), and licorice (*Glycyrrhiza glabra*).
- **BALANCING KAPHA.** Do daily vigorous exercise. Go out in nature. Do daily dry brushing. Eat warming, bitter foods that are drying such as dandelion greens or baked kale chips. Use kapha-balancing herbs such as Curcumin (*Curcuma longa*), Cinnamon (*Cinnamomum verum*), and black pepper (*Piper nigrum*).

PROTOCOLS

Chest Anxiety Protocol

IDENTIFY ROOT CAUSES. Refer to the discussion of Chest Anxiety in Chapter 4. In the space below, write notes about concepts that you resonated with that may be worth further exploration. Consider root causes, testing, and mindfulness strategies.

____

____

____

____

CHEST ANXIETY SUPPLEMENTS

- Taurine (1.5 g/day) lowers blood pressure and is good for chronic stress on the heart.
- L-theanine (400 mg per day) is especially useful for fluttering palpitations with anxiety.
- COQ10 (100 mg each morning) is great for heart health. It is an antioxidant and can be energizing.

HERBAL RECIPES. HERE ARE some ideas to get you started. Pick one from below, or consider formulating your own! For ideas for making your own tincture, check out the section "Herbal Medicine for Panic Relief" later in this chapter.

CHEST ANXIETY SOOTHER FOR EACH DOSHA

VATA	PITTA	KAPHA
40% motherwort (*Leonurus cardiaca*) 30% valerian root (*Valeriana officinalis*) 25% lemon balm (*Melissa officinalis*) 5% ginger (*Zingiber officinale*)	40% motherwort (*Leonurus cardiaca*) 30% hawthorn (*Crataegus oxyacantha*) 25% lemon balm (*Melissa officinalis*) 5% peppermint (*Mentha piperita*)	40% motherwort (*Leonurus cardiaca*) 30% hawthorn (*Crataegus*) 25% chamomilla (*Matricaria chamomilla*) 5% cinnamon (*Cinnamomum verum*)
How to take: Mix 1-3 big squeezes into tea or water once or twice per day.	**How to take:** Mix 1-3 big squeezes into tea or water once or twice per day.	**How to take:** Mix 1-3 big squeezes into tea or water once or twice per day.

Nervous System Anxiety Protocol

IDENTIFY ROOT CAUSES. Refer to the discussion of Nervous System Anxiety in Chapter 3. To build your protocol, start with Nervous System Anxiety basics:

- **SUPPLEMENTS:**
    - Acetyl L-carnitine (1–3 g in the morning) is good for sluggishness, numbness, and tingling nerves.
    - Alpha-lipoic acid (100–600 mg per day) helps with sugars, numbness, and tingling nerves.
    - B-complex vitamins are great for your nerves. If you'd like more specific information, check out the Histamine Detox Protocol on page 319 for details on specific B vitamins and how to dose them.

- **CALMING HABITS.** Refer back to Chapter 9 where we explored bottom-up techniques, and remind yourself of what you committed to practicing.
- **HERBAL RECIPES.** Here are some ideas to get you started. Pick one of the soothers below, or consider formulating your own!

NERVOUS SYSTEM ANXIETY SOOTHER FOR EACH DOSHA

VATA	PITTA	KAPHA
40% California poppy (*Eschscholtzia californica*) 30% passionflower (*Passiflora incarnata*) 25% valerian root (*Valeriana officinalis*) 5% ginger (*Zingiber officinale*)	40% valerian root (*Valeriana officinalis*) 30% passionflower (*Passiflora incarnata*) 25% kava kava (*Piper methysticum*) 5% peppermint (*Mentha piperita*)	40% saffron (*Crocus sativus*) 30% chamomilla (*Matricaria chamomilla*) 25% turmeric (*Curcuma longa*) 5% cayenne (*Capsicum annuum*)
How to take: Mix 1-3 big squeezes into tea or water once or twice per day.	**How to take:** Mix 1-3 big squeezes into tea or water once or twice per day.	**How to take:** Mix 1-3 big squeezes into tea or water once or twice per day.

ZERO IN ON NEUROTRANSMITTERS

SPECIFIC NEUROTRANSMITTER HACKS. If after a week or two on the Nervous System Anxiety Protocol you are looking for additional support, you may consider incorporating neurotransmitter-specific strategies.

To know where to start, refer to the neurotransmitter checklists from Chapter 6. In the space below, write down the neurotransmitters (high or low) where you checked more than two boxes.

____

____

____

____

As you know, checklists are not diagnoses, but they're a place to start. Functional testing, if you opt to go in that direction, can help you to get more information.

Next, refer to your list of neurotransmitters, and circle the three most important. These may be the ones that have the highest scores, or cause the most bothersome symptoms, or maybe you've already had testing done supporting your self-assessment results.

Next up, circle the three you're going to start with in the table below. Select the supplements, herbs, and remedies you want to start with and add them to your Panic Proof Protocol in Appendix A.

NEUROTRANSMITTER SOLUTIONS

NEUROTRANSMITTER	TESTING AND SOLUTIONS
Serotonin	**MARKER:** 5-HIAA, kynurenine, quinolinic acid **TEST:** Organic Acids Test **FOR LOW SEROTONIN: (ONLY IF YOU ARE NOT ON AN SSRI)** **PICK ONE FROM THESE THREE OPTIONS:** • 5-hydroxytryptophan (100–200 mg in the morning) helps with lethargy, depression, and anxiety. • L-tryptophan (500–2000 mg at bedtime) helps with anxiety and restlessness. • St. John's wort tincture (3 big squeezes in morning and at night), if you prefer to go the herbal route. **ALSO INCLUDE:** • A multivitamin with B6 (P5P), vitamin D, B3 (niacinamide), magnesium, and B1 (thiamine) **FOR HIGH SEROTONIN: GETTING HIGH SEROTONIN DOWN IS TRICKY. IF YOUR SEROTONIN IS ELEVATED, TALK TO YOUR DOCTOR.**

NEUROTRANSMITTER	TESTING AND SOLUTIONS
Dopamine	**Marker:** HVA, DOPAC **Test:** Organic Acids Test **FOR LOW DOPAMINE, CONSIDER A PRODUCT THAT CONTAINS A MIXTURE OF THE FOLLOWING:** • L-tyrosine (250–500 mg at bedtime) • DL-phenylalanine (250–1000 mg at bedtime) **ALSO:** • Eat foods that contain tyrosine: meat, fish, dairy, pumpkin seeds. • Lion's Mane mushroom (1–2 g in the morning) • Take a multivitamin with vitamins C and B6, copper, zinc, and, if needed, iron. **FOR HIGH DOPAMINE:** • Tincture: bacopa (*Bacopa monnieri*) (3 big squeezes in the morning and at night) • Probiotic containing *Lactobacillus plantarum*
Adrenaline	**Marker:** VMA **Test:** DUTCH **Marker:** Catecholamine levels and metanephrine levels **Test:** Blood testing **FOR LOW ADRENALINE:** • Tincture: 40% ashwagandha (*Withania somnifera*), 30% shatavari (*Asparagus racemosus*), and 30% licorice (*Glycyrrhiza glabra*). Take 3 big squeezes in the morning and at bedtime, to boost adrenaline. **FOR HIGH ADRENALINE:** • Tincture: kava kava (*Piper methysticum*) (3 big squeezes in juice or water) to reduce acute adrenaline anxiety • L-theanine (200–800 mg) for acute adrenaline anxiety • Taurine (1.5 g) for acute anxiety

NEUROTRANSMITTER	TESTING AND SOLUTIONS
GABA	**MARKER:** 4-hydroxybutyric acid (GHB) and succinic semialdehyde (SSA) **TEST:** Neurotransmitter testing **FOR LOW GABA, START WITH:** • Happy Sleepy Powder (as directed at drnicolecain.com) **IF NEEDED, ADD IN THE ORDER LISTED:** • B6 (P5P) (50–200 mg per day), to support GABA production • Tincture: 40% valerian (*Valeriana officinalis*), 30% passionflower (*Passiflora incarnata*), 25% hops (*Humulus lupulus*), 5% rosemary (*Salvia rosmarinus*), to reduce GABA. Take 3 big squeezes for anxiety relief. • Eat fermented foods like yogurt. • Psychobiotic blend: a mix of *Lactobacillus brevis, Lactococcus lactis*, and *Bifidobacterium dentium*.
Glutamate	**TEST:** There aren't super-helpful tests for glutamate levels. **FOR HIGH GLUTAMATE:** • L-theanine (200–800 mg) • Magnesium (L-threonate or glycinate) (400 mg) • Alpha-lipoic acid (400–600 mg in the morning) • Inhaling lavender, which blocks glutamate receptors
Histamine	**Marker:** N-methyl-histamine **Test:** 23-hour urine test **Marker:** Whole blood histamine **Test:** Blood test **Solution:** Histamine Detox Protocol

TARGETING SYMPTOMS. If you don't resonate with neurotransmitter-specific symptoms and would prefer to target the symptoms themselves, here are some protocols that I have used with success. Do keep in mind, however, that you will get better results by personalizing your protocol to your body's unique needs.

- **MIGRAINES.** Magnesium L-threonate (400–1000 mg), plus an herbal combination containing herbal butterbur (*Petasites hybridus*) and feverfew (*Tanacetum parthenium*), as directed on the bottle.

- **BRAIN ZAPS.** Fish oil containing at least 1000 mg eicosapentaenoic acid and 1000 mg docosahexaenoic acid plus B vitamin complex containing folinic acid, hydroxocobalamin, and thiamine.
- **MUSCLE TENSION.** Herbal mixture containing equal parts of vervain (*Verbena officinalis*), hops (*Humulus lupulus*), valerian (*Valeriana officinalis*), skullcap (*Scutellaria lateriflora*), and passionflower (*Passiflora incarnata*). Take 3 big squeezes every 4–6 hours.
- **HYPERSENSITIVITY.** Mix ¼ teaspoon nutmeg into warm milk (whatever kind you'd like), and sip before you go to sleep. Some providers also suggest selecting a homeopathic remedy based on what best fits your symptoms:
  - Phosphorus 30C. For those sensitive to noise, light, and odors, with cravings for ice cold water, and with desire for company when feeling unwell.
  - Nux Vomica 30C. For those sensitive to noise, light, and odors, very chilly, irritable, and perfectionistic, who prefer to be alone when unwell.
  - Belladonna 30C. For those who are extremely sensitive to noise, light, odors, and movement, who may experience throbbing pains, and who when unwell desire to be alone and in the dark.
- **BURNING PAIN WHEN PANICKING.** Fire Soother Flower Essence Blend (see page 330) (5 drops per day with extra doses as needed).
- **NERVE PAINS, NUMBNESS, AND/OR TINGLING.** Consider a product containing a mixture of L-carnitine, alpha-lipoic acid, and B vitamins.

Histamine Detox Protocol

Here are some general instructions for following a low-histamine diet. The exact foods and supplements that you need to take or avoid will vary depending on your individual circumstances. You may also want to adjust the timing of these steps based on how you feel.

STEP 1: Identify your suspected sources of histamine. Here are some common high-histamine foods and beverages to get you started:

- Aged cheese
- Fermented food (such as yogurt, sauerkraut, and kimchi)
- Dried fruit
- Avocado
- Spinach
- Tomato
- Citrus fruit
- Alcoholic beverages
- Smoked or processed meat
- Fish and shellfish

For a more complete list of histamine-boosting foods that you want to avoid, check out my website, drnicolecain.com, and type the word *histamine* in the search bar.

STEP 2: Remove all these foods and beverages from your diet for one month. This will help to reduce the amount of histamine in your body.

STEP 3: Support the methylation histamine detox pathway in order as listed:

Vitamin B1 (Thiamine)

- Start with a trial dose of 50–100 mg per day for one week.
- If well-tolerated, increase to a replenishment dose of 500–1000 mg per day for one month.
- Then reduce to a maintenance dose of 100–300 mg per day.

Vitamin B12

- Start with a trial dose of 200–500 mcg per day for one week.
- If well-tolerated, increase to a replenishment dose of 1–15 mg per day for one month.

- Then reduce to 400 mcg–5 g per day going forward.
- Try the methylcobalamin form first, but if you feel anxious or agitated on this form, consider switching to hydroxocobalamin.

Vitamin B9

- Start with a trial dose of 200–500 mcg per day for one week.
- If well tolerated, increase to a replenishment dose of 1–15 mg per day for one month.
- Then reduce to a maintenance dose of 400 mcg–5 g per day.
- Try methylfolate first, but if you feel anxious or agitated on this form, consider switching to folinic acid.

Vitamin B6 (use the P5P form)

- Start with a trial dose of 10–50 mg per day for one week.
- If well tolerated, increase to a replenishment dose of 70–300 mg per day for one month.
- Then reduce to a maintenance dose of 15–50 mg per day.

Vitamin C

- Start with a trial dose of 500–1000 mg per day for one week.
- If well tolerated, increase to a replenishment dose of 1000 mg twice per day for one month.
- Then reduce to a maintenance dose of 500 mg per day.

Magnesium

- Start with a trial dose of 400 mg per day for one week.
- If well tolerated, increase to a replenishment dose of 800 mg twice per day for one month.
- Then reduce to a maintenance dose of 400 mg per day.

STEP 4: Next, add supportive trace minerals. I like liquid trace minerals because you can control them by the drop, and they're easy to add into water. Another option is pink Himalayan sea salt.

STEP 5: Support acetylation histamine detox pathway

- Eat lots of foods that are rich in calcium D-glucarate and that boost liver health, all while lowering histamine: Brussels sprouts, red and green cabbage, cauliflower, collard greens, kale, bok choy, broccoli and arugula, apples, and bean sprouts.

STEP 6: Support diamine oxidase (DAO) histamine detox pathway

- Diamine oxidase (DAO) is the main enzyme responsible for breaking down histamine in the gut. If DAO levels are low, or if DAO is not functioning properly, histamine can accumulate in the body. My favorite way to increase DAO is to take it as a supplement with meals.

BONUS: HISTAMINE-LOWERING HERBAL TEAS

- Chamomilla (*Matricaria chamomilla*). This is the plant you may recognize as chamomile. In addition to being very effective at reducing anxiety, chamomilla flowers reduce histamine release from mast cells. A cup of chamomilla tea at night can help calm allergies and mood in one delicious swoop.
- Turmeric (*Curcuma longa*). This delicious spice has many health-promoting benefits. Turmeric blocks mast cells from releasing histamine, combats allergies, and is a powerful antioxidant. It improves mood and is "tridoshic" in Ayurvedic medicine, which means it balances all dosha types.
- Stinging nettle (*Urtica dioica*). You can eat this tasty treat as a salad (properly prepared!), drink it in a tea, or take it as a tincture. Nettle is included in many antihistamine formulas because it reduces histamine release from mast cells and is packed full of calcium, magnesium, iron, and vitamins A and C.

Gut Anxiety Protocol

IDENTIFY ROOT CAUSES. Refer to Chapter 5, which is all about the gut-brain axis, and Gut Anxiety. In the space below, write notes about concepts that you resonated with that might be worth further exploration. Consider root causes, testing, or mindfulness strategies.

____

____

____

____

GUT ANXIETY SUPPLEMENTS

- **NAUSEA.** Here is my favorite anti-nausea recipe: 35% lemon balm (*Melissa officinalis*), 20% raspberry (*Rubus idaeus*), 25% lavender (*Lavandula officinalis*), 5% ginger (*Zingiber officinale*), 5% peppermint (*Mentha piperita*). Take 1–3 big squeezes in chamomilla or fennel tea for calming and relief of anxiety and nausea.
- **HEARTBURN.** Deglycyrrhizinated licorice (DGL) Chewable: Take 50–100 mg up to three times per day.
- **DIARRHEA.** The probiotic yeast *Saccharomyces boulardii* (250 mg per day) plus soluble fiber powder (6–8 g per day).
- **CONSTIPATION.** Increase vitamin C and magnesium until stools soften.
- **GAS AND BLOATING.** Tincture mix 50% gentian root (*Gentiana lutea*) plus 50% skullcap (*Scutellaria lateriflora*), 5 drops in warm water with lemon before meals or apple cider vinegar, 20–30 drops (1 big squeeze) in a small amount of water before meals.

HERBAL RECIPES

Remember the "Self-Assessment Checklist: Gut Anxiety Subtypes" in Chapter 5? This is where that information will come in useful. Pick one of the following tinctures based on your subtype (or of course you can make your own!). For example, if your subtype was Vata Gut, select the Vata Gut Anxiety Soother. That will help you zero in on what herbs will get you the best results.

GUT ANXIETY SOOTHER FOR EACH DOSHA

VATA	PITTA	KAPHA
40% lemon balm (*Melissa officinalis*) 30% skullcap (*Scutellaria lateriflora*) 25% fennel (*Foeniculum vulgare*) seeds 5% ginger (*Zingiber officinale*)	40% skullcap (*Scutellaria lateriflora*) 30% gentian root (*Gentiana lutea*) 25% gotu kola (*Centella asiatica*) 5% peppermint (*Mentha piperita*)	40% chamomilla (*Matricaria chamomilla*) 30% gentian root (*Gentiana lutea*) 25% fenugreek (*Trigonella foenum-graecum*) 5% ginger (*Zingiber officinale*)
How to take: Mix 1–3 big squeezes into tea or water 1–2 times per day.	**How to take:** Mix 1 big squeeze into tea or water 2–3 times per day.	**How to take:** Mix 1 big squeeze into tea or water 2–3 times per day.

Gut Healing Protocol

MORNING

- **GUT HEALING EYE-OPENER.** Mix the following into 8 ounces of warm water: 1 tablespoon apple cider vinegar, 1 big squeeze of ginger (*Zingiber officinale*) tincture, and lemon to taste. Take before each meal, ideally three times per day.

BEFORE MEALS

- **ENZYME-BALANCING BLEND.** Mix as a tincture: 50% skullcap (*Scutellaria lateriflora*) and 50% gentian root (*Gentiana lutea*). Take 5–20 drops in a small amount of tea or water before each meal to retrain your gut to digest optimally.

EVENING

- **GUT-NOURISHING BLEND.** Mix the following into 8 ounces of warm water: 2500 mg slippery elm powder (*Ulmus rubra*), 1000 mg turmeric root (*Curcuma longa*), and 1 g marshmallow root (*Althaea officinalis*).
- **PROBIOTIC.** For best results, take your probiotic near bedtime with a small snack such as yogurt. You can find and order my favorite up-to-date probiotics in the shop at my website.
- **FIBER.** Consider taking a mix of soluble and insoluble fiber. Soluble fiber can help to slow down digestion, promote the growth of beneficial bacteria, and lower the risk of constipation, heart disease, and type 2 diabetes. Insoluble fiber can help to keep the digestive system healthy, prevent constipation, and lower the risk of colon cancer. Oats are a good source of both soluble and insoluble fiber. They are also a good source of beta-glucan, a type of soluble fiber that has been shown to have many health benefits, including lowering cholesterol and blood sugar levels.

EAT LESS:

HARMFUL FOOD ADDITIVES AND INGREDIENTS

- **PRESERVATIVES.** Butylated hydroxyanisole (BHA), butylated hydroxytoluene (BHT), benzoates (such as sodium benzoate), sulfites, carrageenan, sodium nitrites, and nitrates
- **THICKENERS.** Guar gum, xanthan gum
- **YEAST EXTRACT.** Autolyzed yeast, hydrolyzed yeast
- **FLAVOR ENHANCERS.** Monosodium glutamate (MSG), salicylates, all enhancers with the word *artificial*
- **ARTIFICIAL DYES.** FD&C Blue Nos. 1 and 2, FD&C Green No. 3, FD&C Yellow Nos. 5 (tartrazine) and 6, and Red Dye No. 3
- **TRANS FATS.** Partially hydrogenated oils, fully hydrogenated oils

- **HIGH FRUCTOSE CORN SYRUP.** Also avoid its rebranding as corn syrup, maize syrup, glucose syrup, glucose-fructose syrup, tapioca syrup, crystalline fructose, isoglucose, fructose, fruit fructose, and dahlia syrup.
- **ARTIFICIAL SWEETENERS.** The label "sugar free" usually means a food contains an artificial sugar such as aspartame (Equal, NutraSweet), sucralose (Splenda), acesulfame K (Sunett and Sweet One), advantame, neotame (Newtame), or saccharin (Sweet 'N Low and Sugar Twin).

INFLAMMATORY FOODS

- **SMOKED FOODS.** Packaged or cooked in a smoker
- **PROCESSED FOODS.** Typically packaged and altered for shelf life
- **RED MEAT.** Beef, pork, lamb
- **FRIED FOODS.** Frying oils cause the formation of trans fats and can also increase pro-inflammatory omega-6 fat formation
- **SUGARY FOODS.** Cakes, cookies, prepackaged sweets
- **PACKAGED SNACKS.** Typically high in unhealthy fats, sugar, and preservatives
- **REFINED GRAINS.** White rice and white bread are stripped of their nutrients during processing
- **PROCESSED MEATS.** Bacon, ham, sausage are often high in nitrates and nitrites
- **OMEGA-6 FATTY ACIDS.** Found in some vegetable oils such as corn oil and soybean oil

KNOWN FOOD REACTIONS

Elimination and reintroduction testing is significantly more accurate than blood testing. The best way to know if you are reactive to a food is by doing an elimination and reintroduction challenge. You eliminate a particular food group for several weeks, then add in each category of food one at a time and observe your response.

For example, let's say you eliminate dairy, wheat, and eggs, and over time your symptoms improve. Maybe you experience less brain fog, your sleep is better, and your gas and bloating lessen.

Pick one food category to reintroduce first. If you soon experience an intensification in your symptoms, remove that food again, and then move on to try the next food item.

Thought Anxiety Protocol

IDENTIFY ROOT CAUSES. Refer to the discussion of Thought Anxiety in Chapter 3. In the space below, write notes about concepts that you resonated with that might be worth further exploration. Consider root causes, testing, and mindfulness strategies.

____

____

____

____

THOUGHT ANXIETY SUPPLEMENTS AND TINCTURES

Here are some ideas for supplements and tinctures that I have found to be helpful for the different types of Thought Anxiety.

THOUGHT ANXIETY SUBTYPE	SUPPLEMENTS AND TINCTURES
The Auctioneer	**SUPPLEMENTS:** • L-theanine (200–400 mg up to 3 times per day) slows racing thoughts • White Chestnut Flower Essence clears your mind, calms thoughts, and supports sleep. Take 5 drops under the tongue several times a day. **TINCTURE RECIPE:** 40% California poppy (*Eschscholtzia californica*) 30% kava kava (*Piper methysticum*) 20% hops (*Humulus lupulus*) 10% lavender (*Lavandula officinalis*) **HOW TO TAKE:** Mix 1–3 big squeezes into tea or water once or twice per day.
The Ruminator	**SUPPLEMENTS:** • Magnesium L-threonate (400 mg per day) relaxes obsessive thoughts • Red Chestnut Flower Essence helps release worries and focus on what you can control. Place 5 drops under the tongue several times per day. **TINCTURE RECIPE:** 40% milk thistle (*Silybum marianum*) 30% gotu kola (*Centella asiatica*) 20% kava kava (*Piper methysticum*) 10% licorice (*Glycyrrhiza glabra*) **HOW TO TAKE:** Mix 1–3 big squeezes into tea or water once or twice per day.

THOUGHT ANXIETY SUBTYPE	SUPPLEMENTS AND TINCTURES
The Broken Record	**SUPPLEMENTS:** • Omega-3 fatty acids (500 EPA/500 DHA) can help reduce obsessive thoughts. • Crab Apple Flower Essence helps reduce the stickiness of repetitive thoughts and worries. Place 5 drops under the tongue several times per day. **TINCTURE RECIPE:** 40% ashwagandha (*Withania somnifera*) 30% passionflower (*Passiflora incarnata*) 20% valerian (*Valeriana officinalis*) 10% turmeric (*Curcuma longa*) **HOW TO TAKE:** Mix 1–3 big squeezes into tea or water once or twice per day.
The Fog	**SUPPLEMENTS:** • Acetyl L-carnitine (1–3 g in the morning) • Clematis Flower Essence helps ground you out of dissociation and brings you back to the present. Place 5 drops under the tongue several times per day. **TINCTURE RECIPE:** 40% kava kava (*Piper methysticum*) 30% ginkgo (*Ginkgo biloba*) 20% bacopa (*Bacopa monnieri*) 10% rosemary (*Rosmarinus officinalis*) **HOW TO TAKE:** Mix 1–3 big squeezes into tea or water once or twice per day.

Anger Anxiety Protocol

IDENTIFY ROOT CAUSES. Refer to the discussion of Anger Anxiety in Chapter 3. Also refer to Chapter 10, where we learned about Parts Work. Oftentimes when we are angry and frustrated, a part is expressing an unmet need. In the space below, write notes about concepts that you resonated with that might be worth further exploration, thoughts, feelings, or beliefs that come up for you. Also make notes regarding root causes, testing, and mindfulness strategies that you might consider.

____

____

____

____

STRATEGIES TO CALM THE FIRE

- Most of the time Anger Anxiety is due to excess pitta, so be sure to check out the pitta-calming strategies elsewhere in this chapter.
- Apply a cold pack to the neck, face, or chest for 30 seconds on, then 30 seconds off. Repeat as needed.
- Use a fidget. Different fidgets have different benefits—experiment and find the one that works best for you.
- Create a playlist of choice to help regulate your nervous system. Check out my Spotify, which you can find under my name, for some of my anxiety-reducing playlists, including Alpha Waves and Pink Noise tracks.

FIRE SOOTHER FLOWER ESSENCE BLEND

- Holly: Encourages generosity of spirit and love toward others.
- Crabapple: Reduces overwhelm and stickiness of thoughts and worries.
- Walnut: Improves focus, reduces distractibility, helps with overwhelm.
- Impatiens: Helps us slow down and be patient.
- Elm: Helps give strength and energy and lifts our mood so we can carry on.

Mix equal parts of these five ingredients. Take 5 drops at least once per day, with extra doses as needed.

PITTA'S ANGER ANXIETY SOOTHER BLEND

40% vervain (*Verbena officinalis*)
30% kava kava (*Piper methysticum*)
25% passionflower (*Passiflora incarnata*)
5% peppermint (*Mentha piperita*)

Mix 1–3 big squeezes into tea or water once or twice per day.

Depressive Anxiety Protocol

IDENTIFY ROOT CAUSES. Refer to the discussion of Depressive Anxiety in Chapter 3. Sometimes when we are extremely overwhelmed, we become depressed and hopeless.

In the space below, write notes about concepts that you resonated with from the section about your origin story from Chapter 1. Be sure to also include notes regarding root causes, testing, and mindfulness strategies that stuck out to you as you read the other chapters in this book.

____

____

____

____

STRATEGIES TO BOOST MOOD

- **ESSENTIAL OILS.** Many different essential oils have been studied for their effectiveness at reducing depression and calming anxiety.
  - My favorites are rose, lavender, bergamot, orange, and lemon.
  - Mix your essential oil of choice with a small amount of sunflower or safflower oil for kapha types, sesame or almond for vata types, and coconut for pitta.
  - Apply to your wrists (which are along the heart merid-

ian in Traditional Chinese Medicine), temples, or the bottoms of your big toes.

- **MUSIC.** Emerging research from *PLOS* on Music Medicine suggests that listening to music can lift depression and calm anxiety. Listening to music can stimulate the vagus nerve, inducing relaxation. Music also stimulates dopamine release in the brain, causing feelings of happiness. From folk to classical, baroque, and binaural beats, create your playlist, and enjoy! The type of music that was studied to be the worst for your anxiety and mood was heavy metal, so maybe hold off on that if you're feeling particularly stressed and depressed.

MOOD UPLIFT FLOWER ESSENCE BLEND. Mix 5 drops from each of the following into a mixture that contains 50% water and 50% alcohol of choice, e.g., Everclear:

- Star of Bethlehem: Helps cope with bad news, disappointment, and grief.
- Elm: For exhaustion and overwhelm with life. Gives you strength and lifts your mood.
- Sweet Chestnut: Helps with despair and hopelessness; gives endurance and strength.
- Willow: Helps you overcome, be goal directed, and feel optimistic.
- Mustard: Dispels feelings of gloom—as a great "Eeyore" essence, it brings joy and happiness.

Mix equal parts of these five ingredients. Take 5 drops at least once per day, with extra doses as needed.

MOOD-BOOSTING BLEND FOR EACH DOSHA

VATA	PITTA	KAPHA
40% shatavari (*Asparagus racemosus*) 30% saffron (*Crocus sativus*) 25% oats (*Avena sativa*) 5% cinnamon (*Cinnamomum verum*)	40% lemon balm (*Melissa officinalis*) 30% hawthorn (*Cratae-gus*) 25% rhodiola (*Rhodiola rosea*) 5% lavender (*Lavandula officinalis*)	40% St. John's wort (*Hypericum perforatum*) 30% ashwagandha (*Withania somnifera*) 25% rose petals (*Rosa spp.*) 5% ginger (*Zingiber officinale*)
How to take: Mix 1–3 big squeezes into tea or water once or twice per day.	**How to take:** Mix 1–3 big squeezes into tea or water once or twice per day.	**How to take:** Mix 1–3 big squeezes into tea or water once or twice per day.

Trauma Anxiety Protocol

You will get best results treating Trauma Anxiety when your protocol addresses the trauma itself, while supporting your body, mind, and nervous system in healing from the effects of trauma. For example, if one of your Trauma Anxiety symptoms includes racing thoughts, while you do the trauma-healing work, you may also glean from your Thought Anxiety protocol.

Hormone Anxiety Protocol

Once you've identified if and how your endocrine system is a part of your story of panic and anxiety, you can create a protocol that not only promotes calm and control but actually restores balance to your hormones. Below are some of my favorite protocols for the most commonly observed anxiety-producing hormone imbalances I see in my clients.

HORMONE ANXIETY SOLUTIONS

HORMONE ANXIETY TYPE	SOLUTIONS
Thyroid	**TESTING:** When the thyroid is out of balance, consider the following tests: • Comprehensive thyroid panel, including thyroid antibodies • Testing for food sensitivity, especially to wheat • Screen for too-low vitamin D and iron • Screen for iodine deficiency with an iodine patch test or iodine blood test • Stool testing, to evaluate for dysbiosis • Environmental toxin testing including metals and nonmetal testing **CALMING AN OVERACTIVE THYROID:** My favorite blend contains 50% lemon balm (*Melissa officinalis*) and 50% motherwort (*Leonurus cardiaca*). Take 3 big squeezes in tea or water in the morning and again at night. **BOOSTING AN UNDERACTIVE THYROID:** Take a multivitamin containing zinc, selenium, and iodine. Consider a thyroid-boosting blend containing equal parts of licorice (*Glycyrrhiza glabra*), magnolia berry (*Schisandra chinensis*), oats (*Avena sativa*), and ashwagandha (*Withania somnifera*). Take 3 big squeezes in tea or water in the morning and again at night. **BRINGING DOWN REVERSE T3:** Take COQ10 (100 mg per day) and a multivitamin that contains iodine, selenium, zinc, and vitamin B12.

HORMONE ANXIETY TYPE	SOLUTIONS
Adrenal	**TESTING:** If you suspect imbalances in cortisol or other adrenal hormones, consider the following tests: • Cortisol test. Ideally, try to collect several samples (urine/blood/saliva) to be tested for cortisol levels throughout the day: first in the morning upon waking, then at noon, then around 3:00 P.M., then at bedtime, and again if you wake up in the middle of the night. A blood test will more likely be covered by insurance. • Serum sex-hormone testing. Testing for estradiol, progesterone, free and total testosterone, DHT, SHBG, DHEA-S, FSH, and LH is often covered by insurance. • Specialty cash-based functional tests. Include comprehensive stool analysis and environmental toxicity testing if warranted. **REDUCING CORTISOL:** • Phosphatidylserine (100 mg) capsule and ashwagandha (*Withania somnifera*) herbal tincture dosed at 3 big squeezes in tea or water at bedtime. • Consume high-protein, low-carb meals. • Avoid caffeine and other stimulants. **BOOSTING CORTISOL:** Any of the herbs in the *adaptogen* category in "Herbal Medicine for Panic Relief" can help balance adrenal health and normalize cortisol. For example, for fatigue and high stress, you might make a mixture containing equal parts Siberian ginseng (*Eleutherococcus senticosus*), cordyceps mushroom (*Cordyceps sinensis*), shatavari (*Asparagus racemosus*), and licorice (*Glycyrrhiza glabra*). Take 3 big squeezes in the morning and again at lunch. (Do not take the tincture in the afternoon or evening because it may be somewhat energizing.)
Estrogen	**TESTING:** If you suspect an estrogen imbalance, here are some suggestions for testing: • Serum testing: Testing for estradiol, progesterone, free and total testosterone, DHT, SHBG, DHEA-S, FSH, and LH is often covered by insurance. • Consider screening for cortisol levels, too. • Consider specialty cash-based functional tests, including comprehensive stool analysis and environmental toxicity testing if warranted. **REDUCING ESTROGEN:** Start with flaxseeds (2 tablespoons per day). If you need further support (based on follow-up testing or symptoms), add a supplement that contains this mix: • Calcium D-glucarate (1–5 g per day), found in oranges, apples, etc.

HORMONE ANXIETY TYPE	SOLUTIONS
Estrogen	• Indole-3-carbinol (I3C) (200–600 mg per day), found in cruciferous veggies. • Diindolylmethane (DIM) (50–100 mg per day), found in broccoli and Brussels sprouts. **ALSO CONSIDER:** • Liver support. Eat a whole foods diet that includes 3–4 servings of cruciferous vegetables per day. • Eat fiber-rich foods. Fruits, veggies, whole grains, and legumes can bind up excess estrogen from the gut and remove it from the body. **OPTIMIZING ESTROGEN METABOLITES:** Add flaxseeds (2 tablespoons of ground golden flax) and maca (2 teaspoons) to your smoothies.
Progesterone	**TESTING:** Testing is the same as for estrogen. **REDUCING PROGESTERONE:** • Exercise. Exercise can increase your metabolism, which results in more testosterone, which can combat excess progesterone levels. • Avoid alcohol and tobacco. Alcohol and tobacco can disrupt hormone balance and contribute to high levels of progesterone. • Support estrogen levels. Typically, as estrogen rises, progesterone will go down. **INCREASING PROGESTERONE:** • Supplement with magnesium, zinc, and vitamin B6. • Eat a healthy diet rich in fiber, veggies, whole grains, and brightly colored fruits. • Consider an herbal tincture mixture, such as: 30% chaste tree berry (*Vitex agnus-castus*), 20% black cohosh (*Actaea racemosa*), 20% dong quai (*Angelica sinensis*), 20% wild yam (*Dioscorea villosa*), and 10% licorice (*Glycyrrhiza glabra*). Take 3 big squeezes in tea or water in the morning and again in the evening.
Testosterone	**TESTING.** Testing is the same as for estrogen. In addition, consider gluten testing: • Celiac panel • Gluten and wheat food sensitivity testing

HORMONE ANXIETY TYPE	SOLUTIONS
Testosterone	• Consider a testosterone-lowering tincture, such as 30% chaste tree berry (*Vitex agnus-castus*), 30% green tea (*Camellia sinensis*), 30% licorice (*Glycyrrhiza glabra*), and 10% peppermint (*Mentha piperita*). Take 3 big squeezes in the morning and again at lunch. **INCREASING TESTOSTERONE:** • Get plenty of exercise, including a mix of cardio and resistance training. • Consider an herbal tincture, such as 30% ashwagandha (*Withania somnifera*), 30% fenugreek (*Trigonella foenum-graecum*), 30% maca (*Lepidium meyenii*), and 10% rosemary (*Salvia rosmarinus*). Take 3 big squeezes in the morning and at lunchtime. • Supplement with D-aspartic acid (2000–3000 mg in the morning).

Environmental Detox Protocol

It is important to always do testing to ensure that your body is equipped to meet the demands of a detox, especially for your liver and kidneys. Depending on the type of toxicity you are aiming to remove, your exact protocol will vary.

STEP 1: BUILD UP THE BODY.

The first step to detoxification is to build up the body's detoxification organs, such as the liver, bowels, and kidneys, with a variety of supplements and herbs and a healthy diet. Here are some options to consider:

- **SUPPLEMENTS:** Probiotics, apple pectin, and activated charcoal
- **HERBS:** Milk thistle, dandelion root, burdock root, ginger, and turmeric
- **FOODS:** Brightly colored organic berries, leafy green vegetables, and whole grains

STEP 2: OPEN YOUR EMUNCTORIES.

The second step is to open your emunctories every day. Emunctories are the channels through which the body eliminates toxins. They include the skin, bowels, kidneys, lungs, and lymphatic system.

You can open your emunctories to drain out toxins with sweating, bowel movements, crying, urinating, and deep breathing. Sweating eliminates toxins through the skin. Bowel movements remove toxins through the stool. Drinking fluids helps to flush toxins out of the body via the bladder. And deep breathing helps to move toxins out of the lungs.

DAILY DETOX ROUTINE

- **CLEANSING DRINK.** Mix 1 teaspoon each of turmeric powder, dandelion root powder, and organic milk thistle powder in 8–10 ounces of warm water or juice. If you tend to be on the warmer side, add lemon and peppermint to taste. If you tend to be chilly, add lemon and ginger to taste.
- **DETOX SUPPLEMENTS.** Take a detox supplement that is appropriate for your individual needs. Some good options include chelated minerals, chlorella, cilantro, and spirulina.
- **DETOX DIET.** Eat an anti-inflammatory diet that is rich in fruits, vegetables, and whole grains. Avoid processed foods, sugary drinks, and alcohol.
- **HYDRATION.** Drink plenty of water throughout the day. Aim for half your body weight in ounces of water daily. You can add minerals to your water to support detoxification pathways.
- **DETOX HABITS.** Pick one to do each day.
    - Lymphatic brushing. Do lymphatic brushing in the shower to help move lymph fluid through the body. Start at your feet and brush upward toward your heart, using long, sweeping strokes. Be sure to brush all the major lymph nodes.
    - Castor oil packs. Apply a castor oil pack to your abdomen or liver to help detoxify these organs. Soak a flannel or wool cloth in castor oil, wring it out, and place it on

the desired area. Cover the cloth with a heating pad and relax for 30 to 60 minutes.

- Warming compress. Apply a cool compress to an area of your body that is sore or inflamed. Soak a washcloth in cool water, wring it out, and place it on the desired area. Cover the cloth with a towel and relax for 20 to 30 minutes.
- Epsom salt bath. An Epsom salt bath can help detoxify your body and relax your muscles. Add 2 cups of Epsom salts to a hot bath and soak for 20 to 30 minutes.

DAILY SCHEDULE

Follow this schedule for the first three weeks:

- Morning: Drink your cleansing drink before you eat or drink anything else. Then empty your bowels and bladder and take a shower. Do lymphatic brushing while you are in the shower.
- Noon: Eat lunch, your main meal of the day.
- Afternoon: Drink your cleansing drink and get some movement, such as stretching or walking.
- Dinner: Eat a light dinner that is well-balanced, with lean protein, fat, and whole grains.
- Evening: Drink your cleansing drink and take a sauna, use a warming compress, apply a castor oil pack, or take an Epsom salt bath.

BOTANICAL AND HERBAL REMEDIES

I love using botanical medicines for anxiety and panic because they are effective, safe, and generally well tolerated. Some botanicals work quickly, such as kava kava (*Piper methysticum*), while others work better over time, like oats (*Avena sativa*). The best part of herbal medicine is you can customize herbal remedies and dosages to fit your unique needs.

In this chapter, you will learn about some of my favorite herbs for anxiety and panic. We will explore some of the ways they work, and I will help you zero in on what types of anxiety they are best for.

KEY CATEGORIES OF HERBS

- **ADAPTOGENS.** Adaptogens are herbs that can help you adapt to stress. Some are better for the adrenal glands, while others are effective for supporting the thyroid, brain, and other organ systems.
- **ANTI-INFLAMMATORIES.** Herbs can be powerful anti-inflammatories. For example, turmeric (*Curcuma longa*) can reduce histamine. Generally speaking, reducing inflammation will be your most powerful tool in healing mind and body.
- **CARMINATIVES.** Carminatives are herbs that support digestion and dispel gas and bloating. I always include an herb from this category to reduce Gut Anxiety and promote gut healing.
- **NOOTROPICS.** Nootropics support memory, focus, concentration, intelligence, creativity, and learning. They protect the brain from cognitive degeneration. Use them when you want to improve cognitive function or have signs and symptoms of Thought Anxiety.
- **RELAXING NERVINES.** Relaxing nervines are nature's tranquilizers. In higher doses they can also be quite sedating. Use them if you are looking for natural ways to calm your mind and body.
- **STIMULATING NERVINES.** Generally, I stay away from stimulating nervines in treating anxiety and panic. But if you experience the Fog subtype of Thought Anxiety, you might consider incorporating a little bit of a stimulating nervine.
- **TONIFYING NERVINES.** Tonifying nervines are also called restoratives or trophorestoratives. They can nourish and restore health to the brain and nervous system. Use them if you have undergone a lot of stress, have a history of environmental toxicity or inflammation, or if you feel like you have lost function or vitality.

How to Make an Herbal Tincture

An herbal tincture is a concentrated liquid extract made from plants that can be used as medicine. You can make tinctures from scratch—planting, growing, nurturing, and harvesting your herbs and extracting the active ingredients into teas, tinctures, or other types of mixtures. Or you can buy pre-made tinctures or teas and mix them to your heart's content.

I personally love using tinctures because they tend to have a longer shelf life than teas or infusions. All the mixtures you'll learn about will include four parts.

MY TEMPLATE FOR HERBAL TINCTURES

1. **START WITH A LEAD HERB.** Typically, the lead herb will be 40% of your blend. Pick an herb that has the action that you are looking for, such as a nootropic or nervine. It should suit your type of anxiety and any root causes you have identified. For example, if you experience Depressive Anxiety from chronic stress, you might choose St. John's wort (*Hypericum perforatum*) because it helps lift mood and calm anxiety and it is a tonifying nervine. You could also choose lemon balm (*Melissa officinalis*), which is a nootropic that is also antidepressant and anti-anxiety and can help combat stress.
2. **ADD A SECONDARY HERB.** This herb should make up around 30% of your blend. It will complement the lead herb and provide support. For example, if you are also experiencing Gut Anxiety, you might add chamomilla (*Matricaria chamomilla*) or skullcap (*Scutellaria lateriflora*).
3. **TERTIARY HERB.** The tertiary herb will be 25% of your blend. It will further round out the formula and provide even more support. For example, lavender (*Lavandula officinalis*) is good for lifting the mood, it can soothe the gut, and it's generally cooling.
4. **DRIVER HERB.** Round out your blend with 5% of a fourth herb. It should be a driver herb, one that will synergize the

blend and help it work more effectively. For example, if you are generally a person who runs hot, you might add a cooling driver herb like peppermint (*Mentha piperita*).

Let's walk through two examples of herbal tinctures:

EXAMPLE 1: Here is a tincture for Depressive Anxiety with some Gut Anxiety, for a person who is generally on the warmer side. It uses herbs that can reduce anxiety, improve mood, soothe the gut, and be generally cooling:

- Lead herb (40%): St. John's wort (*Hypericum perforatum*)
- Secondary herb (30%): lemon balm (*Melissa officinalis*)
- Tertiary herb (25%): kava kava (*Piper methysticum*)
- Driver herb (5%): lavender (*Lavandula officinalis*)

EXAMPLE 2: Let's say you have anxiety that causes difficulty sleeping, you get chills with stress, and your stress causes brain fog. You want to calm your nervous system while feeling sharper and crisper mentally while being generally warmed.

- Lead herb (40%): chamomilla (*Matricaria chamomilla*)
- Secondary herb (30%): ginkgo (*Ginkgo biloba*)
- Tertiary herb (25%): passionflower (*Passiflora incarnata*)
- Driver herb (5%): rosemary (*Salvia rosmarinus*)

Dosage

Start with a low dose of your tincture, and increase gradually as needed. Typically, the herbs I use can be dosed at 1–4 ml (1 ml is 1 big squeeze or dropperful, which is 20–30 drops) one to three times per day. But you should refer to each herb's monograph for specific dosing. See Appendix B for my favorite herbal monograph resource.

HERBAL MEDICINE FOR PANIC RELIEF

This table contains some of my favorite herbs and botanicals that can help with symptoms of panic and anxiety. I have arranged them in categories, but feel free to read more about them. Mix and match them as you see fit.

ADAPTOGENS	HERBS FOR THE FOG	HERBS FOR MUSCLE TENSION	HERBS FOR STOMACH ANXIETY	HERBS FOR GUT ANXIETY	HERBS FOR ANGER ANXIETY
Siberian ginseng (*Eleutherococcus senticosus*)	Kava kava (*Piper methysticum*)	Skullcap (*Scutellaria lateriflora*)	Chamomilla (*Matricaria recutita*)	Chamomilla (*Matricaria recutita*)	Vervain (*Verbena officinalis*)
Cordyceps mushroom (*Cordyceps sinensis*)	Ginkgo (*Ginkgo biloba*)	Hops (*Humulus lupulus*)	Lemon balm (*Melissa officinalis*)	Skullcap (*Scutellaria lateriflora*)	Passionflower (*Passiflora incarnata*)
Ashwagandha (*Withania somnifera*)	Rosemary (*Rosmarinus officinalis*)	Valerian (*Valeriana officinalis*)	Peppermint (*Mentha piperita*)	Ginger (*Zingiber officinale*)	Chamomilla (*Matricaria recutita*)
Shatavari (*Asparagus racemosus*)	Rhodiola (*Rhodiola rosea*)	Lemon balm (*Melissa officinalis*)	Valerian (*Valeriana officinalis*)	Spearmint (*Mentha spicata*)	Kava kava (*Piper methysticum*)
Licorice (*Glycyrrhiza glabra*)	Bacopa (*Bacopa monnieri*)	Peppermint (*Mentha piperita*)	Kava kava (*Piper methysticum*)	Peppermint (*Mentha piperita*)	Peppermint (*Mentha piperita*)

HERBS FOR THE AUCTIONEER	HERBS FOR THE RUMINATOR	HERBS FOR THE BROKEN RECORD	HERBS FOR CHEST ANXIETY	ANTI-INFLAMMATORY HERBS	QUICK-ACTING HERBS
California poppy (*Eschscholtzia californica*)	Kava kava (*Piper methysticum*)	Passionflower (*Passiflora incarnata*)	Hawthorn (*Crataegus oxycantha*)	Turmeric (*Curcuma longa*)	Kava kava (*Piper methysticum*)

ADAPTOGENS	HERBS FOR THE FOG	HERBS FOR MUSCLE TENSION	HERBS FOR STOMACH ANXIETY	HERBS FOR GUT ANXIETY	HERBS FOR ANGER ANXIETY
Kava kava (*Piper methysticum*)	St. John's wort (*Hypericum perforatum*)	Indian gooseberry (*Phyllanthus emblica*)	Motherwort (*Leonurus cardiaca*)	Ginger (*Zingiber officinale*)	Lavender (*Lavandula officinalis*)
Hops (*Humulus lupulus*)	Gotu kola (*Centella asiatica*)	Turmeric (*Curcuma longa*)	Linden tree (*Tilia europaea*)	Licorice (*Glycyrrhiza glabra*)	Valerian (*Valeriana officinalis*)
Valerian (*Valeriana officinalis*)	Milk thistle (*Silybum marianum*)	Ashwagandha (*Withania somnifera*)	Lemon balm (*Melissa officinalis*)	Skullcap (*Scutellaria lateriflora*)	Chamomilla (*Matricaria recutita*)

BRAIN HEALING HERBS (NOOTROPICS)	SEDATING HERBS (NERVINES)	TONIFYING HERBS (TROPHORESTORATIVES)	HERBS FOR DEPRESSIVE ANXIETY	DRIVER HERBS THAT ARE COOLING	DRIVER HERBS THAT ARE WARMING
Ginkgo (*Ginkgo biloba*)	Passionflower (*Passiflora incarnata*)	Oats (*Avena sativa*)	Lemon balm (*Melissa officinalis*)	Lavender (*Lavandula officinalis*)	Ginger (*Zingiber officinale*)
Siberian ginseng (*Eleutherococcus senticosus*)	Lavender (*Lavandula officinalis*)	Gotu kola (*Centella asiatica*)	Hawthorn (*Crataegus oxyacantha*)	Peppermint (*Mentha piperita*)	Cayenne (*Capsicum annuum*)
Ashwagandha (*Withania somnifera*)	Chamomilla (*Matricaria recutita*)	St. John's wort (*Hypericum perforatum*)	St. John's wort (*Hypericum perforatum*)	Bacopa (*Bacopa monnieri*)	Cinnamon (*Cinnamomum verum*)
Magnolia berry (*Schisandra chinensis*)	Hops (*Humulus lupulus*)	Lion's mane (*Hericium erinaceus*)	Saffron (*Crocus sativus*)	Licorice (*Glycyrrhiza glabra*)	Black pepper (*Piper nigrum*)

SUPPLEMENTS

In all the protocols in this chapter, you'll see different types of supplements. But before we jump straight into "just tell me what to take so my panic goes away," we need to discuss what supplements are and when they should be used. There are a couple of points I want to touch on.

- **QUALITY MATTERS.** Back in Chapter 5, we talked about how the details matter when selecting strains and brands of psychobiotics. The same goes for supplements. If you're going to spend the money on something, you deserve to know that you're getting what you think you're getting. It should be good quality, have actual therapeutic doses, and contain no harmful ingredients such as titanium dioxide or artificial colors.
- **SUPPLEMENTS ARE NOT REGULATED BY THE FDA.** This means that the FDA has not evaluated whether what's on the herb's label reflects what's *in* the bottle. Upward of 25 percent of the supplements sold on major retailer sites are counterfeit, which means they may have mislabeled ingredients, toxic additives, or impurities that can cause illness, such as mold or bacteria. So it is important for you to do your research before taking any supplements. A great resource for learning more about ingredients and additives is the Environmental Working Group, which has a website at EWG.org.

When in doubt, try to stick with reputable physician-grade brands that have been third-party tested. Because brands and their products are always changing, I have more up-to-date information about my favorite supplements on my website.

MICRODOSING PSYCHEDELICS

Okay, let's talk about psychedelics. Are they the next big thing in mental health? One of the most common questions I'm asked nowadays is "Can magic mushrooms help with my anxiety?" In order to answer that, I have to talk a little bit about what these substances are and how we think they work.

Psychedelic substances, also known as hallucinogens, are a class of compounds that can trigger nonordinary states of consciousness. They fall into three chemical classes: tryptamines (e.g., psilocybin and Dimethyltryptamine), phenethylamines (MDMA and mescaline), and lysergamides (LSD and its derivatives).

Indigenous cultures have used psychedelics for centuries for spiritual and healing purposes, with the goal of attaining greater awareness of self and one's role in the connected universe. After decades of being classified as Schedule 1 drugs and stigmatized due to the war on drugs, psychedelics are now undergoing a renaissance of research into their potential therapeutic benefits for conditions such as treatment-resistant anxiety, depression, substance-use disorders, and trauma.

What Is Psilocybin?

Psilocybin, nicknamed the "magic mushroom," is a naturally occurring psychedelic compound found in more than 200 species of fungi from the mushroom genus *Psilocybe*. In the human body, the liver and gut microbiota convert it into its active form, psilocin.

Human beings have used psilocybin for thousands of years. One of the earliest records of its use was found on a mural in northern Australia dating back to 10,000 BCE, depicting subjects in a trance under the influence of "magic mushrooms."

In recent years, psilocybin mushrooms have been in the spotlight, with hundreds of thousands of individuals microdosing every year. The National Institutes of Health have invested nearly $4 million in research at Johns Hopkins into the efficacy of psychedelic use in psychiatric conditions.

Progressive private drug companies have raised millions of dollars to develop targeted psilocybin molecules for psychiatric use. Additionally, public and private entities are working to legitimize the therapeutic use of psychedelics like psilocybin through FDA consideration and local legislative action.

How Psilocybin Works

Psilocybin is thought to act on the insula, the part of the brain that is involved in our sense of self or ego. It also acts on the prefrontal cortex and hippocampus, which are involved in decision-making, memory, and learning. Its effects may increase the brain's neuroplasticity, its ability to change and adapt. Increased neuroplasticity can lead to the release of old, intractable thought patterns and the formation of new, more helpful connections.

One of psilocybin's primary mechanisms of action is to affect serotonin, a neurotransmitter involved in mood, perception, and cognition (see Chapter 6). This may underlie some of its therapeutic benefits, such as its potential to treat depression, anxiety, and addiction.

Microdosing

When taken in significant quantities (typically 1 gram or more), psilocybin can alter consciousness and perception, producing visual and auditory hallucinations, shifts in spiritual awareness and connectivity, mystical or religious experiences, an expanded mental state, or a dissolution of the ego.

Eckhart Tolle describes the ego as a protective shell that isolates us from others and creates a sense of separation from our true self and the world around us. As the ego diminishes or dissolves, we can become more present and feel more connected to the reality around us. This allows for a broader perception and a more holistic, bottom-up interpretation of reality.

A microdosing regimen uses a tiny dosage (less than 0.5 grams) taken on a cyclic schedule. It is thought to work by opening the doors of perception and disrupting chronic dysfunctional thought patterns without any hallucinogenic effect.

Potential Benefits of Microdosing Psilocybin

The beneficial effects of microdosing psilocybin are being actively investigated now due to the promising results of earlier research. Some preliminary findings suggest that it may be helpful for a variety of mental health conditions, including:

- Improving brain connectivity by laying down new neural patterns and allowing for the dissolution of old, problematic ones.
- Increasing brain-derived neurotrophic factor, which supports learning, memory, and brain cell growth.
- Balancing the brain areas associated with the default mode network, which can reduce ruminative and self-concerned thoughts.
- Improving mental wellness, including the potential resolution of chronic anxiety, depression, obsessive-compulsive disorder, addiction, and trauma response.
- Improving memory and cognition, which can lead to increased confidence and competence in daily tasks.
- Aiding in recovery from substance dependence.
- Reducing chronic pain in cases of injury and inflammatory disease.
- Combating neurodegenerative disorders such as Alzheimer's disease by enhancing neuronal activity and possibly abating plaque buildup.

Risks of Psilocybin Use

The effects of psilocybin vary based on a lot of individualizing factors such as how much you take, your mental state, and the setting you are in when you take it, as well as certain medical conditions.

Most adverse experiences are transient and have been associated with macrodosing, or the high-dose, recreational use of psilocybin in an uncontrolled setting. These experiences can take the form of extreme anxiety, paranoia, and even psychotic manifestations. Episodes typically resolve as the psilocin is completely processed by the body (six to eight hours).

Although it's relatively uncommon, some people who take psilocybin may experience persistent and upsetting changes in how they see themselves or the world. Physicians refer to this experience as hallucinogen-persisting perception disorder. It may largely be avoided if the person consumes the substance under the guidance of an experienced professional in the right emotional state and setting. In fact, researchers at Harvard Health assert that psilocybin is generally thought to be safe in low dosages.

The Verdict: Is Microdosing Right for You?

Ultimately the choice of whether to try microdosing comes down to you. Key considerations should always include the source and quality of the psilocybin product; a properly vetted microdosing regimen; awareness of supportive (healthy diet, exercise, sunshine, restful sleep) and unsupportive (poor diet, excessive alcohol, toxic relationships, inadequate hydration) practices; and an integrated environment, including a healthful setting, strong relationships, and a supportive community.

If microdosing psilocybin is something you'd like to learn more about, check out the Multidisciplinary Association for Psychedelic Studies. MAPS is the go-to resource on all things related to the research and development of psychedelic drugs, including clinical trials, news, and educational resources. Psychedelic Alpha is another good resource for up-to-date information on laws regarding possession and use of psilocybin.

CONCLUSION

Imagine a house that has weathered many seasons. It has witnessed the blackest of nights and the most enchanting of sunrises. If its walls could speak, they would tell the story of your life.

This house has been with you since the very beginning. It has sheltered you through everything you've ever experienced. No matter what happens, it will always be there for you.

In reading this book, you have learned about the hands that constructed your house. You have learned about the foundation on which it was built, the marks others have left and how they have impacted you, and the many different ways your house speaks. You have learned how to understand what it needs and the many ways you can tend to it.

You have learned about anatomy, physiology, biochemistry, and neuropsychology, and you have dived into trauma-informed therapy, the science of herbs and mushrooms, environmental medicine and detoxification, diet, lifestyle, psychobiotics, supplements, and medications.

You have bravely waded through the nuances of Ayurvedic theory and practice, the art and science of how the gut-brain axis communicates with your brain, hormones, and complex organ systems.

You've met some of the most incredible people I've had the pleasure of working with, walking alongside them through their very intimate journeys of becoming panic proof.

The last time I saw Aria, I was given the gift of remembering exactly why I do this work. It was a sunny day in Phoenix, and she was sitting on the couch across from me, just as she had done at our very first meeting.

On her lap rested a manila envelope. "I don't think I need to see you anymore," she said.

While a patient graduating from care is the ultimate goal, I felt a twinge of sadness.

"Do you remember when we first met?" she asked. "You told me my brain was capable of 'incredible healing.'"

"I remember that." Aria had been skeptical at best, I recalled. But she had continued showing up and doing the work.

"That night when I went home, I remember feeling equal parts terrified and doubtful. I didn't really believe that I could get better, but for the first time in a long time, I had a glimmer of hope."

Aria turned her attention to the envelope. "I've been keeping notes every day since we started. You'll notice that in the beginning, there are a lot of expletives." She grinned. "But as you read on, you'll see how the way I thought about my symptoms and the way I thought about this process changed."

She unwound the string that was holding it shut and pulled out a stack of papers. She began reading aloud from the first page.

"July 6, 2016: I saw Dr. Cain for the first time today. She told me that *the episode* was my body trying to give me information. She has me writing down everything I'm noticing when I feel stressed. I don't think there's enough paper in the world for that. But here goes." Aria holds up a wad of papers. "I typed in an extremely small font."

I laughed. "I know the feeling."

She continued reading. "July 6, 2017: Last night I had the best sex of my life. No fear, no stress, no visits to lobby bathrooms. I felt completely empowered, beautiful, and powerful.

"Over the past 365 days, I have come to cherish my body. I have learned that my emotions are valid, and that feeling them is not a sign of weakness, but of strength. I have discovered that I am worthy of pleasure and that I have the choice to do what I want, be with who I want, and that all the answers I need are within me.

"One year ago today, I was hoping to not have panic attacks at best.

But I've gotten so much more than that: I've gotten myself back. All of myself."

She put the papers back into the envelope and handed it to me, saying, "In case you ever decide to write a book."

And so I did.

I'll write this one more time: You are capable of incredible healing. By listening to the wisdom of your mind and body, you can truly heal. Not just get by—you can thrive. And be strong. And be amazing. And be the glorious, sparkly soul that you are.

Be Panic Proof.

ACKNOWLEDGMENTS

This book exists because of the many people who have shared their stories, wisdom, and vulnerabilities, and because they believed in my work.

To all the clients who have allowed me to be a part of their lives: It is an honor to hold space with you and to be a part of your transformation.

To the Holistic Wellness Collective community: Thank you for joining together in a mission to spread the hope of holistic and trauma-informed practices. You inspire me every single day.

To my team of clinicians: Thank you for helping me throughout my healing journey, especially during the times when it has been really dark and scary: Lisa Rathbun, Henry Schulte, MD, and Ana Gomez.

To my beloved mentors: Thank you for your unconditional care, for being my best cheerleaders, and for reminding me of my higher truth: Rafe Adams, Pam Conboy, George Poszywak, James Sensenig, ND, and Randy Webb.

To my beta readers, who read pages upon pages of drafts of this book: You gave me honest feedback and pushed me to be a better teacher (in alphabetical order), thank you: Paul Anderson, ND, Megan Chance, Michele Figuereo, Ashley Khaja, Camille Martin, Richelle Mickle, Kristyn Stankiewicz, and Christina Wyman, PhD.

To Hadlee Garrison: Thank you for your wisdom regarding all things Ayurveda.

To Haylee Masteller: You took my ideas and made them into the beautiful images woven throughout this book. Thank you.

To Susan Shapiro whose online classes paved my way into the writing world.

To my agents Wendy Sherman and Laura Mazer: Thank you for your unwavering support for me in writing my first book and making it possible for it to get out into the world.

To my incredible editor, Donna Loffredo (and her best furry friend, Ozzy): Thank you for coaching me through the process of taking decades of information out of my brain and transforming it into this absolutely amazing book you're reading right now.

To Craig Adams, whose keen eye for detail transformed my sometimes incoherent paragraphs into works of grammatical art. And to the rest of the outstanding team at Rodale: Thank you for bringing this book to life. I am so grateful for your hard work and dedication, and I'm proud to be published by Rodale: Diana Baroni, Gail Gonzales, Marnie Cochran, Christina Foxley, and Katherine Leak.

And to Paul, my best friend, partner, and inspiration: Thank you for being by my side every step of the way. I couldn't have done any of this without you.

And to my sweet cavapoo, Sheva: Your snuggles are magic for the soul.

APPENDIX A

MY PANIC PROOF PROTOCOL

My Stoplight Strategies: ______________________________

Habits that keep me in the Green Light Zone: ______________________________

Signs I am transitioning into the Yellow Light Zone: ______________________________

Signs I am in the Yellow Light Zone: ______________________________

Habits, supplements, and medicines to get me back
into the Green Light Zone: ______________________________

____

____

Signs I am transitioning into the Red Light Zone: ______________________________

Signs I am in the Red Light Zone: ______________________________

My crisis resources: ______________________________

____

____

My Dosha: ______________________________

Signs and symptoms indicating my dosha is out of balance: ______________________________

____

____

Foods to balance my dosha: ______

Spices to balance my dosha: ______

Habits to balance my dosha: ______

The Panic Reset:

STEP 1: Nervous System Calming Habits:

______

______

______

STEP 2: Wise Mind Habits:

______

______

______

STEP 3: Reintegrating Habits:

______

______

______

STEP 4: Restructuring Habits:

______

______

______

NUTRITION: Panic Proof foods I am emphasizing:

______

______

______

MY EXERCISE GOALS: Pick three forms of exercise you are committed to doing.

Activity 1: I will (list first activity) _________ for a duration of (list amount of time) _________ on (list specific days) _________

Activity 2: I will (list next activity) _________ for a duration of (list amount of time) _________ on (list specific days) _________

Activity 3: I will (list next activity) _________ for a duration of (list amount of time) _________ on (list specific days) _________

My Panic Proof Herbal Recipe:

____

My Panic Proof Supplements:

____

____

____

APPENDIX B

RESOURCES FOR FURTHER READING

Crisis Resources:

- The suicide crisis hotline: Call or text 988 or chat 988lifeline.org
- LGBTQ+ National Hotline: 1-888-843-4564
- Black Emotional and Mental Health Collective: https://beam.community/
- National Domestic Violence Hotline: 1-800-799-7233 or text LOVEIS to 22522
- Veterans Crisis Line: Call 988, then select 1, or text 838255
- To find a treatment facility in your local area: https://www.findtreatment.gov/

Trauma-Informed Therapy Resources:

- Book to learn more about Parts Work: *No Bad Parts* by Richard Schwartz
- Book to learn more about EMDR: *Every Memory Deserves Respect: EMDR, the Proven Trauma Therapy with the Power to Heal* by Deborah Korn and Michael Baldwin
- To find a therapist that takes your insurance: https://www.psychologytoday.com

Book on Herbalism:

- Rosemary Gladstar's *Medicinal Herbs: A Beginner's Guide* at https://scienceandartofherbalism.com

Genetic Testing:

- *Dirty Genes* by Dr. Ben Lynch at https://www.seekinghealth.com

Environmental Toxins:

- The Environmental Protection Agency https://www.epa.gov/environmental-topics

Mold:

- *Break the Mold* by Dr. Jill Crista at https://drcrista.com/break-the-mold/
- The Environmental Protection Agency, *A Brief Guide to Mold, Moisture and Your Home* at https://www.epa.gov/mold/brief-guide-mold-moisture-and-your-home

Finding a Trauma-Informed Therapist:

- Go to emdria.org and search for a clinician in your area

Community Mental Health Programs/Sliding Scale Resource:

- Mental Health America at https://www.mhanational.org/local-resources

Psychedelic Research:

- Multidisciplinary Association for Psychedelic Studies (MAPS) at https://maps.org
- Johns Hopkins Psychedelics Research at https://www.hopkinsmedicine.org/psychiatry/research/psychedelics-research
- Stanford Psychedelic Science Group at https://med.stanford.edu/spsg.html

BIBLIOGRAPHY

Akarsu, K., A. Koç, and N. Ertuğ. "The Effect of Nature Sounds and Earplugs on Anxiety in Patients Following Percutaneous Coronary Intervention: A Randomized Controlled Trial." *European Journal of Cardiovascular Nursing 18(8)*. June 23, 2019. https://doi.org/10.1177/1474515119858826.

Akdis, C. A., MD, and K. Blaser, PhD. "Histamine in the Immune Regulation of Allergic Inflammation." *Journal of Allergy and Clinical Immunology 112(1)*. July 2003. https://doi.org/10.1067/mai.2003.1585.

Akpinar, Ş., and M. G. Karadağ. "Is Vitamin D Important in Anxiety or Depression? What Is the Truth?" *Current Nutrition Reports 11*. September 13, 2022. https://doi.org/10.1007/s13668-022-00441-0.

Albarran, A. "How Gluten Induced Malnutrition Affects Testosterone Levels." Gluten Free Society. April 9, 2013. https://www.glutenfreesociety.org/how-gluten-induced-malnutrition-effects-testosterone-levels/.

Alok, S., S. K. Jain, A. Verma, et al. "Plant Profile, Phytochemistry and Pharmacology of *Asparagus racemosus* (Shatavari): A Review." *Asian Pacific Journal of Tropical Disease 3(3)*. 2013. https://doi.org/10.1016%2FS2222-1808(13)60049-3.

"Alpha-Lipoic Acid." Mount Sinai. Accessed January 29, 2024. https://www.mountsinai.org/health-library/supplement/alpha-lipoic-acid.

"Amino Acids Support Guide." Genova Diagnostics. 2020. https://www.gdx.net/core/support-guides/Amino-Acids-Support-Guide.pdf.

Anderson, F. G. " 'Who's Taking What?' Connecting Neuroscience, Psychopharmacology and Internal Family Systems for Trauma." In *Internal Family Systems Therapy: New Dimensions,* edited by M. Sweezy and E. L. Ziskind. 1st ed. New York: Routledge, 2013.

Anderson, S. C., J. F. Cryan, PhD, and T. G. Dinan, MD, PhD. *The Psychobiotic Revolution: Mood, Food, and the New Science of the Gut-Brain Connection*. Washington, D.C.: National Geographic, 2017.

Anderson, T., R. Petranker, A. Christopher, et al. "Psychedelic Microdosing Benefits and Challenges: An Empirical Codebook." *Harm Reduction Journal 16*. July 10, 2019. https://doi.org/10.1186/s12954-019-0308-4.

Andrews, A. M. "Celebrating Serotonin." *ACS Chemical Neuroscience 3(9)*. September 19, 2012. https://www.ncbi.nlm.nih.gov/pmc/articles/PMC3447390/.

Appel, K., T. Rose, B. Fiebich, et al. "Modulation of the γ-Aminobutyric Acid (GABA) System by *Passiflora incarnata* L." *Phytotherapy Research 25(6)*. June 2011. https://doi.org/10.1002/ptr.3352.

Armanini, D., G. Bonanni, M. J. Mattarello, et al. "Licorice Consumption and Serum Testosterone in Healthy Man." *Experimental and Clinical Endocrinology & Diabetes 111(6)*. September 2003. https://doi.org/10.1055/s-2003-42724.

Ashok, T., N. Patni, M. Fatima, et al. "Celiac Disease and Autoimmune Thyroid Disease: The Two Peas in a Pod." *Cureus 14(6)*. June 23, 2022. https://doi.org/10.7759%2Fcureus.26243.

Bagga, D., J. L. Reichert, K. Koschutnig, et al. "Probiotics Drive Gut Microbiome Triggering Emotional Brain Signatures." *Gut Microbes 9(6)*. June 14, 2018. https://www.ncbi.nlm.nih.gov/pmc/articles/PMC6287679/.

Balali-Mood, M., K. Naseri, Z. Tahergorabi, et al. "Toxic Mechanisms of Five Heavy Metals: Mercury, Lead, Chromium, Cadmium, and Arsenic." *Frontiers in Pharmacology 12*. April 13, 2021. https://doi.org/10.3389%2Ffphar.2021.643972.

Balogh, K. "Endocrinologists' Take on the Accuracy of the At-Home Iodine Test." Healthnews. January 17, 2024. https://healthnews.com/longevity/biohacking/endocrinologists-take-on-the-accuracy-of-the-at-home-iodine-test/.

Barati, F., A. Nasiri, N. Akbari, and G. Sharifzadeh. "The Effect of Aromatherapy on Anxiety in Patients." *Nephro-Urology Monthly 8(5)*. July 31, 2016. https://doi.org/10.5812%2Fnumonthly.38347.

Barone, M., S. Tanzi, K. Lofano, et al. "Dietary-Induced Erβ Upregulation Counteracts Intestinal Neoplasia Development in Intact Male ApcMin/+ Mice." *Carcinogenesis 31(2)*. November 27, 2009. https://doi.org/10.1093/carcin/bgp275.

Barrett, F. S., M. K. Doss, N. D. Sepeda, et al. "Emotions and Brain Function Are Altered up to One Month After a Single High Dose of Psilocybin." *Scientific Reports*. February 10, 2020. https://doi.org/10.1038%2Fs41598-020-59282-y.

Bathla, M., M. Singh, and P. Relan. "Prevalence of Anxiety and Depressive Symptoms Among Patients with Hypothyroidism." *Indian Journal of Endocrinology and Metabolism 20(4)*. July–August 2016. https://doi.org/10.4103%2F2230-8210.183476.

Batman, D. C. "Hippocrates: 'Walking Is Man's Best Medicine!'" *Occupational Medicine 62(5)*. July 2012. https://doi.org/10.1093/occmed/kqs084.

"Be Your Own Best Advocate: How to Stand Up for Yourself, Find a Therapist." *Psychology Today*. Accessed January 25, 2024. https://www.psychologytoday.com/us/blog/fulfillment-at-any-age/202401/how-to-become-your-own-best-advocate.

Bektas, A., H. Erdal, M. Ulusoy, et al. "Does Serotonin in the Intestines Make You

Happy?" *Turkish Journal of Gastroenterology 31(10)*. October 1, 2020. https://doi.org/10.5152%2Ftjg.2020.19554.

Bengston Nash, S. M., M. Schlabach, and P. D. Nichols. "A Nutritional-Toxicological Assessment of Antarctic Krill Oil Versus Fish Oil Dietary Supplements." *Nutrients 6(9)*. August 28, 2014. https://doi.org/10.3390%2Fnu6093382.

"Benzodiazepines: More Quotations." Benzo.org.uk. Accessed January 14, 2024. https://www.benzo.org.uk/kwotez.htm.

Bernal, J. "Deiodinase: Deiodinases (Dio) Are Selenocysteine-Containing Enzymes Capable of Removing Iodide from Iodothyronines (Bianco, Salvatore, Gereben, Berry & Larsen, 2002). *ScienceDirect: Encyclopedia of Hormones/Vitamins and Hormones, 2018*. https://www.sciencedirect.com/topics/biochemistry-genetics-and-molecular-biology/deiodinase.

Bertoni, A.P.S., I. S. Brum, A. C. Hillebrand, et al. "Progesterone Upregulates Gene Expression in Normal Human Thyroid Follicular Cells." *International Journal of Endocrinology 2015*. May 21, 2015. https://doi.org/10.1155%2F2015%2F864852.

Bikle, D. D. "The Free Hormone Hypothesis: When, Why, and How to Measure the Free Hormone Levels to Assess Vitamin D, Thyroid, Sex Hormone, and Cortisol Status." *JBMR Plus 5(1)*. October 1, 2020. https://doi.org/10.1002/jbm4.10418.

"The Biogenic Amines." In *Neuroscience,* edited by D. Purves, G. J. Augustine, D. Fitzpatrick, et al. 2nd ed. Sunderland, Mass.: Sinauer Associates. 2001.

Blankespoor, J. "Introduction to Immune Stimulants, Immunomodulators, and Antimicrobials." Chestnut School of Herbal Medicine. September 25, 2023. https://chestnutherbs.com/blog-herbs-for-the-immune-system/.

Bly, R. *Iron John: A Book About Men*. Boston: Da Capo Press, 2015. https://catalog.cadl.org/Record/.b21715464.

Bocchio, M., S. B. McHugh, D. M. Bannerman, et al. "Serotonin, Amygdala and Fear: Assembling the Puzzle." *Frontiers in Neural Circuits 10*. April 5, 2016. https://doi.org/10.3389/fncir.2016.00024.

Bogadi, M., and S. Kaštelan. "A Potential Effect of Psilocybin on Anxiety in Neurotic Personality Structures in Adolescents." *Croation Medical Journal 62(5)*. October 2021. https://doi.org/10.3325%2Fcmj.2021.62.528.

Bonaz, B., T. Bazin, and S. Pellissier. "The Vagus Nerve at the Interface of the Microbiota-Gut-Brain Axis." *Frontiers in Neuroscience 12*. February 7, 2018. https://www.ncbi.nlm.nih.gov/pmc/articles/PMC5808284/.

Bonds, R. S., and T. Midoro-Horiuti. "Estrogen Effects in Allergy and Asthma." *Current Opinion in Allergy and Clinical Immunology 13(1)*. February 1, 2013. https://doi.org/10.1097%2FACI.0b013e32835a6dd6.

Bravo, J. A., P. Forsythe, M. V. Chew, et al. "Ingestion of Lactobacillus Strain Regulates Emotional Behavior and Central GABA Receptor Expression in a Mouse Via the Vagus Nerve." *Proceedings of the National Academy of Sciences 108(38)*. September 20, 2011. https://doi.org/10.1073/pnas.1102999108.

Breit, S., A. Kupferberg, G. Rogler, and G. Hasler. "Vagus Nerve as Modulator of the Brain-Gut Axis in Psychiatric and Inflammatory Disorders." *Frontiers in Psychiatry 9*. March 13, 2018. https://www.frontiersin.org/articles/10.3389/fpsyt.2018.00044/full.

Bren, G. A. "Environmental Exposures and Autoimmune Thyroid Disease." *Thyroid 20(7)*. July 2010. https://doi.org/10.1089%2Fthy.2010.1636.

Brosnan, M. E., and J. T. Brosnan. "Histidine Metabolism and Function." *Journal of Nutrition 150(Suppl 1)*. October 1, 2020. https://doi.org/10.1093/jn/nxaa079.

Bruni, O., L. Ferini-Strambi, E. Giacomoni, et al. "Herbal Remedies and Their Possible Effect on the GABAergic System and Sleep." *Nutrients 13(2)*. February 6, 2021. https://doi.org/10.3390%2Fnu13020530.

Bruta, K., Vanshika, K. Bhasin, et al. "The Role of Serotonin and Diet in the Prevalence of Irritable Bowel Syndrome: A Systematic Review." *Translational Medicine Communications 6(1)*. January 5, 2021. https://transmedcomms.biomedcentral.com/articles/10.1186/s41231-020-00081-y.

Buczynski, R., PhD, and B. van der Kolk, MD. "A QuickStart Guide: How to Work with the Traumatized Brain." National Institute for the Clinical Application of Behavioral Medicine (NICABM). Accessed January 5, 2024. https://www.ncbi.nlm.nih.gov/pmc/articles/PMC7176178/.

Buha, A., V. Matovic, B. Antonijevic, et al. "Overview of Cadmium Thyroid Disrupting Effects and Mechanisms." *International Journal of Molecular Sciences 19(5)*. May 17, 2018. https://doi.org/10.3390%2Fijms19051501.

Burgess, L. "What Is Hallucinogen-Persisting Perception Disorder?" MedicalNewsToday. April 14, 2023. https://www.medicalnewstoday.com/articles/320181#what-is-hppd.

Burns, D., N. Shin, R. Jalluri, et al. "H4 Receptor Antagonists and Their Potential Therapeutic Applications." In *Annual Reports in Medicinal Chemistry*, edited by M. C. Desai. Vol. 49. Cambridge, Mass.: Academic Press, 2014.

Cadegiani, F. A., and C. E. Kater. "Adrenal Fatigue Does Not Exist: A Systematic Review." *BMC Endocrine Disorders 16(1)*. August 24, 2016. https://doi.org/10.1186/s12902-016-0128-4.

Cain, N., ND, MA. "Dare To: Trauma Informed Holistic Medicine." Dr. Nicole Cain. Accessed January 13, 2024. www.drnicolecain.com.

———. "Dr. Nicole Cain's Specialty Test Ordering Platform." Dr. Nicole Cain. Accessed January 11, 2024. https://labs.rupahealth.com/store/storefront_J64eW7r?fbclid=IwAR0Z-QtbQJrNfVpmOds5xy2WrxythPOxyZLStfwJpZ8F69htKedpOBmDTTM.

———. "Happy Healthy with Hadlee." Dr. Nicole Cain. Accessed January 29, 2024. https://drnicolecain.com/welcome-dosha-quiz/.

———. "Histamine 101: Histamine Intolerance and Mental Health (What You Need to Know)." Dr. Nicole Cain. Accessed January 29, 2024. https://drnicolecain.com/histamine-intolerance-and-mental-health/.

———. "The One About Poop—Constipation Cures & Gut Anxiety." Dr. Nicole Cain. December 6, 2022. https://drnicolecain.podbean.com/e/the-one-about-poop/.

———. "Radical Acknowledgement Guided Meditation." Insight Timer. Accessed January 5, 2024. https://insighttimer.com/drnicolecain/guided-meditations/radical-acknowledgement-guided-meditation/.

———. "Spotify/4 Public Playlists." Dr. Nicole Cain. Accessed January 25, 2024. https://open.spotify.com/user/nicole.a.cain.

———. "Which of the 8 Types of Anxiety Do You Experience?" Dr. Nicole Cain. Accessed January 5, 2024. https://drnicolecain.com/anxiety-quiz/.

Campbell, J. *The Hero's Journey: Joseph Campbell on His Life & Work*. Novato, Calif.: New World Library, 2014.

Carpenter, S., PhD. "That Gut Feeling." *Monitor on Psychology 43(8)*. September 2012. https://www.apa.org/monitor/2012/09/gut-feeling.

Carthy, E., and T. Ellender. "Histamine, Neuroinflammation and Neurodevelopment: A Review." *Frontiers in Neuroscience 15*. July 14, 2021. https://doi.org/10.3389%2Ffnins.2021.680214.

Cavanna, F., S. Muller, L. A. de la Fuente, et al. "Microdosing with Psilocybin Mushrooms: A Double-Blind Placebo-Controlled Study." *Translational Psychiatry 12*. August 2, 2022. https://doi.org/10.1038%2Fs41398-022-02039-0.

Chandrashekhar, V. M., K. S. Halagali, R. B. Nidavani, et al. "Anti-allergic Activity of German Chamomile (*Matricaria recutita* L.) in Mast Cell Mediated Allergy Model." *Journal of Ethnopharmacology 137(1)*. September 1, 2011. https://doi.org/10.1016/j.jep.2011.05.029.

"Chaste Tree Berry (*Vitex agnus castus* 2)." Association for the Advancement of Restorative Medicine (AARM™). Accessed January 22, 2024. https://restorativemedicine.org/library/monographs/chaste-tree-berry-vitex-agnus-castus-2/.

Chen, D., T. Aihara, C.-M. Zhao, et al. "Differentiation of the Gastric Mucosa I. Role of Histamine in Control of Function and Integrity of Oxyntic Mucosa: Understanding Gastric Physiology Through Disruption of Targeted Genes." *American Journal of Physiology: Gastrointestinal and Liver Physiology*. October 1, 2006. https://doi.org/10.1152/ajpgi.00178.2006.

Cherry, K., MSEd. "10 Cool Optical Illusions and How They Work." Verywell Mind. March 3, 2023. https://www.verywellmind.com/cool-optical-illusions-2795841.

Childre, L. "Introducing . . . Inner Balance™ Coherence Plus." HeartMath. Accessed January 26, 2024. https://www.heartmath.com/.

Chimakurthy, J., MPharm, and T.E.G.K. Murthy, PhD. "Effect of Curcumin on Quinpirole Induced Compulsive Checking: An Approach to Determine the Predictive and Construct Validity of the Model." *North American Journal of Medical Sciences 2(2)*. 2010. https://www.ncbi.nlm.nih.gov/pmc/articles/PMC3354439/.

Chinta, S. J., and J. K. Anderson. "Dopaminergic Neurons." *International Journal of Biochemical Cellular Biology 37(5)*. May 2005. https://doi.org/10.1016/j.biocel.2004.09.009.

Choi, J. Y., D.-A. Huh, and K. W. Moon. "Association Between Blood Lead Levels and Metabolic Syndrome Considering the Effect of the Thyroid-Stimulating Hormone Based on the 2013 Korea National Health and Nutrition Examination Survey." *PLOS One*. December 31, 2020. https://doi.org/10.1371/journal.pone.0244821.

Cohen, S. "If You Want to Boost Immunity, Look to the Gut." UCLA Health. March 19, 2021. https://www.uclahealth.org/news/want-to-boost-immunity-look-to-the-gut.

Comas-Basté, O., S. Sánchez-Pérez, M. T. Veciana-Nogués, et al. "Histamine Intolerance: The Current State of the Art." *Biomolecules 10(8)*. August 10, 2020. https://doi.org/10.3390%2Fbiom10081181.

"Concerned About Contaminants in Your Tap Water?" Environmental Working Group (EWG). Accessed January 29, 2024. https://www.ewg.org/.

"Conquer Your Fear of Flying." Phoenix Sky Harbor International Airport. Accessed January 5, 2024. https://www.skyharbor.com/at-the-airport/services/fear-of-flying-classes/.

Cooper, G. M. *The Cell: A Molecular Approach*. 2nd ed. Sunderland, Mass.: Sinauer Associates, 2000. https://www.ncbi.nlm.nih.gov/books/NBK9907/.

"Cordyceps (*Cordyceps militaris*)." Association for the Advancement of Restorative Medicine (AARM™). Accessed January 25, 2024. https://restorativemedicine.org/library/monographs/cordyceps/#sd.

Costas-Ferreira, C., R. Durán, and L.R.F. Faro. "Toxic Effects of Glyphosate on the Nervous System: A Systematic Review." *International Journal of Molecular Sciences 23(9)*. April 21, 2022. https://doi.org/10.3390%2Fijms23094605.

Cronkleton, E., and O. Walters. "What Are the Benefits and Risks of Alternate Nostril Breathing?" Healthline. May 24, 2023. https://www.healthline.com/health/alternate-nostril-breathing#takeaway.

Davis, K., FNP. "Psilocybin (Magic Mushrooms): What It Is, Effects and Risks." MedicalNewsToday. October 31, 2023. https://www.medicalnewstoday.com/articles/308850.

Daws, R. E., C. Timmermann, B. Giribaldi, et al. "Increased Global Integration in the Brain After Psilocybin Therapy for Depression." *Nature Medicine 28*. April 11, 2022. https://doi.org/10.1038/s41591-022-01744-z.

Deen, M., H. D. Hansen, A. Hougaard, et al. "High Brain Serotonin Levels in Migraine Between Attacks: A 5-HT4 Receptor Binding PET Study." *NeuroImage: Clinical 18*. January 28, 2018. https://doi.org/10.1016%2Fj.nicl.2018.01.016.

Del Rio, J. P., M. I. Alliende, N. Molina, et al. "Steroid Hormones and Their Action in Women's Brains: The Importance of Hormonal Balance." *Frontiers in Public Health 6*. May 23, 2018. https://doi.org/10.3389/fpubh.2018.00141.

de Vos, C.M.H., N. L. Mason, and K.P.C. Kuypers. "Psychedelics and Neuroplasticity: A Systematic Review Unraveling the Biological Underpinnings of Psychedelics." *Frontiers in Psychiatry 12*. September 10, 2021. https://doi.org/10.3389/fpsyt.2021.724606.

Dhaliwal, S., MD, and D. Dugdale, MD. "Adrenal Glands." MedlinePlus. April 29, 2022. https://medlineplus.gov/ency/article/002219.htm#:~:text=Each%20adrenal%20gland%20is%20about,gland%20is%20called%20the%20medulla.

———. "Hyperthyroidism (Overactive Thyroid)." Penn Medicine. August 12, 2022. https://www.pennmedicine.org/for-patients-and-visitors/patient-information/conditions-treated-a-to-z/hyperthyroidism-overactive-thyroid#:~:text=Graves%20disease%20(most%20common%20cause,gland%20or%20pituitary%20gland%20(rare).

Dhaliwal, S., and A. P. Kalogeropoulos. "Markers of Iron Metabolism and Outcomes in Patients with Heart Failure: A Systematic Review." *International Journal of Molecular Sciences 24(6)*. March 2023. https://doi.org/10.3390/ijms24065645.

Di Stefano, G., A. Di Lionardo, E. Galosi, et al. "Acetyl-L-Carnitine in Painful Peripheral Neuropathy: A Systematic Review." *Journal of Pain Research 12*. April 26, 2019. https://doi.org/10.2147%2FJPR.S190231.

Doss, M. K., M. Považan, M. D. Rosenberg, et al. "Psilocybin Therapy Increases Cognitive and Neural Flexibility in Patients with Major Depressive Disorder." *Translational Psychiatry 11*. November 8, 2021. https://doi.org/10.1038/s41398-021-01706-y.

"Drug Fact Sheet: Ketamine." Department of Justice, Drug Enforcement Administration. April 2020. https://www.dea.gov/sites/default/files/2020-06/Ketamine-2020.pdf.

Duek, O., Y. Li, B. Kelmendi, et al. "Modulating Amygdala Activation to Traumatic Memories with a Single Ketamine Infusion." medRxiv. Accessed January 16, 2024. https://doi.org/10.1101/2021.07.07.21260166.

Duranti, S., L. Ruiz, G. A. Lugli, et al. "*Bifidobacterium adolescentis* as a Key Member of the Human Gut Microbiota in the Production of GABA." *Scientific Reports 10*. August 24, 2020. https://doi.org/10.1038/s41598-020-70986-z.

Durrani, D., R. Idrees, H. Idrees, and A. Ellahi. "Vitamin B6: A New Approach to Lowering Anxiety, and Depression?" *Annals of Medicine & Surgery*. September 15, 2022. https://doi.org/10.1016%2Fj.amsu.2022.104663.

Eijsbouts, C., T. Zheng, N. A. Kennedy, et al. "Genome-Wide Analysis of 53,400 People with Irritable Bowel Syndrome Highlights Shared Genetic Pathways with Mood and Anxiety Disorders." *Nature Genetics 53*. November 5, 2021. https://doi.org/10.1038/s41588-021-00950-8.

Emmerson, G., PhD, and P. Federn. "What Is Ego State Therapy?" and "Where Does Ego State Therapy Come From?" Ego State Therapy International (ESTI). Accessed January 26, 2024. https://www.egostateinternational.com/ego-state-therapy.php.

English, A., E. McKibben, D. Sivaramakrishnan, et al. "A Rapid Review Exploring the Role of Yoga in Healing Psychological Trauma." *International Journal of Environmental Research and Public Health 19(23)*. December 3, 2022. https://doi.org/10.3390%2Fijerph192316180.

"Epinephrine (Adrenaline)." Cleveland Clinic. March 27, 2022. https://my.clevelandclinic.org/health/articles/22611-epinephrine-adrenaline.

Ergang, P., K. Vagnerová, P. Hermanová, et al. "The Gut Microbiota Affects Corticosterone Production in the Murine Small Intestine." *International Journal of Molecular Sciences 22(8)*. April 19, 2021. https://www.ncbi.nlm.nih.gov/pmc/articles/PMC8073041/.

Erol, N., A. T. Karaagac, and N. G. Kounis. "Dangerous Triplet: Polycystic Ovary Syndrome, Oral Contraceptives and Kounis Syndrome." *World Journal of Cardiology 6(12)*. December 26, 2014. https://doi.org/10.4330%2Fwjc.v6.i12.1285.

"Facts About Dietary Supplements." U.S. Food and Drug Administration (FDA). May 16, 2023. https://www.fda.gov/news-events/rumor-control/facts-about-dietary-supplements.

Fedurco, M., J. Gregorová, K. Šebrlová, et al. "Modulatory Effects of *Eschscholzia californica* Alkaloids on Recombinant GABAA Receptors." *Biochemistry Research International 2015*. October 5, 2015. https://doi.org/10.1155/2015/617620.

Fei, C., MD. "Iron Deficiency Anemia: A Guide to Oral Iron Supplements." *Clinical Correlations*. March 26, 2015. https://www.clinicalcorrelations.org/2015/03/26/iron-deficiency-anemia-a-guide-to-oral-iron-supplements/.

Felmingham, K. L., J. M. Caruana, L. N. Miller, et al. "Lower Estradiol Predicts Increased Reinstatement of Fear in Women." *Behavior Research and Therapy 142*. July 2021. https://doi.org/10.1016/j.brat.2021.103875.

Feyzollahi, Z., H. M. Kouchesfehani, H. Jalali, et al. "Effect of *Vitex agnus-castus* Ethanolic Extract on Hypothalamic *KISS-1* Gene Expression in a Rat Model of Polycystic Ovary Syndrome." *Avicenna Journal of Phytomedicine 11(3)*. May–June 2021. https://www.ncbi.nlm.nih.gov/pmc/articles/PMC8140208/.

Field, D. "Vitamin B6 May Reduce Anxiety Symptoms, Study Shows." MedicalNewsToday. July 20, 2022. https://www.medicalnewstoday.com/articles/vitamin-b6-may-reduce-anxiety-symptoms-study-shows.

Fierascu, R. C., I. Fierascu, A. Ortan, et al. "*Leonurus cardiaca* L. as a Source of Bioactive Compounds: An Update of the European Medicines Agency Assessment Report (2010)." *BioMed Research International*. April 17, 2019. https://doi.org/10.1155%2F2019%2F4303215.

"Find Drugs & Conditions." Drugs.com. Accessed January 25, 2024. https://www.drugs.com/.

Finlayson, A.J.R., J. Macoubrie, C. Huff, et al. "Experiences with Benzodiazepine Use, Tapering, and Discontinuation: An Internet Survey." *Therapeutic Advances in Psychopharmacology 12*. April 25, 2022. https://doi.org/10.1177%2F20451253221082386.

Fulghum B. D. "Normal Testosterone and Estrogen Levels in Women." WebMD. May 4, 2022. https://www.webmd.com/women/normal-testosterone-and-estrogen-levels-in-women.

"Functional Neurologic Disorder/Conversion Disorder." Mayo Clinic. January 11, 2022. https://www.mayoclinic.org/diseases-conditions/conversion-disorder/symptoms-causes/syc-20355197.

"Gamma-Aminobutyric Acid (GABA)." Cleveland Clinic. April 25, 2022. https://my.clevelandclinic.org/health/articles/22857-gamma-aminobutyric-acid-gaba.

Ganesan, K., C. Anastasopoulou, and K. Wadud. "Euthyroid Sick Syndrome." StatPearls—NCBI Bookshelf. December 8, 2023. https://www.ncbi.nlm.nih.gov/books/NBK482219/.

Gao, J. "Correlation Between Anxiety-Depression Status and Cytokines in Diarrhea-Predominant Irritable Bowel Syndrome." *Experimental and Therapeutic Medicine*. May 8, 2013. https://doi.org/10.3892/etm.2013.1101.

Gautam, S., A. Jain, M. Gautam, et al. "Clinical Practice Guidelines for the Management of Depression." *Indian Journal of Psychiatry 59(Suppl 1)*. January 2017. https://www.ncbi.nlm.nih.gov/pmc/articles/PMC5310101/.

"Generalized Anxiety Disorder." Mayo Clinic. October 13, 2017. https://www.mayoclinic.org/diseases-conditions/generalized-anxiety-disorder/symptoms-causes/syc-20360803.

Gepp, K., PsyD, and Z. Villines. "What to Know About Anxiety and Numbness." MedicalNewsToday. September 4, 2023. https://www.medicalnewstoday.com/articles/can-anxiety-cause-numbness.

Gilfarb, R. A., and B. Leuner. "GABA System Modifications During Periods of Hormonal Flux Across the Female Lifespan." *Frontiers in Behavioral Neuroscience 16*. June 16, 2022. https://doi.org/10.3389%2Ffnbeh.2022.802530.

Glover, E. M., PhD, T. Jovanovic, PhD, and S. D. Norrholm, PhD. "Estrogen and Extinction of Fear Memories: Implications for Posttraumatic Stress Disorder Treatment." *Biological Psychiatry 78(3)*. August 1, 2015. https://doi.org/10.1016%2Fj.biopsych.2015.02.007.

Glover, E. M., PhD, K. B. Mercer, MPH, S. D. Norrholm, PhD, et al. "Inhibition of Fear Is Differentially Associated with Cycling Estrogen Levels in Women." *Journal of Psychiatry & Neuroscience 38(5)*. September 2013. https://doi.org/10.1503%2Fjpn.120129.

"Glutamate Receptors." In *Neuroscience,* edited by D. Purves, G. J. Augustine, D. Fitzpatrick, et al. 2nd ed. Sunderland, Mass.: Sinaur Associates, 2001.

Gocki, J., and Z. Bartuzi. "Role of Immunoglobulin G Antibodies in Diagnosis of Food Allergy." *Advances in Dermatology and Allergology 33(4)*. August 16, 2016. https://doi.org/10.5114%2Fada.2016.61600.

Godek, D., and A. M. Freeman. "Physiology, Diving Reflex." StatPearls—NCBI Bookshelf. September 26, 2022. https://www.ncbi.nlm.nih.gov/books/NBK538245/.

Goldman, B. "Sense of Self: The Brain Structure That Holds Key to 'I.'" *Neuroscience News*. June 22, 2023. https://neurosciencenews.com/self-awareness-brain-23515/.

Golthe, N. P., I. Khan, J. Hayes, et al. "Yoga Effects on Brain Health: A Systematic Review of the Current Literature." *Brain Plasticity 5(1)*. December 26, 2019. https://doi.org/10.3233%2FBPL-190084.

Goodman, Ken, LCSW. "How to Calm an Anxious Stomach: The Brain-Gut Connection." Anxiety & Depression Association of America (ADAA). September 19, 2018. https://adaa.org/learn-from-us/from-the-experts/blog-posts/consumer/how-calm-anxious-stomach-brain-gut-connection.

"GPL-TOX Profile: Assess Environmental Toxic Burden." Mosaic Diagnostics. Accessed January 25, 2024. https://mosaicdx.com/test/gpl-tox-profile/.

Green, R. A., C. A. Marsden, and E. J. Mylecharane. "The Serotonin Club: Coming of Age." *Trends in Pharmacological Sciences 29(9)*. September 2008. https://www.cell.com/trends/pharmacological-sciences/fulltext/S0165-6147(08)00161-2.

Grinspoon, P., MD. "The Popularity of Microdosing of Psychedelics: What Does the Science Say?" Harvard Health Publishing. September 19, 2022. https://www.health.harvard.edu/blog/the-popularity-of-microdosing-of-psychedelics-what-does-the-science-say-202209192819.

"The Gut-Brain Connection." Cleveland Clinic. September 20, 2023. https://my.clevelandclinic.org/health/body/the-gut-brain-connection.

Halford, J. C., J. A. Harrold, E. J. Boyland, et al. "Serotonergic Drugs: Effects on Appetite Expression and Use for the Treatment of Obesity." *Drugs 67(1)*. 2007. https://doi.org/10.2165/00003495-200767010-00004.

Hamamah, S., A. Aghazarian, A. Nazaryan, et al. "Role of Microbiota-Gut-Brain Axis in Regulating Dopaminergic Signaling." *Biomedicines 10(2)*. February 13, 2022. https://doi.org/10.3390%2Fbiomedicines10020436.

Hass-Cohen, N., and R. Carr. *Art Therapy and Clinical Neuroscience*. London: Jessica Kingsley, 2008.

Healy, D. "Serotonin and Depression." *The BMJ 350* (apr21 7): h1771. 2015. https://doi.org/10.1136/bmj.h1771.

Heisler, L. K., N. Pronchuk, K. Nonogaki, et al. "Serotonin Activates the Hypothalamic-Pituitary-Adrenal Axis via Serotonin 2C Receptor Stimulation." *Journal of Neuroscience 27(26)*. June 27, 2007. https://doi.org/10.1523/JNEUROSCI.2584-06.2007.

Henz, D., and W. I. Schöllhorn. "EEG Brain Activity in Dynamic Health Qigong Training: Same Effects for Mental Practice and Physical Training?" *Frontiers in Psychology 8*. February 7, 2017. https://doi.org/10.3389%2Ffpsyg.2017.00154.

"The Hidden Dangers in Your Dietary Supplements." American College of Healthcare Sciences. December 2, 2016. https://achs.edu/blog/2016/12/02/dangerous-supplement-ingredients/.

Hillhouse, T. M., and J. H. Porter. "A Brief History of the Development of Antidepressant Drugs: From Monoamines to Glutamate." *Experimental and Clinical Psychopharmacology 23(1)*. February 2015. https://www.ncbi.nlm.nih.gov/pmc/articles/PMC4428540/.

Hodges, R. E., and D. M. Minich. "Modulation of Metabolic Detoxification Pathways Using Foods and Food-Derived Components: A Scientific Review with Clinical Application." *Journal of Nutrition and Metabolism 2015*. June 16, 2015. https://doi.org/10.1155%2F2015%2F760689.

Holick, M. F., PhD, MD. "Vitamin D Helps You Live Longer! World Vitamin D Day—November 2nd." The Vitamin D Society. October 25, 2022. https://www.vitamindsociety.org/.

Holick, M. F., PhD, MD, et al. "Evaluation, Treatment, and Prevention of Vitamin D Deficiency: An Endocrine Society Clinical Practice Guideline." *Journal of Clinical Endocrinology & Metabolism 96(7)*. July 2011. https://pubmed.ncbi.nlm.nih.gov/21646368.

Holman, E. A., and R. C. Silver. "Getting 'Stuck' in the Past: Temporal Orientation and Coping with Trauma." *Journal of Personality and Social Psychology 74(5)*. May 1998. https://doi.org/10.1037//0022-3514.74.5.1146.

"Hormones and Endocrine System." Johns Hopkins Medicine. Accessed January 11, 2024. https://www.hopkinsmedicine.org/health/conditions-and-diseases/hormones-and-the-endocrine-system.

Hussain, T., G. Murtaza, D. H. Kalhoro, et al. "Relationship Between Gut Microbiota and Host-Metabolism: Emphasis on Hormones Related to Reproductive Function." *Animal Nutrition 7(1)*. January 4, 2021. https://doi.org/10.1016%2Fj.aninu.2020.11.005.

"Imagine a World Where There Are No Barriers to Black Healing." Black Emotional and Mental Health Collective (BEAM). Accessed January 25, 2024. https://beam.community/.

"Inflammation: A Unifying Theory of Disease?" Harvard Health Publishing, March 29, 2023. https://www.health.harvard.edu/staying-healthy/inflammation-a-unifying-theory-of-disease#:~:text=Chronic%20inflammation%20plays%20an%20important,cause%20of%20major%20degenerative%20diseases.

Institute for Quality and Efficiency in Health Care (IQWiG). "Depression: How Effective Are Antidepressants?" InformedHealth.org—NCBI Bookshelf. June 18, 2020. https://www.ncbi.nlm.nih.gov/books/NBK361016/.

"Insulin Resistance." Cleveland Clinic. December 16, 2021. https://my.clevelandclinic.org/health/diseases/22206-insulin-resistance.

"The Internal Family Systems Model Outline." IFS Institute. Accessed January 26, 2024. https://ifs-institute.com/resources/articles/internal-family-systems-model-outline.

"Iron." The Nutrition Source. March 2023. https://www.hsph.harvard.edu/nutritionsource/iron/.

Ito, C. "The Role of Brain Histamine in Acute and Chronic Stresses." *Biomedicine &*

Pharmacotherapy 54(5). June 2000. https://doi.org/10.1016/S0753-3322(00)80069-4.

Jahanbakhsh, S. P., A. A. Manteghi, S. A. Emami, et al. "Evaluation of the Efficacy of *Withania somnifera* (Ashwagandha) Root Extract in Patients with Obsessive-Compulsive Disorder: A Randomized Double-Blind Placebo-Controlled Trial." *Complementary Therapies in Medicine 27*. April 9, 2016. https://doi.org/10.1016/j.ctim.2016.03.018.

"Johns Hopkins Medicine Receives First Federal Grant for Psychedelic Treatment Research in 50 Years." Johns Hopkins Medicine. October 18, 2021. https://www.hopkinsmedicine.org/news/newsroom/news-releases/2021/10/johns-hopkins-medicine-receives-first-federal-grant-for-psychedelic-treatment-research-in-50-years.

Johnson-Wimbley, T. D. "Diagnosis and Management of Iron Deficiency Anemia in the 21st Century." *Therapeutic Advances in Gastroenterology 4(3)*. May 2011. https://doi.org/10.1177%2F1756283X11398736.

Jung, C. *C. G. Jung Letters, Volume 2: 1951–1961*. Bollingen Series, vol. 72. Princeton, N.J.: Princeton University Press, 1976.

———. *Consciousness and the Unconscious: Lectures Delivered at ETH Zurich, Volume 2: 1934*. Philemon Foundation Series, vol. 23. Princeton, N.J.: Princeton University Press, 2022.

Kachanathu, S. J., S. K. Verma, and G. L. Khanna. "Effect of Music Therapy on Heart Rate Variability: A Reliable Marker to Pre-competition Stress in Sports Performance." *Journal of Medical Sciences 13(6)*. 2013. https://doi.org/10.3923/jms.2013.418.424.

Kajimura, S., N. Masuda, J.K.L. Lau, and K. Murayama. "Focused Attention Meditation Changes the Boundary and Configuration of Functional Networks in the Brain." *Scientific Reports 10*. October 28, 2020. https://doi.org/10.1038/s41598-020-75396-9.

Kakuda, T. "Neuroprotective Effects of Theanine and Its Preventive Effects on Cognitive Dysfunction." *Pharmacological Research 64(2)*. April 6, 2011. https://doi.org/10.1016/j.phrs.2011.03.010.

Kalra, B., S. Kalra, and J. B. Sharma. "The Inositols and Polycystic Ovary Syndrome." *Indian Journal of Endocrinology and Metabolism 20(5)*. September–October 2016. https://doi.org/10.4103%2F2230-8210.189231.

Kaplan, D., MD, and C. Dosiou, MD. "Two Cases of Graves' Hyperthyroidism Treated with Homeopathic Remedies Containing Herbal Extracts from *Lycopus spp*. and *Melissa officinalis*." *Journal of the Endocrine Society 5(Suppl 1)*. May 3, 2021. https://doi.org/10.1210%2Fjendso%2Fbvab048.1984.

Kapur, J., and S. Joshi. "Progesterone Modulates Neuronal Excitability Bidirectionally." *Neuroscience Letters 744*. January 23, 2022. https://doi.org/10.1016%2Fj.neulet.2020.135619.

Karci, C. K., and G. G. Celik. "Nutritional and Herbal Supplements in the Treatment of Obsessive-Compulsive Disorder." *General Psychiatry 33(2)*. March 11, 2020. https://doi.org/10.1136%2Fgpsych-2019-100159.

Kennedy, K. M. "Prescribing Benzodiazepines in General Practice." *British Journal of General Practice*. March 2019. https://doi.org/10.3399%2Fbjgp19X701753.

Kenny, J. B., and B. Bordoni. "Neuroanatomy, Cranial Nerve 10 (Vagus Nerve)." StatPearls—NCBI Bookshelf. November 7, 2022. https://www.ncbi.nlm.nih.gov/books/NBK537171/.

Kim, S., K. Jo, K.-B. Hong, et al. "GABA and L-Theanine Mixture Decreases Sleep Latency and Improves NREM Sleep." *Pharmaceutical Biology 57(1)*. December 2019. https://doi.org/10.1080/13880209.2018.1557698.

Kluziak, M., and D. Śmiałek. "Fiber Calculator." Omni Calculator. Accessed January 12, 2024. https://www.omnicalculator.com/health/fiber.

Knezevic, J., C. Starchl, A. T. Berisha, et al. "Thyroid-Gut-Axis: How Does the Microbiota Influence Thyroid Function?" *Nutrients 12(6)*. June 12, 2020. https://doi.org/10.3390%2Fnu12061769.

Knigge, U., and J. Warberg. "The Role of Histamine in the Neuroendocrine Regulation of Pituitary Hormone Secretion." *Acta Endocrinologica 124(6)*. June 1991. https://doi.org/10.1530/acta.0.1240609.

Kofler, L., H. Ulmer, and H. Kofler. "Histamine 50-Skin-Prick Test: A Tool to Diagnose Histamine Intolerance." *International Scholarly Research Notices*. February 22, 2011. https://doi.org/10.5402%2F2011%2F353045.

Komori, T. "The Relaxation Effect of Prolonged Expiratory Breathing." *Mental Illness 10(1)*. May 15, 2018. https://www.ncbi.nlm.nih.gov/pmc/articles/PMC6037091/.

Kong, Z.-L., S. Sudirman, H.-J. Lin, and W.-N. Chen. "In Vitro Anti-inflammatory Effects of Curcumin on Mast Cell–Mediated Allergic Responses via Inhibiting FcεRI Protein Expression and Protein Kinase C Delta Translocation." *Cytotechnology 72(1)*. November 26, 2019. https://doi.org/10.1007/s10616-019-00359-6.

Koopman, N., D. Katsavelis, A. S. Ten Hove, et al. "The Multifaceted Role of Serotonin in Intestinal Homeostasis." *International Journal of Molecular Sciences 22(17)*. September 22, 2021. https://doi.org/10.3390%2Fijms22179487.

Kozlowska, K., MBBS, FRANZCP, PhD, P. Walker, BSc Psych, Mpsychol, L. McLean, MBBS, FRANZCP, PhD, and P. Carrive, PhD. "Fear and the Defense Cascade: Clinical Implications and Management." *Harvard Review of Psychiatry 23(4)*. July 8, 2015. https://doi.org/10.1097%2FHRP.0000000000000065.

Kozlowska, U., C. Nichols, K. Wiatr, and M. Figiel. "From Psychiatry to Neurology: Psychedelics as Prospective Therapeutics for Neurodegenerative Disorders." *Journal of Neurochemistry 162(1)*. October 22, 2021. https://doi.org/10.1111/jnc.15509.

Kriegel, D. L., II, MD, FAAFP, and A. Azrak, DO. "Benzodiazepines for Panic Disorder in Adults." *American Family Physician 101(7)*. April 1, 2020. https://www.aafp.org/pubs/afp/issues/2020/0401/od1.html.

Krupa, A., and I. Kowalska. "The Kynurenine Pathway—New Linkage Between Innate and Adaptive Immunity in Autoimmune Endocrinopathies." *International Journal of Molecular Sciences 22(18)*. September 13, 2021. https://doi.org/10.3390%2Fijms22189879.

Kurdi, M. S., K. A. Theerth, and R. S. Deva. "Ketamine: Current Applications in Anesthesia, Pain, and Critical Care." *Anesthesia: Essays and Researches 8(3)*. September–December 2014. https://doi.org/10.4103%2F0259-1162.143110.

Kutlikova, H. H., J. B. Durdiaková, B. Wagner, et al. "The Effects of Testosterone on the Physiological Response to Social and Somatic Stressors." *Psychoneuroendocrinology 117*. July 2020. https://doi.org/10.1016/j.psyneuen.2020.104693.

Laskowski, E. R., MD. "What's a Normal Resting Heart Rate?" Mayo Clinic. October 8, 2022. https://www.mayoclinic.org/healthy-lifestyle/fitness/expert-answers/heart-rate/faq-20057979.

"Lead in Cosmetics." U.S. Food and Drug Administration (FDA). February 25, 2022. https://www.fda.gov/cosmetics/potential-contaminants-cosmetics/lead-cosmetics.

Lestari, M.P.L., D. Wanda, and H. Hayati. "The Effectiveness of Distraction (Cartoon-Patterned Clothes and Bubble-Blowing) on Pain and Anxiety in Preschool Children During Venipuncture in the Emergency Department." *Comprehensive Child and Adolescent Nursing 40(Suppl 1)*. 2017. https://doi.org/10.1080/24694193.2017.1386967.

Li, C., C. Xing, J. Zhang, et al. "Eight-Hour Time-Restricted Feeding Improves Endocrine and Metabolic Profiles in Women with Anovulatory Polycystic Ovary Syndrome." *Journal of Translational Medicine 19(1)*. April 13, 2021. https://doi.org/10.1186/s12967-021-02817-2.

Li, H.-B., Y. Jiang, and F. Chen. "Separation Methods Used for *Scutellaria baicalensis* Active Components." *Journal of Chromatography B 812(1–2)*. December 5, 2004. https://doi.org/10.1016%2Fj.jchromb.2004.06.045.

Liang, S., X. Wu, and F. Jin. "Gut-Brain Psychology: Rethinking Psychology from the Microbiota-Gut-Brain Axis." *Frontiers in Integrative Neuroscience 12*. September 11, 2018. https://www.frontiersin.org/articles/10.3389/fnint.2018.00033/full.

Lim, T. K. "*Glycyrrhiza glabra*." *Edible Medicinal and Non-medicinal Plants*. October 22, 2015. https://doi.org/10.1007%2F978-94-017-7276-1_18.

Lin, Y.-Y., J.-S. Chen, W.-B. Wu, et al. "Combined Effects of 17β-estradiol and Exercise Training on Cardiac Apoptosis in Ovariectomized Rats." *PLOS One 13(12)*. December 20, 2018. https://doi.org/10.1371%2Fjournal.pone.0208633.

Linehan, M. "Distress Tolerance: TIPP Skills; To Reduce Extreme Emotion Mind *Fast*. Change Your Body Chemistry." *DBT Skills Training Handouts and Worksheets*. 2nd ed. New York: The Guilford Press, 2014. https://modlab.yale.edu/sites/default/files/files/TIPPSkills1.pdf.

———. "M8: Wise Mind." DBT: Dialectical Behavioral Therapy. Accessed January 26, 2024. https://dialecticalbehaviortherapy.com/mindfulness/wise-mind/.

"The Link Between Dental Health and Mental Health: What You Need to Know." Cleveland Clinic. May 26, 2022. https://health.clevelandclinic.org/link-between-dental-health-and-mental-health/.

Liu, A., S. Menon, N. J. Colson, et al. "Analysis of the MTHFR C677T Variant with Migraine Phenotypes." *BMC Research Notes 3*. July 28, 2010. https://doi.org/10.1186%2F1756-0500-3-213.

Liu, P., Ú. C. McMenamin, B. T. Johnston, et al. "Use of Proton Pump Inhibitors and Histamine-2 Receptor Antagonists and Risk of Gastric Cancer in Two Population-Based Studies." *British Journal of Cancer.* May 5, 2020. https://doi.org/10.1038/s41416-020-0860-4.

López, V., B. Nielsen, M. Solas, et al. "Exploring Pharmacological Mechanisms of Lavender (*Lavandula angustifolia*) Essential Oil on Central Nervous System Targets." *Frontiers in Pharmacology 8*. May 19, 2017. https://doi.org/10.3389%2Ffphar.2017.00280.

Lopresti, A. L., P. D. Drummond, and S. J. Smith. "A Randomized, Double-Blind, Placebo-Controlled, Crossover Study Examining the Hormonal and Vitality Effects of Ashwagandha (*Withania somnifera*) in Aging, Overweight Males." *American Journal of Men's Health 13(2)*. March 10, 2019. https://doi.org/10.1177%2F1557988319835985.

Ma, X., Y.-J. Shin, H.-S. Park, et al. "*Lactobacillus casei* and Its Supplement Alleviate Stress-Induced Depression and Anxiety in Mice by the Regulation of BDNF Expression and NF-κB Activation." *Nutrients 15(11)*. May 26, 2023. https://pubmed.ncbi.nlm.nih.gov/37299451/.

Malcolm, B. J., PharmD, MPH, and K. Tallian. "Essential Oil of Lavender in Anxiety Disorders: Ready for Prime Time?" *Mental Health Clinician 7(4)*. March 26, 2018. https://doi.org/10.9740%2Fmhc.2017.07.147.

Mancini, A., C. Di Segni, S. Raimondo, et al. "Thyroid Hormones, Oxidative Stress, and Inflammation." *Mediators of Inflammation 2016*. March 8, 2016. https://doi.org/10.1155%2F2016%2F6757154.

Mansoori, A., S. Hosseini, M. Zilaee, et al. "Effect of Fenugreek Extract Supplement on Testosterone Levels in Male: A Meta-analysis of Clinical Trials." *Phytotherapy Research 34(7)*. February 11, 2020. https://doi.org/10.1002/ptr.6627.

Marchand, W. R. "Neural Mechanisms of Mindfulness and Meditation: Evidence from Neuroimaging Studies." *World Journal of Radiology 6(7)*. July 28, 2014. https://doi.org/10.4329%2Fwjr.v6.i7.471.

Markowsky, G. "Information Theory: Physiology, Physics." Britannica. Accessed January 5, 2024. https://www.britannica.com/science/information-theory/Physiology.

Marzbani, H., H. R. Marateb, and M. Mansourian. "Neurofeedback: A Comprehensive Review on System Design, Methodology and Clinical Applications." *Basic and Clinical Neuroscience 7(2)*. April 2016. https://doi.org/10.15412%2FJ.BCN.03070208.

"Mast Cell Activation Syndrome (MCAS)." American Academy of Allergy, Asthma & Immunology (AAAAI). Accessed January 16, 2024. https://www.aaaai.org/conditions-treatments/related-conditions/mcas.

McFarland, L. V., C. T. Evans, and E.J.C. Goldstein. "Strain-Specificity and Disease-Specificity of Probiotic Efficacy: A Systematic Review and Meta-analysis." *Frontiers in Medicine 5*. 2018. https://doi.org/10.3389/fmed.2018.00124.

McVean, A., BSc. "Rabbits Eat Their Own Poop." McGill University, Office for Science and Society. March 31, 2018. https://www.mcgill.ca/oss/article/did-you-know/rabbits-eat-their-own-poop.

Mei, N., B. Lai, J. Liu, et al. "Speciation of Trace Mercury Impurities in Fish Oil Supplements." *Food Control 84*. February 2018. https://doi.org/10.1016/j.foodcont.2017.08.001.

Meikle, A. W. "The Interrelationships Between Thyroid Dysfunction and Hypogonadism in Men and Boys." *Thyroid: Review 14(Suppl 1)*. 2014. https://doi.org/10.1089/105072504323024552.

Mesa, N., PhD. "Eight Weeks of Meditation Doesn't Change the Brain, Study Finds." *The Scientist*. May 20, 2022. https://www.the-scientist.com/news-opinion/eight-weeks-of-meditation-doesn-t-change-the-brain-study-finds-70042.

Messaoudi, M., R. Lalonde, N. Violle, et al. "Assessment of Psychotropic-Like Properties of a Probiotic Formulation (*Lactobacillus helveticus* R0052 and *Bifidobacterium longum* R0175) in Rats and Human Subjects." *British Journal of Nutrition 105*. 2011. https://doi.org/10.1017/s0007114510004319.

Messaoudi, M., N. Violle, J.-F. Bisson, et al. "Beneficial Psychological Effects of a Probiotic Formulation (*Lactobacillus helveticus* R0052 and *Bifidobacterium longum* R0175) in Healthy Human Volunteers." *Gut Microbes 2(4)*. July–August 2011. https://pubmed.ncbi.nlm.nih.gov/21983070/.

"Microbiomix™ Clinical Reference Guide." Genova Diagnostics. 2022. https://www.gdx.net/core/interpretive-guides/Microbiomix-Metabolites-Interp-Chart.pdf.

"Millions of Americans Have Mental and Substance Use Disorders. Find Treatment Here." FindTreatment.gov. Accessed January 25, 2024. https://www.findtreatment.gov/.

Mittal, R., L. H. Debs, A. P. Patel, et al. "Neurotransmitters: The Critical Modulators Regulating Gut-Brain Axis." *Journal of Cellular Physiology*. April 10, 2017. https://www.ncbi.nlm.nih.gov/pmc/articles/PMC5772764/.

Möller, H.-J., B. Bandelow, H.-P. Volz, et al. "The Relevance of 'Mixed Anxiety and Depression' as a Diagnostic Category in Clinical Practice." *European Archives of Psychiatry and Clinical Neuroscience*. March 22, 2016. https://www.ncbi.nlm.nih.gov/pmc/articles/PMC5097109/.

Mombereau, C., K. Kaupmann, W. Froestl, et al. "Genetic and Pharmacological Evidence of a Role for GABAB Receptors in the Modulation of Anxiety- and Antidepressant-Like Behavior." *Neuropsychopharmacology 29(6)*. June 2004. https://doi.org/10.1038/sj.npp.1300413.

Moncrieff, J., R. E. Cooper, T. Stockman, et al. "The Serotonin Theory of Depression: A Systematic Umbrella Review of the Evidence." *Molecular Psychiatry 28*. July 20, 2022. https://doi.org/10.1038/s41380-022-01661-0.

Mor, F., M. A. Kilik, O. Ozmen, et al. "A Role for Testosterone in the Toxicity of Ochratoxin A in Male Rats." *Toxicology Letters 211*. June 2012. http://dx.doi.org/10.1016/j.toxlet.2012.03.438.

Multidisciplinary Association for Psychedelic Studies (MAPS). Website. Accessed January 29, 2024. https://maps.org/.

Murray, V. "Toxic Plants (Excluding Fungi)." 1996. Elsevier eBooks. https://doi.org/10.1016/b978-044481557-6/50033-2.

Muscaritoli, M. "The Impact of Nutrients on Mental Health and Well-Being: Insights from the Literature." *Frontiers in Nutrition 8*. March 8, 2021. https://doi.org/10.3389/fnut.2021.656290.

Musey, P. I., J. A. Lee, C. A. Hall, et al. "Anxiety About Anxiety: A Survey of Emergency Department Provider Beliefs and Practices Regarding Anxiety-Associated Low Risk Chest Pain." *BMC Emergency Medicine 18*. March 14, 2018. https://bmcemergmed.biomedcentral.com/articles/10.1186/s12873-018-0161-x.

"Mushroom Laws by State." Wisevoter. Accessed January 29, 2024. https://wisevoter.com/state-rankings/mushroom-laws-by-state/.

Naidoo, U., MD. "Gut Feelings: How Food Affects Your Mood." Harvard Health Publishing. December 7, 2018. https://www.health.harvard.edu/blog/gut-feelings-how-food-affects-your-mood-2018120715548.

Nasir, M., D. Trujillo, J. Levine, et al. "Glutamate Systems in DSM-5 Anxiety Disorders: Their Role and a Review of Glutamate and GABA Psychopharmacology." *Frontiers in Psychiatry*. November 19, 2020. https://doi.org/10.3389/fpsyt.2020.548505.

Neal, A., B. A. Moffat, J. M. Stein, et al. "Glutamate Weighted Imaging Contrast in Gliomas with 7 Tesla Magnetic Resonance Imaging." *NeuroImage: Clinical*. January 29, 2019. https://doi.org/10.1016%2Fj.nicl.2019.101694.

Niazi, I. K., M. S. Navid, J. Bartley, et al. "EEG Signatures Change During Unilateral Yogi Nasal Breathing." *Scientific Reports 12*. January 11, 2022. https://doi.org/10.1038/s41598-021-04461-8.

Nielsen, S. E., A. Y. Herrera, et al. "Hypothalamic-Pituitary-Gonadal Axis: Puberty Is Defined as the Short Period Between Childhood and Adulthood During Which Reproductive Competence Is Attained by the Awakened Hypothalamic-

Pituitary-Gonadal (HPG) Axis." *Peptides*. 2009. https://www.sciencedirect.com/topics/neuroscience/hypothalamic-pituitary-gonadal-axis.

Nordio, M., P. Kumanov, A. Chiefari, and G. Puliani. "D-Chiro-Inositol Improves Testosterone Levels in Older Hypogonadal Men with Low-Normal Testosterone: A Pilot Study." *Basic and Clinical Andrology 31*. November 12, 2021. https://doi.org/10.1186%2Fs12610-021-00146-4.

Nuguru, S. P., S. Rachakonda, S. Sripathi, et al. "Hypothyroidism and Depression: A Narrative Review." *Cureus 14(8)*. August 20, 2022. https://doi.org/10.7759%2Fcureus.28201.

Obrenovich, E. M. "Leaky Gut, Leaky Brain?" *Microorganisms 6(4)*. October 18, 2018. https://www.ncbi.nlm.nih.gov/pmc/articles/PMC6313445/.

Ohta, Y., K. Yoshida, S. Kamiya, et al. "Feeding Hydroalcoholic Extract Powder of *Lepidium meyenii* (maca) Increases Serum Testosterone Concentration and Enhances Steroidogenic Ability of Leydig Cells in Male Rats." *Andrologia 48(3)*. April 2016. https://doi.org/10.1111/and.12453.

O'Mahony, S. M., G. Clarke, Y. E. Borre, et al. "Serotonin, Tryptophan Metabolism and the Brain-Gut-Microbiome Axis." *Behavioral Brain Research 277*. January 15, 2015. https://doi.org/10.1016/j.bbr.2014.07.027.

Opal, S. M. "A Brief History of Microbiology and Immunology." In *Vaccines: A Biography*, edited by A. Artenstein. New York: Springer, 2009. https://www.ncbi.nlm.nih.gov/pmc/articles/PMC7176178/.

Ousdal, O. T., A. M. Milde, A. R. Craven, et al. "Prefrontal Glutamate Levels Predict Altered Amygdala-Prefrontal Connectivity in Traumatized Youths." *Psychological Medicine 49(11)*. September 18, 2019. https://doi.org/10.1017%2FS0033291718002519.

Pamphlett, R., P. A. Doble, and D. P. Bishop. "Mercury in the Human Thyroid Gland: Potential Implications for Thyroid Cancer, Autoimmune Thyroiditis, and Hypothyroidism." *PLOS One 16(2)*. February 9, 2021. https://doi.org/10.1371%2Fjournal.pone.0246748.

"Panic Disorder." National Health Service (NHS). August 22, 2023. https://www.nhs.uk/mental-health/conditions/panic-disorder/.

Parikh, N., H. Cruickshank, and S. Waserman. "Epinephrine for Food-induced Anaphylaxis: Dose, Route, and Timing of Administration." n.d. Elsevier eBooks. https://www.sciencedirect.com/topics/agricultural-and-biological-sciences/epinephrine.

Pasteur, L. *The Physiological Theory of Fermentation and the Germ Theory and Its Application to Medicine and Surgery*. Whitefish, Mont.: Kessinger Publishing, 2010.

Pearson, K., PhD, RD. "Is Pink Himalayan Salt Better Than Regular Salt?" Healthline. February 9, 2023. https://www.healthline.com/nutrition/pink-himalayan-salt.

Pennisi, E. "Meet the Psychobiome." *Science*. May 7, 2020. https://www.science.org/content/article/meet-psychobiome-gut-bacteria-may-alter-how-you-think-feel-and-act.

Perakis, C. R. "Soul Sickness: A Frequently Missed Diagnosis." *Journal of the American Osteopathic Association 110(6)*. June 2010. https://pubmed.ncbi.nlm.nih.gov/20606242/.

Pereira, J. C., Jr., M. Pradella-Hallinan, and H. de Lins Pessoa. "Imbalance Between Thyroid Hormones and the Dopaminergic System Might Be Central to the Pathophysiology of Restless Legs Syndrome: A Hypothesis." *Clinics 65(5)*. May 2010. https://doi.org/10.1590%2FS1807-59322010000500013.

Perry, B. D., MD, PhD, and O. Winfrey. *What Happened to You? Conversations on Trauma, Resilience, and Healing*. New York: Flatiron Books, 2021.

Petra, A., MS, RD, and R. Ajmera, MS, RD. "4 Potential Side Effects of Too Much Folic Acid." Healthline. March 31, 2023. https://www.healthline.com/nutrition/folic-acid-side-effects.

Pettigrew, J. D. "Iconography in Bradshaw Rock Art: Breaking the Circularity." *Clinical and Experimental Optometry 94(5)*. September 2011. http://dx.doi.org/10.1111/j.1444-0938.2011.00648.x.

Pinto-Sanchez, M. I., G. B. Hall, K. Ghajar, et al. "Probiotic *Bifidobacterium longum* NCC3001 Reduces Depression Scores and Alters Brain Activity: A Pilot Study in Patients with Irritable Bowel Syndrome." *Gastroenterology 153(2)*. May 5, 2017. https://doi.org/10.1053/j.gastro.2017.05.003.

Pizer, A., RYT. "Sun Salutation Illustrated Step-by-Step Instructions." Verywell Fit. July 13, 2022. https://www.verywellfit.com/illustrated-stepbystep-sun-salutation-3567187.

"Post-acute Withdrawal Syndrome (PAWS): What Is PAWS?" American Addiction Centers. January 3, 2024. https://americanaddictioncenters.org/withdrawal-timelines-treatments/post-acute-withdrawal-syndrome.

Poulia, N., F. Delis, C. Brakatselos, et al. "CBD Effects on Motor Profile and Neurobiological Indices Related to Glutamatergic Function Induced by Repeated Ketamine Pre-administration." *Frontiers in Pharmacology 12*. October 27, 2021. https://doi.org/10.3389/fphar.2021.746935.

"Psilocybin." Department of Justice, Drug Enforcement Administration. Accessed January 29, 2024. https://www.dea.gov/sites/default/files/2020-06/Psilocybin-2020_0.pdf.

"Psychedelic Legalization & Decriminalization Tracker." Psychedelic Alpha. 2024. https://psychedelicalpha.com/data/psychedelic-laws.

"Psychedelics and Cognition: A New Look." Cognitive Neuroscience Society. March 28, 2023. https://www.cogneurosociety.org/psychedelics-and-cognition-a-new-look/.

Radboud University. "New Vision on Amygdala After Study on Testosterone and Fear." Science*Daily*. June 12, 2015. www.sciencedaily.com/releases/2015/06/150612143027.htm.

Radwan, A., I. M. El-Sewify, and H. M. El-Said Azzazy. "Monitoring of Cobalt and Cadmium in Daily Cosmetics Using Powder and Paper Optical Chemosensors."

ACS Omega 7(18). May 10, 2022. https://doi.org/10.1021%2Facsomega.2c00730.

Rahrig, H., D. R. Vago, M. A. Passarelli, et al. "Meta-analytic Evidence That Mindfulness Training Alters Resting State Default Mode Network Connectivity." *Scientific Reports*. July 18, 2022. https://www.nature.com/articles/s41598-022-15195-6.

Rehfeld, J. F. "Cholecystokinin and Panic Disorder: Reflections on the History and Some Unsolved Questions." *Molecules 18*. September 26, 2021. https://www.ncbi.nlm.nih.gov/pmc/articles/PMC8469898/.

"Relaxation Techniques: Breath Control Helps Quell Errant Stress Response." Harvard Health Publishing. July 6, 2020. https://www.health.harvard.edu/mind-and-mood/relaxation-techniques-breath-control-helps-quell-errant-stress-response.

"Reminiscing Can Help Boost Mental Performance." *Neuroscience News*. October 23, 2014. https://neurosciencenews.com/psychology-mental-task-reminiscing-1471/.

"Researchers Identify Area of the Brain That Processes Empathy." Mount Sinai. September 1, 2012. https://www.mountsinai.org/about/newsroom/2012/researchers-identify-area-of-the-brain-that-processes-empathy.

Ribeiro, M.K.A., T.R.M. Alcântara-Silva, J.C.M. Oliveira, et al. "Music Therapy Intervention in Cardiac Autonomic Modulation, Anxiety, and Depression in Mothers of Preterms: Randomized Controlled Trial." *BMC Psychology 6(1)*. December 13, 2018. https://doi.org/10.1186/s40359-018-0271-y.

Riezzo, G., G. Chimienti, A. Orlando, et al. "Effects of Long-Term Administration of *Lactobacillus reuteri* DSM-17938 on Circulating Levels of 5-HT and BDNF in Adults with Functional Constipation." *Beneficial Microbes 10(2)*. March 13, 2019. https://pubmed.ncbi.nlm.nih.gov/30574801/.

Rose-Francis, K., RDN, CDCES, LD, and R. Ajmera, MS, RD. "The 7 Best Plant Sources of Omega-3 Fatty Acids." Healthline. October 30, 2023. https://www.healthline.com/nutrition/7-plant-sources-of-omega-3s#TOC_TITLE_HDR_4.

Roshanzamir, F., PhD, and S. M. Safavi, MSc. "The Putative Effects of D-Aspartic Acid on Blood Testosterone Levels: A Systematic Review." *International Journal of Reproductive BioMedicine 15(1)*. January 2017. https://pubmed.ncbi.nlm.nih.gov/28280794/.

Rotimi, O. A., C. D. Onuzulu, A. L. Dewald, et al. "Early Life Exposure to Aflatoxin B1 in Rats: Alterations in Lipids, Hormones, and DNA Methylation Among the Offspring." *International Journal of Environmental Research and Public Health 18(2)*. January 12, 2021. https://doi.org/10.3390%2Fijerph18020589.

Rousmans, S., O. Robin, A. Dittmar, and E. Vernet-Maury. "Autonomic Nervous System Responses Associated with Primary Tastes." *Chemical Senses 25(6)*. December 2000. https://doi.org/10.1093/chemse/25.6.709.

Saccaro, L. F., Z. Schilliger, A. Dayer, et al. "Inflammation, Anxiety, and Stress in Bipolar Disorder and Borderline Personality Disorder: A Narrative Review."

Neuroscience & Biobehavioral Reviews 127. August 2021. https://www.sciencedirect.com/science/article/pii/S014976342100172X.

Santin, A. P., and T. W. Furlanetto. "Role of Estrogen in Thyroid Function and Growth Regulation." *Journal of Thyroid Research 2011*. May 4, 2011. https://doi.org/10.4061%2F2011%2F875125.

Santini, F., P. Vitti, G. Ceccarini, et al. "Lemon Balm (Melissa Officinalis 2)." Restorative Medicine. n.d. https://restorativemedicine.org/library/monographs/lemon-balm-melissa-officinalis-2/.

Sareddy, G. R., and R. K. Vadlamudi. "Cancer Therapy Using Ligands That Target Estrogen Receptor Beta." *Chinese Journal of Natural Medicines 13(11)*. November 1, 2015. https://doi.org/10.1016%2FS1875-5364(15)30083-2.

Sargis, R. M., MD, PhD. "An Overview of the Testes." HealthCentral. January 2015. https://www.healthcentral.com/mens-health/overview-testes.

Sarris, J., E. LaPorte, and I. Schweitzer. "Kava: A Comprehensive Review of Efficacy, Safety, and Psychopharmacology." *Australian & New Zealand Journal of Psychiatry*. November 15, 2010. https://doi.org/10.3109/00048674.2010.522554.

Sattar, Y., J. Wilson, A. M. Khan, et al. "A Review of the Mechanism of Antagonism of N-methyl-D-aspartate Receptor by Ketamine in Treatment-Resistant Depression. *Cureus 10(5)*. May 18, 2018. https://www.cureus.com/articles/12447-a-review-of-the-mechanism-of-antagonism-of-n-methyl-d-aspartate-receptor-by-ketamine-in-treatment-resistant-depression#!/.

Sawchuk, C., PhD, LP. "Depression (Major Depressive Disorder)." Mayo Clinic. October 14, 2022. https://www.mayoclinic.org/diseases-conditions/depression/symptoms-causes/syc-20356007.

Scheer, R., and D. Moss. "Dirt Poor: Have Fruits and Vegetables Become Less Nutritious?" *Scientific American*. April 27, 2011. https://www.scientificamerican.com/article/soil-depletion-and-nutrition-loss/.

Shaffer, F., and J. P. Ginsberg. "An Overview of Heart Rate Variability Metrics and Norms." *Frontiers in Public Health 5*. September 28, 2017. https://doi.org/10.3389%2Ffpubh.2017.00258.

Shahrajabian, M. H. "Powerful Stress Relieving Medicinal Plants for Anger, Anxiety, Depression, and Stress During Global Pandemic." *Recent Patents on Biotechnology 16(4)*. 2022. https://doi.org/10.2174/1872208316666220321102216.

Sharma, A., P. K. Menon, R. Patnaik, et al. "Novel Treatment Strategies Using TiO2-Nanowired Delivery of Histaminergic Drugs and Antibodies to Tau with Cerebrolysin for Superior Neuroprotection in the Pathophysiology of Alzheimer's Disease." In *International Review of Neurobiology,* edited by H. S. Sharma and A. Sharma. Vol. 137. Cambridge, Mass.: Academic Press, 2017.

Sharma, H., et al. "Histaminergic Receptors Modulate Spinal Cord Injury-Induced Neuronal Nitric Oxide Synthase Upregulation and Cord Pathology: New Roles of Nanowired Drug Delivery for Neuroprotection." *International Review of Neurobiology*. 2017. https://doi.org/10.1016/bs.irn.2017.09.001.

Shaukat, A., MD, MPH, FACG, C. J. Kahi, MD, MSc, FACG, C. A. Burke, MD, FACG, et al. "ACG Clinical Guidelines: Colorectal Cancer Screening 2021." *American Journal of Gastroenterology 116(3)*. March 2021. https://journals.lww.com/ajg/fulltext/2021/03000/acg_clinical_guidelines__colorectal_cancer.14.aspx.

Shenoy, A. R., T. Dehmel, M. Stettner, et al. "Citalopram Suppresses Thymocyte Cytokine Production." *Journal of Neuroimmunology 262(1–2)*. September 15, 2013. https://doi.org/10.1016/j.jneuroim.2013.06.006.

Shepard, W. "Amazon.com: The Place Where American Dreams Are Stolen by Chinese Counterfeiters." Forbes Asia. September 27, 2017. https://www.forbes.com/sites/wadeshepard/2017/09/27/amazon-com-the-place-where-american-dreams-are-stolen-by-chinese-counterfeiters/?sh=2e67fc8c4c72.

Shoib, S., J. Ahmad, M. A. Wani, et al. "Depression and Anxiety Among Hyperthyroid Female Patients and Impact of Treatment." *Middle East Current Psychiatry 28*. June 8, 2021. https://doi.org/10.1186/s43045-021-00107-7.

Siddiqui, I. A., M. Asim, B. B. Hafeez, et al. "Green Tea Polyphenol EGCG Blunts Androgen Receptor Function in Prostate Cancer." *FASEB Journal 25(4)*. April 2011. https://doi.org/10.1096%2Ffj.10-167924.

Smausz, R., J. Neill, and J. Gigg. "Neural Mechanisms Underlying Psilocybin's Therapeutic Potential—The Need for Preclinical In Vivo Electrophysiology." *Journal of Psychopharmacology 36(7)*. May 30, 2022. https://doi.org/10.1177%2F02698811221092508.

Smeland, O. B., T. W. Meisingset, K. Borges, and U. Sonnewald. "Chronic Acetyl-L-Carnitine Alters Brain Energy Metabolism and Increases Noradrenaline and Serotonin Content in Healthy Mice." *Neurochemistry International 61(1)*. April 23, 2012. https://doi.org/10.1016/j.neuint.2012.04.008.

Smiley, C. E., B. S. Pate, S. J. Bouknight, et al. "Estrogen Receptor Beta in the Central Amygdala Regulates the Deleterious Behavioral Neuronal Consequences of Repeated Social Stress in Female Rats." bioRxiv. October 4, 2022. https://doi.org/10.1101/2022.10.03.509933.

Soares, C. N., and B. Zitek. "Reproductive Hormone Sensitivity and Risk for Depression Across the Female Life Cycle: A Continuum of Vulnerability?" *Journal of Psychiatry & Neuroscience 33(4)*. July 2008. https://www.ncbi.nlm.nih.gov/pmc/articles/PMC2440795/.

Sochacka-Tatara, E., R. Majewska, F. P. Perera, et al. "Urinary Polycyclic Aromatic Hydrocarbon Metabolites Among 3-Year-Old Children from Krakow, Poland." *Environmental Research 164*. July 2018. https://doi.org/10.1016/j.envres.2018.02.032.

Song, C., W.-H. Zhang, X.-H. Wang, et al. "Acute Stress Enhances the Glutamatergic Transmission onto Basoamygdala Neurons Embedded in Distinct Microcircuits." *Molecular Brain 3*. January 9, 2017. https://doi.org/10.1186/s13041-016-0283-6.

Song, N.-N., Y.-F. Jia, L. Zhang, et al. "Reducing Central Serotonin in Adulthood

Promotes Hippocampal Neurogenesis." *Scientific Reports 6*. February 3, 2016. https://doi.org/10.1038/srep20338.

Stein, M., PsyD. "Thoughts Are Just Thoughts: How to Stop Worshiping Your Anxious Mind." Anxiety & Depression Association of America (ADAA). August 21, 2019. https://adaa.org/learn-from-us/from-the-experts/blog-posts/consumer/thoughts-are-just-thoughts.

Steinmaus, C. M., MD, MPH. "Perchlorate in Water Supplies: Sources, Exposures, and Health Effects." *Current Environmental Health Reports 3(2)*. June 2016. https://doi.org/10.1007%2Fs40572-016-0087-y.

Stolk R. F., E. van der Pasch, F. Naumann, et al. "Norepinephrine Dysregulates the Immune Response and Compromises Host Defense During Sepsis." *American Journal of Respiratory and Critical Care Medicine 202(6)*. September 15, 2020. https://pubmed.ncbi.nlm.nih.gov/32520577/.

"Stress & Smoking." Smokefree.gov. Accessed January 26, 2024. https://smokefree.gov/challenges-when-quitting/stress/stress-smoking.

Su, K.-P., P.-T. Tseng, P.-Y. Lin, et al. "Association of Use of Omega-3 Polyunsaturated Fatty Acids with Changes in Severity of Anxiety Symptoms: A Systematic Review and Meta-analysis." *JAMA Network Open 1(5)*. September 7, 2018. https://doi.org/10.1001/jamanetworkopen.2018.2327.

Tan, Y. Z., S. Ozdemir, A. Temiz, and F. Celik. "The Effect of Relaxing Music on Heart Rate and Heart Rate Variability During ECG GATED-Myocardial Perfusion Scintigraphy." *Complementary Therapies in Clinical Practice 21(2)*. February 14, 2015. https://doi.org/10.1016/j.ctcp.2014.12.003.

Tang, Q., Z. Huang, H. Zhou, and P. Ye. "Effects of Music Therapy on Depression: A Meta-analysis of Randomized Controlled Trials." *PLOS One 15(11)*. November 18, 2020. https://doi.org/10.1371%2Fjournal.pone.0240862.

"Taurine—Uses, Side Effects, and More." WebMD. Accessed January 29, 2024. https://www.webmd.com/vitamins/ai/ingredientmono-1024/taurine.

Terry, N., and K. G. Margolis. "Serotonergic Mechanisms Regulating the GI Tract: Experimental Evidence and Therapeutic Relevance." In *Gastrointestinal Pharmacology,* edited by Beverley Greenwood-Van Meerveld. *Handbook of Experimental Pharmacology,* vol. 239. Cham, Switzerland: Springer, 2017.

Thakker, D., A. Raval, I. Patel, and R. Walia. "N-Acetylcysteine for Polycystic Ovary Syndrome: A Systematic Review and Meta-analysis of Randomized Controlled Clinical Trials." *Obstetrics and Gynecology International 2015*. January 8, 2015. https://doi.org/10.1155%2F2015%2F817849.

Thangam, E. B., E. A. Jemima, H. Singh, et al. "The Role of Histamine and Histamine Receptors in Mast Cell–Mediated Allergy and Inflammation: The Hunt for New Therapeutic Targets." *Frontiers in Immunology 9*. August 13, 2018. https://doi.org/10.3389/fimmu.2018.01873.

"Thyroid Testing Example Results." Testing.com. November 11, 2022. https://www.testing.com/thyroid-testing-example-results/.

Tian, P., K. J. O'Riordan, Y.-K. Lee, et al. "Towards a Psychobiotic Therapy for Depression: *Bifidobacterium breve* CCFM1025 Reverses Chronic Stress–Induced Depressive Symptoms and Gut Microbial Abnormalities in Mice." *Neurobiology of Stress 12*. May 2020. https://www.sciencedirect.com/science/article/pii/S2352289520300060.

Tinsley, G., PhD, CSCS,*D, CISSN. "Glutamine: Benefits, Uses and Side Effects." Healthline. January 13, 2018. https://www.healthline.com/nutrition/glutamine.

Tolle, E. "Dissolving the Ego." YouTube. Accessed January 29, 2024. https://www.youtube.com/watch?v=pEnjM1jC1Rw.

"The Top 300 of 2021." ClinCalc.com. Accessed March 25, 2024. https://clincalc.com/DrugStats/Top300Drugs.aspx.

Torres-Altoro, M. I., B. N. Mathur, J. M. Drerup, et al. "Organophosphates Dysregulate Dopamine Signaling, Glutamatergic Neurotransmission, and Induce Neuronal Injury Markers in Striatum." *Journal of Neurochemistry 119(2)*. September 20, 2011. https://doi.org/10.1111%2Fj.1471-4159.2011.07428.x.

Totten, M. S., T. S. Davenport, L. F. Edwards, and J. M. Howell. "Trace Minerals and Anxiety: A Review of Zinc, Copper, Iron, and Selenium." *Dietetics 2(1)*. February 20, 2023. https://doi.org/10.3390/dietetics2010008.

Trauner, G., S. Khom, I. Baburin, et al. "Modulation of GABAA Receptors by Valerian Extracts Is Related to the Content of Valerenic Acid." *Planta Medica 74(1)*. December 19, 2008. https://doi.org/10.1055/s-2007-993761.

Ueland, P. M., A. Ulvik, L. Rios-Avila, et al. "Direct and Functional Biomarkers of Vitamin B6 Status." *Annual Review of Nutrition 35*. May 13, 2015. https://doi.org/10.1146%2Fannurev-nutr-071714-034330.

Ulrich, K., C. Ngnoumen, A. Clausel, et al. "Effects of Three Genres of Focus Music on Heart Rate Variability and Sustained Attention." *Journal of Cognitive Enhancement 6*. September 28, 2021. https://doi.org/10.1007/s41465-021-00226-3.

Vanderhout, S. M., M. R. Panah, B. Garcia-Bailo, et al. "Nutrition, Genetic Variation and Male Fertility." *Translational Andrology and Urology 10(3)*. March 2021. https://doi.org/10.21037%2Ftau-20-592.

van der Kolk, B., MD. *The Body Keeps the Score: Brain, Mind, and Body in the Healing of Trauma*. New York: Penguin Books, 2015.

———. "How Drama and Theater Can Rewire Limiting Beliefs." National Institute for the Clinical Application of Behavioral Medicine (NICABM). Accessed January 26, 2024. https://www.nicabm.com/trauma-how-drama-and-theater-can-rewire-limiting-beliefs/.

van der Weiden, A., J. Benjamins, M. Gillebaart, et al. "How to Form Good Habits? A Longitudinal Field Study on the Role of Self-Control in Habit Formation." *Frontiers in Psychology 11*. March 27, 2020. https://doi.org/10.3389/fpsyg.2020.00560.

Verma, K. C., Col., and A. S. Kushwaha, Lt. Col. "Demineralization of Drinking

Water: Is It Prudent?" *Medical Journal Armed Forces India 70(4)*. March 6, 2014. https://doi.org/10.1016%2Fj.mjafi.2013.11.011.

Vignes, M., and G. L. Collingridge. "The Synaptic Activation of Kainate Receptors." *Nature 388*. July 10, 1997. https://doi.org/10.1038/40639.

Villines, Z. "What to Know About Facial Numbness and Anxiety." MedicalNewsToday. September 21, 2023. https://www.medicalnewstoday.com/articles/facial-numbness-and-anxiety.

Vingren, J. L., W. J. Kraemer, N. A. Ratamess, et al. "Testosterone Physiology in Resistance Exercise and Training: The Up-Stream Regulatory Elements." *Sports Medicine 40(12)*. December 2010. https://doi.org/10.2165/11536910-000000000-00000.

Virit, O., S. Selek, M. Bulut, et al. "High Ceruloplasmin Levels Are Associated with Obsessive Compulsive Disorder: A Case Control Study." *Behavioral and Brain Functions 4*. November 18, 2008. https://doi.org/10.1186%2F1744-9081-4-52.

Visconti A., C. Le Roy, F. Rosa, et al. "Interplay Between the Human Gut Microbiome and Host Metabolism." *Nature Communications 10(1)*. October 3, 2019. https://pubmed.ncbi.nlm.nih.gov/31582752/.

Voss, R., MD, and M. Zhou, MD. "Improvement in Neuropsychiatric Symptoms with the Addition of Nortriptyline in the Context of Mast Cell Activation Syndrome." *American Journal of Psychiatry: Residents' Journal*. December 2, 2022. https://doi.org/10.1176/appi.ajp-rj.2022.180206.

Waheed, N. *Salt*. CreateSpace. 2013. https://www.goodreads.com/quotes/7685383-and-i-said-to-my-body-softly-i-want-to.

Walker, W. H., II, J. C. Walton, A. C. DeVries, et al. "Circadian Rhythm Disruption and Mental Health." *Translational Psychiatry*. January 23, 2020. https://doi.org/10.1038/s41398-020-0694-0.

Walter, K. N., E. J. Corwin, J. Ulbrecht, et al. "Elevated Thyroid Stimulating Hormone Is Associated with Elevated Cortisol in Healthy Young Men and Women." *Thyroid Research 5*. October 30, 2012. https://doi.org/10.1186%2F1756-6614-5-13.

Wang, C., H. Liu, K. Li, et al. "Tactile Modulation of Memory and Anxiety Requires Dentate Granule Cells Along the Dorsoventral Axis." *Nature Communications 11(1)*. November 27, 2020. https://doi.org/10.1038/s41467-020-19874-8.

Wang, H., PhD, C. Braun, PhD, E. F. Murphy, et al. "*Bifidobacterium longum* 1714™ Strain Modulates Brain Activity of Healthy Volunteers During Social Stress." *American Journal of Gastroenterology 114(7)*. July 2019. https://www.ncbi.nlm.nih.gov/pmc/articles/PMC6615936/.

Wang, Y. "Leaky Blood-Brain Barrier: A Double Whammy for the Brain." *Epilepsy Currents 20(3)*. April 29, 2020. https://journals.sagepub.com/doi/10.1177/1535759720917920.

Ware, M., RDN, LD. "What Are the Benefits of Cod Liver Oil?" MedicalNewsToday. June 8, 2023. https://www.medicalnewstoday.com/articles/270071.

Watson, S. "Dopamine: The Pathway to Pleasure." Harvard Health Publishing. July 20, 2021. https://www.health.harvard.edu/mind-and-mood/dopamine-the-pathway-to-pleasure.

Weinberg L. S. "Iron Deficiency's Unseen Impact on Mental Health." *Neuroscience News*. May 30, 2023. https://neurosciencenews.com/iron-deficiency-mental-health-23368/#:~:text=Specifically%2C%20iron%20plays%20an%20important,schizophrenia%2C%20Levin%20and%20Gattari%20write.

"Welcome to IEATA." International Expressive Arts Therapy Association (IEATA). Accessed January 26, 2024. https://www.ieata.org/.

"What Is Benzodiazepine Protracted Withdrawal?" Benzodiazepine Information Coalition. Accessed January 14, 2024. https://www.benzoinfo.com/protracted-withdrawal-syndrome/.

"What Is Dysbiosis?" WebMD. December 6, 2022. https://www.webmd.com/digestive-disorders/what-is-dysbiosis.

"What Is Ketamine?" Alcohol and Drug Foundation (ADF). December 7, 2023. https://adf.org.au/drug-facts/ketamine/.

"What to Know About Diamine Oxidase (DAO) for Histamine Intolerance." WebMD. July 13, 2023. https://www.webmd.com/allergies/what-to-know-about-diamine-oxidase-histamine-intolerance.

Winstone, J. K., K. V. Pathak, W. Winslow, et al. "Glyphosate Infiltrates the Brain and Increases Pro-Inflammatory Cytokine TNFa: Implications for Neurodegenerative Disorders." *Journal of Neuroinflammation 19(193)*. July 28, 2022. https://doi.org/10.1186/s12974-022-02544-5.

Wong, K. H., MD, PhD. "Urticaria Medication." Medscape. September 16, 2020. https://emedicine.medscape.com/article/762917-medication?form=fpf.

Wu, C.-H., Y.-H. Hsueh, J.-M. Kuo, and S.-J. Liu. "Characterization of Probiotic *Lactobacillus brevis* RK03 and Efficient Production of γ-Aminobutyric Acid in Batch Fermentation." *International Journal of Molecular Sciences 19(1)*. January 4, 2018. https://doi.org/10.3390%2Fijms19010143.

Wu, M., H. Liu, J. Zhang, et al. "The Mechanism of *Leonuri Herba* in Improving Polycystic Ovary Syndrome Was Analyzed Based on Network Pharmacology and Molecular Docking." *Journal of Pharmacy & Pharmaceutical Sciences 26*. February 15, 2023. https://doi.org/10.3389%2Fjpps.2023.11234.

Wu, S.-I., C.-C. Wu, P.-J. Tsai, et al. "Psychobiotic Supplementation of PS128™ Improves Stress, Anxiety, and Insomnia in Highly Stressed Information Technology Specialists: A Pilot Study." *Frontiers in Nutrition 8*. March 26, 2021. https://www.frontiersin.org/articles/10.3389/fnut.2021.614105/full.

Xiang, F., L. Lin, M. Hu, and X. Qi. "Therapeutic Efficacy of a Polysaccharide Isolated from *Cordyceps sinensis* on Hypertensive Rats." *International Journal of Biological Macromolecules 82*. September 30, 2015. https://doi.org/10.1016/j.ijbiomac.2015.09.060.

Yang, K., L. Zeng, T. Bao, and J. Ge. "Effectiveness of Omega-3 Fatty Acid for Polycystic Ovary Syndrome: A Systematic Review and Meta-analysis." *Reproductive Biology and Endocrinology 16*. March 27, 2018. https://doi.org/10.1186%2Fs12958-018-0346-x.

Yong, S. J., T. Tong, J. Chew, and W. L. Lim. "Antidepressive Mechanisms of Probiotics and Their Therapeutic Potential." *Frontiers in Neuroscience 13*. January 14, 2020. https://www.ncbi.nlm.nih.gov/pmc/articles/PMC6971226/.

Yoshii, T. "The Role of the Thalamus in Post-traumatic Stress Disorder." *International Journal of Molecular Sciences*. February 9, 2021. https://www.ncbi.nlm.nih.gov/pmc/articles/PMC7915053/.

"Your Health and Hormones: Endocrine System." Endocrine Society. Accessed January 11, 2024. https://www.endocrine.org/patient-engagement.

Zagorski, N. "Finding a Balance in the Chemical Imbalance Theory." *Psychiatric News*. January 27, 2023. https://psychnews.psychiatryonine.org/doi/10.1176/appi.pn.2023.02.12.28.

Zeidan, M. A., BA, S. A. Igoe, BA, C. Linnman, PhD, et al. "Estradiol Modulates Medial Prefrontal Cortex and Amygdala Activity During Fear Extinction in Women and Female Rats." *Biological Psychiatry 70(10)*. November 15, 2011. https://doi.org/10.1016%2Fj.biopsych.2011.05.016.

Zhang, X., T. T. Ge, G. Yin, et al. "Stress-Induced Functional Alterations in Amygdala: Implications for Neuropsychiatric Diseases." *Frontiers in Neuroscience 12*. May 29, 2018. https://doi.org/10.3389%2Ffnins.2018.00367.

Zhang, Y.-X., L.-P. Yang, C. Gai, et al. "Association Between Variants of MTHFR Genes and Psychiatric Disorders: A Meta-analysis." *Frontiers in Psychiatry 13*. August 18, 2022. https://doi.org/10.3389%2Ffpsyt.2022.976428.

Zhao, L., J. Zhang, L. Yang, et al. "Glyphosate Exposure Attenuates Testosterone Synthesis via NR1D1 Inhibition of StAR Expression in Mouse Leydig Cells." *Science of the Total Environment 785*. September 1, 2021. https://doi.org/10.1016/j.scitotenv.2021.147323.

Zheng, K. H., A. Khan, and E. D. Espiridion. "Phenibut Addiction in a Patient with Substance Use Disorder." *Cureus 11(7)*. July 24, 2019. https://doi.org/10.7759%2Fcureus.5230.

Zouboulis, C. C. "The Skin as an Endocrine Organ." *Dermato-Endocrinology 1(5)*. September–October 2009. https://doi.org/10.4161%2Fderm.1.5.9499.

INDEX

About the Author

NICOLE CAIN is a pioneer in integrative approaches for mental and emotional wellness. With a degree in clinical psychology and a license as a Naturopathic Physician in the state of Arizona, her approach to mental health is multidisciplinary: medical, psychological, and holistic.

Instagram: @drnicolecain